ANIMAL WELFARE

This book is dedicated to
Edwin Calvert Appleby (b1925) and
Leslie Edward Hughes (1909–1976)
whose enthusiasm and encouragement helped to
awaken our interest in biology and who have
themselves contributed much to animal welfare.

Animal Welfare

Edited by

Michael C. Appleby

Senior Lecturer in Applied Ethology
Institute of Ecology and Resource Management
University of Edinburgh, UK

and

Barry O. Hughes

Principal Veterinary Research Officer
Roslin Institute (Edinburgh), UK

CAB INTERNATIONAL

CAB INTERNATIONAL
Wallingford
Oxon OX10 8DE
UK
Tel: +44 (0)1491 832111
Fax: +44 (0)1491 833508
E-mail: cabi@cabi.org

CAB INTERNATIONAL
198 Madison Avenue
New York, NY 10016-4314
USA
Tel: +1 212 726 6490
Fax: +1 212 686 7993
E-mail: cabi-nao@cabi.org

A catalogue record for this book is available from the British Library, London, UK.

Library of Congress Cataloging-in-Publication Data
Animal welfare / edited by Mike C. Appleby and Barry O. Hughes.
      p.   cm.
    Includes bibliographical references (p.   ) and index.
    ISBN 0-85199-180-7 (alk. paper)
     1. Animal welfare. I. Appleby, Michael C. II. Hughes, Barry O.
  HV4711.A587   1977   97–12578
                                                          CIP

ISBN 0 85199 180 7

Typeset in Souvenir Light by Advance Typesetting Ltd, Oxford
Printed and bound in the UK by the University Press, Cambridge.

Contents

CONTRIBUTORS

Dr Michael Appleby, *Senior Lecturer in Applied Ethology, Institute of Ecology and Resource Management, University of Edinburgh, West Mains Road, Edinburgh EH9 3JG, UK (mappleby@srv0.bio.ed.ac.uk)*

Dr Rolf Beilharz, *Senior Associate in Animal Breeding, Agriculture and Environmental Management, Department of Agriculture and Resource Management, University of Melbourne, Parkville, Victoria 3052, Australia (rolf_beilharz@muwayf.unimelb.edu.au)*

Dr Richard Bennett, *Lecturer in Agricultural Economics, Department of Agricultural and Food Economics, University of Reading, Reading RG6 6AR, UK (r.m.bennett@rdg.ac.uk)*

Dr Lynda Birke, *Senior Lecturer, Centre for the Study of Women and Gender, University of Warwick, Coventry, Warwickshire, UK (cerae@snow.csv.warwick.ac.uk)*

Dr Roger Crisp, *Fellow and Tutor in Philosophy, St Anne's College, University of Oxford, Oxford OX2 6HS, UK (rcrisp@vax.ox.ac.uk)*

Mr Peter Curtis, *Honorary Senior Fellow, Department of Veterinary Clinical Science and Animal Husbandry, University of Liverpool, Veterinary Field Station, Leahurst, Neston, South Wirral L64 7TE, UK*

Professor Ian Duncan, *Professor of Animal Welfare, Department of Animal and Poultry Science, University of Guelph, Guelph, Ontario N1G 2W1, Canada (iduncan@aps.uoguelph.ca)*

Professor Paul Flecknell, *Professor of Laboratory Animal Science, Comparative Biology Centre, Medical School, University of Newcastle, Framlington Place, Newcastle upon Tyne NE2 4HH, UK (p.a.flecknell@newcastle.ac.uk)*

Professor David Fraser, *Professor of Animal Welfare, Department of Animal Science and Centre for Applied Ethics, University of British Columbia, 2357 Main Hall, Vancouver V6T 1Z4, Canada*

Professor Harold Gonyou, *Research Scientist in Ethology, Prairie Swine Centre, PO Box 21057, 2105-8th Street East, Saskatoon, Saskatchewan S7H 5N9, Canada (gonyou@sask.usask.ca)*

Dr Paul Hemsworth, *Principal Scientist in Animal Production, Victorian Institute of Animal Science, Agriculture Victoria, 475–485 Mickleham Road, Attwood, Victoria 3049, Australia (hemsworthp@woody.agvic.gov.au)*

Dr Paul Hocking, *Principal Investigator, Roslin Institute (Edinburgh), Roslin, Midlothian EH25 9PS, UK (paul.hocking@bbsrc.ac.uk)*

Dr Nils Holtug, *Lecturer in Philosophy, Bioethical Research Group, Department of Education, Philosophy and Rhetorics, University of Copenhagen, Njalsgade 80, DK2300, Copenhagen S, Denmark (nhol@coco.ihi.ku.dk)*

Dr Barry Hughes, *Principal Veterinary Research Officer, Roslin Institute (Edinburgh), Roslin, Midlothian EH25 9PS, UK (barry.hughes@bbsrc.ac.uk)*

Dr Bill Jackson, *Veterinary surgeon, barrister and RCVS Consultant, 19 Raven's Croft, Eastbourne, East Sussex BN20 7HX, UK*

Dr Bryan Jones, *Principal Investigator, Roslin Institute (Edinburgh), Roslin, Midlothian EH25 9PS, UK (bryan.jones@bbsrc.ac.uk)*

Dr Ute Knierim, *Lecturer in Applied Ethology and Animal Welfare, Institute of Animal Hygiene and Welfare, Tieraerztliche Hochschule Hanover, Buenteweg 17p, D-30559 Hanover, Germany (uknierim@itt.tiho-hannover.de)*

Dr Ilias Kyriazakis, *Senior Specialist in Behavioural Nutrition, Genetics and Behavioural Sciences Department, Scottish Agricultural College (Edinburgh), King's Buildings, West Mains Road, Edinburgh EH9 3JG, UK (i.kyriazakis@ed.sac.ac.uk)*

Professor Jan Ladewig, *Professor of Animal Welfare and Ethology, Royal Veterinary and Agricultural University, Department of Forensic and State Veterinary Medicine, 13 Bulowsvej, DK1870, Copenhagen V, Denmark (jan.ladewig@ihh.kvl.dk)*

Dr Georgia Mason, *Lecturer in Vertebrate Biology, Animal Behaviour Research Group, Department of Zoology, University of Oxford, South Parks Road, Oxford OX1 3PS, UK (georgia.mason@zoo.ox.ac.uk)*

Dr Lindsay Matthews, *Senior Scientist and Lecturer in Animal Behaviour and Welfare, Animal Behaviour and Welfare Research Centre, AgResearch Ruakura Agricultural Centre, Private Bag 3123, Hamilton, New Zealand (matthewsl@agresearch.cri.nz)*

Professor Joy Mench, *Professor of Animal Welfare, Departments of Animal Science and Avian Sciences, University of California, Davis, CA 95616, USA (jamench@ucdavis.edu)*

Dr Mike Mendl, *Lecturer in Animal Behaviour, Division of Animal Health and Husbandry, Department of Clinical Veterinary Science, University of Bristol, Langford House, Langford, Bristol BS18 7DU, UK (mike.mendl@bris.ac.uk)*

Dr Andrew Mills, *Research Scientist in Animal Behaviour, Station de Recherches Avicoles, INRA Centre de Tours-Nouzilly, 37380 Nouzilly, France (mills@tours.inra.fr)*

Dr Vince Molony, *Reader in Preclinical Veterinary Science, Royal (Dick) School of Veterinary Studies, University of Edinburgh, Summerhall, Edinburgh EH9 1QH, UK (v.molony@ed.ac.uk)*

Dr Ruth Newberry, *Assistant Professor, Center for the Study of Animal Well-being, Department of Animal Sciences & College of Veterinary Medicine, Washington State University, PO Box 646351, Pullman, WA 99164-6351, USA (rnewberry@wsu.edu)*

Dr Carol Petherick, *Research Scientist in Beef Industry Services, Queensland Department of Primary Industries, Swan's Lagoon Beef Cattle Research Station, Millaroo, via Ayr, Queensland 4807, Australia*

Dr Jeff Rushen, *Research Scientist in Animal Behaviour and Stress Physiology, Agriculture and Agri-Food Canada, PO Box 90, Lennoxville, Quebec J1M 1Z3, Canada (rushenj@em.agr.ca)*

Professor Peter Sandøe, *Associate Professor of Philosophy, Bioethical Research Group, Department of Education, Philosophy and Rhetorics, University of Copenhagen, Njalsgade 80, DK2300, Copenhagen S, Denmark (psand@coco.ihi.ku.dk)*

Dr John Savory, *Principal Investigator, Roslin Institute (Edinburgh), Roslin, Midlothian EH25 9PS, UK (john.savory@bbsrc.ac.uk)*

Dr Willem Schouten, *Senior Lecturer in Applied Ethology and Behavioural Physiology, Department of Animal Hygiene, Section Ethology, Wageningen Agricultural University, PO Box 338, 6700 AH Wageningen, The Netherlands (willem.schouten@etho.vh.wau.nl)*

Dr Claudia Terlouw, *Researcher in Stress Responses of Farm Animals, INRA Station de Recherches sur la Viande, Centre Clermont-Ferrand-Theix, 63122 Saint-Genès-Champanelle, France (terlouw@clermont.inra.fr)*

Dr Natalie Waran, *Course Director, MSc in Applied Animal Behaviour and Animal Welfare, Insititute of Ecology and Resource Management, University of Edinburgh, West Mains Road, Edinburgh EH9 3JG, UK (nwaran@srv0.bio.ed.ac.uk)*

Dr Françoise Wemelsfelder, *Research Scientist, Genetics and Behavioural Sciences Department, Scottish Agricultural College (Edinburgh), Bush Estate, Penicuik, Midlothian EH26 0QE, UK (f.wemelsfelder@ed.sac.ac.uk)*

INTRODUCTION

Michael C. Appleby (University of Edinburgh, UK) and
Barry O. Hughes (Roslin Institute, UK)

Concern for animal welfare is not new and has often been given considerable emphasis, for example by Mahatma Gandhi:

> The greatness of a nation and its moral progress can be judged by the way its animals are treated.

However, it is clear that such concern, particularly for animals in our care, has recently increased and continues to increase in many nations. This book is a response to that public interest. It pulls together diverse approaches to the subject, from philosophy through scientific study and measurement to the implementation of practical solutions to real problems. This will be of benefit to students, to scientists in the field and to others who are increasingly trying to use the information that scientists provide without having been provided with a framework in which to do so. Such people include, for example, agriculturalists, legislators and members of animal protection societies.

What is animal welfare? This is discussed below, especially in Chapter 2, but we should say at this point that 'Welfare is a characteristic of an animal, not something given to it' (Broom and Johnson 1993, p. 75) (although see Chapter 2 and Part III concerning interpretation of this 'characteristic'). This runs counter to a perception held by some people that animal welfare refers only to our effects on animals and that the concept is irrelevant to, for example, wild animals. Thus a group of Edinburgh students (at the beginning of their course on welfare) defined welfare (Appleby 1996, p. 24) as:

> The state of well-being brought about by meeting the physical, environmental, nutritional, behavioural and social needs of the animal or groups of animals under the care, supervision or influence of people.

The perception is further complicated in North America by the use of the word 'welfare' to mean something provided for humans (and by implication animals) in need. Thus A.F. Fraser, writing from Canada (e.g. 1992), uses 'well-being' to refer to endogenous states of being within an animal and 'welfare' to human interventions designed to promote good well-being. This distinction is not widely accepted and the terms welfare and well-being are generally (and certainly in this book) regarded as synonyms. Speaking of synonyms, we acknowledge that humans are animals and that the book is concerned with non-human animals; we hope to be forgiven for not using this clumsy phrase throughout.

Originally 'welfare' meant 'well-being, happiness' (Oxford English Dictionary, 1973) – literally 'a state of faring well' (Chambers Dictionary, 1983) – and animal welfare was defined by Hughes (1976a), for example, as 'A state of complete mental and physical health, where the animal is in harmony with its environment.' Its meaning has gradually changed, however, and it is now generally used to indicate the state of an animal in terms of its position on a scale (although not a simple scale: *see* Part II). Thus:

> Welfare can vary between very poor and very good . . . In order to use the concept of welfare in a scientific way it is necessary always to specify the level of an animal's welfare and not simply to reserve the word to indicate that the animal has, or does not have, problems.
>
> (Broom and Johnson 1993, p. 75)

A bias towards material on farm animals is evident throughout the book. This is because most work has been done on farm animals and a great deal has been written on this group. However, most of the material is relevant to all groups of animals. It is to be hoped that the approaches developed in the active field of farm animal welfare will continue to be applied – or adapted as necessary – to other species. Another evident bias is the emphasis on science, particularly behavioural science: the majority of the authors are behavioural scientists. This is because while it would have been possible to produce a book with more emphasis on other approaches to welfare – sociological or political approaches, for example – we believe that the most important response to increasing public concern for welfare is the attempt to understand animals more fully and to investigate ways of providing for their needs, and these are scientific endeavours. The emphasis on behaviour in the book also reflects the field of animal welfare in general. It has arisen (as we say in Chapter 12) because behaviour is the interface between the animal and most aspects of its environment and may therefore be both the source of some problems and a symptom of other problems such as disease. This is only an emphasis, however, not a monopoly: other aspects of welfare that do not involve behaviour are covered in their place.

The contents are intended to be both accessible and useful. They combine selected readings with critical commentaries from experts in the different fields. The authors of each chapter were encouraged to identify papers that have made influential contributions in the field. Selections from these papers were then incorporated into a commentary that puts the papers into context, explains their importance and reviews current thinking on the topic. In other words many of the chapters are reviews built round the key references rather than articles with references in support. This enables the reader to see how the ideas have developed – including mistakes that have been made – as well as grasping the 'received wisdom' of the present day. The tendency for consensus was further increased by inviting two or more authors to contribute to most chapters. As usual with quotations, both accuracy and readability are important: minor changes that do not affect the sense have sometimes been made without indication (for example, omission of a parenthetical reference) and readers should check the original for a definitive version. Page numbers are given to assist this.

We have tackled the complex subject of animal welfare in what we hope is a systematic fashion. The history, background and philosophy are dealt with under 'Issues' and then the various ways in which animals may suffer are explained under 'Problems', using categories similar to the UK Farm Animal Welfare Council's (1992) Five Freedoms. The various measures used to assess well-being are described under 'Assessment' while the ways in which suffering can be ameliorated and well-being enhanced are explained under 'Solutions'. Finally, the means by which solutions are put into practice are discussed under 'Implementation'. Any division of such subject material into categories is artificial. For example, chapters on Problems will tend to indicate solutions to those problems, so there will be overlap. However, it is our hope and our belief that the chapters are complementary and that the whole is greater than the sum of its parts, to give an overall impression of the active, developing and important field of animal welfare.

We are grateful for invaluable discussion with our co-authors and other colleagues during the planning and throughout the completion of the book, and for their comments on our own contributions.

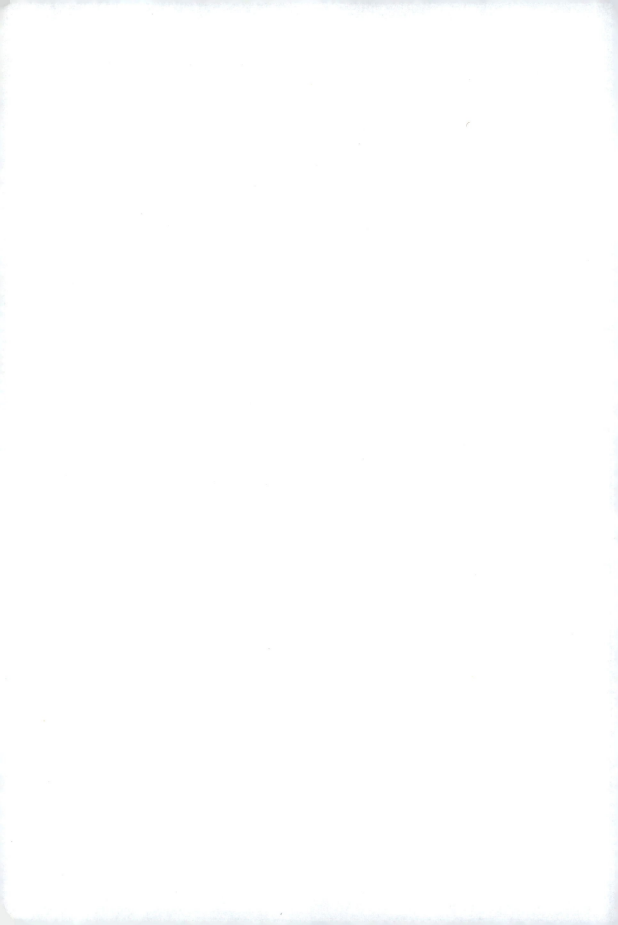

PART I
Issues

We are irretrievably involved with animals. Given this fact, we must address the question of our responsibilities, or animals' rights, associated with such involvement. This is the substance of Chapter 1. That chapter also touches on the question of whether we should use animals at all. The rest of the book tends to assume that we do so, because attempts to minimize use of animals would alter the balance of responsibilities and rights but would not avoid the need to examine them.

Readers will not have uniform views on animal welfare, but most people believe that animals can suffer in ways that in some respects are comparable to human suffering. For practical reasons we need to give more thought to what is understood by the term animal welfare and why this varies between different people; this is discussed in Chapter 2.

CHAPTER 1

Ethics

Peter Sandøe (University of Copenhagen, Denmark),
Roger Crisp (University of Oxford, UK) and Nils Holtug
(University of Copenhagen, Denmark)

Abstract

This is a discussion of views concerning how we ought to treat animals and of
the justifications on which these views are based. First, an account is given of
what it is to justify a moral view. Secondly, the view that animals do not have
moral standing and that therefore we have no direct duties to them is examined.
Thirdly, four different views about the nature of our duties to animals are presented and discussed. They are: utilitarianism, the animal rights view, the species-
integrity view, and the agent-centred view. Finally, it is discussed why it is
important to hold a justified view concerning one's duties to animals.

1.1. Introduction

That humans have ethical duties to animals is an assumption that underlies the
study of animal welfare. There would not be much point in studying how
animals fare in livestock production systems, for example, if we did not think
that humans had any duty to look after the animals in their care.

The aim of this chapter is to present ethical views concerning how
we ought to treat animals and the justifications on which these views are
based.

1.2. Justification of Ethical Views

First, it needs to be explained what is meant by justifying an ethical view. Many
people think that in ethics we simply express our feelings; and since feelings
cannot be justified neither can ethical views.

Against this philosophers have argued that there is more to a justified
moral view than having a feeling. Thus Rachels (1983, pp. 10–11) explains
the difference between a moral judgement and an expression of personal taste:

> If someone says 'I like coffee,' he does not need to have a reason – he is
> merely making a statement about himself, and nothing more. There is no
> such thing as 'rationally defending' one's like or dislike of coffee, and so there

Animal Welfare (eds Michael C. Appleby and Barry O. Hughes)

is no arguing about it. So long as he is accurately reporting his tastes, what he says must be true. Moreover, there is no implication that anyone should feel the same way; if everyone else in the world hates coffee, it doesn't matter. On the other hand, if someone says that something is *morally wrong,* he does need reasons, and if his reasons are sound, other people must acknowledge their force.

When it comes to justifying moral judgements, moral principles play an important role. This may be illustrated by the famous passage, first published in 1789 (p. 283), in which Bentham argued that animals ought to be protected by the law:

> The day *may* come, when the rest of the animal creation may acquire those rights which never could have been withholden from them but by the hand of tyranny. The French have already discovered that the blackness of the skin is no reason why a human being should be abandoned without redress to the caprice of a tormentor. It may come one day to be recognized, that the number of the legs, the villosity of the skin, or the termination of the *os sacrum,* are reasons equally insufficient for abandoning a sensitive being to the same fate. What else is it that should trace the insuperable line? Is it the faculty of reason, or, perhaps, the faculty of discourse? But a full-grown horse or dog is beyond comparison a more rational, as well as a more conversible animal, than an infant of a day, or a week, or even a month, old. But suppose the case were otherwise what would it avail? The question is not, Can they *reason*? nor, Can they *talk*? but, Can they *suffer*?

Bentham asks which justification can be given for saying that unlike humans animals should not be protected by legal rights. One traditional answer to this question is that animals do not possess the ability to reason and to use language. Those who give this answer must accordingly accept the principle that those and only those creatures which can reason and talk should be given rights. However, this means that human infants and some mentally retarded humans should not be awarded rights.

So first, someone who thinks that animals should have no rights has to explain why he thinks so. Secondly, this reason implies a moral principle. Thirdly, this has consequences that to most people are unattractive, i.e. that infants and mentally retarded humans should have no rights. Finally, the person who started out thinking that animals should have no rights may feel that he has to change his view.

1.3. Do Animals Have Moral Standing?

Bentham uses his opponent's way of thinking against that person himself. He also has a positive argument why animals should have rights: that animals can suffer. And since Bentham thinks that the ability to suffer (and feel pleasure) is what matters in our duties to other humans he also thinks that we owe duties to the animals.

Bentham's arguments perhaps do not *prove* beyond all reasonable doubt that humans have duties to animals. However, to deny his conclusion one must answer his arguments. Some modern philosophers have tried to do so. For example, Narveson (1983, pp. 56–58) argues that animals have no rights because they cannot be parties to an agreement:

> On the contract view of morality, morality is a sort of agreement among rational, independent, self-interested persons, persons who have something to gain from entering into such an agreement . . .
>
> A major feature of this view of morality is that it explains why we have it and who is party to it. We have it for reasons of long-run selfinterest, and parties to it include all and only those who have *both* of the following characteristics: (1) they stand to gain by subscribing to it, at least in the long run, compared with not doing so, and (2) they are *capable* of entering into (and keeping) an agreement . . . Given these requirements, it will be clear why animals do not have rights. For there are evident shortcomings on both scores. On the one hand, humans have nothing generally to gain by voluntarily refraining from (for instance) killing animals or 'treating them as mere means.' And on the other, animals cannot generally make agreements with us anyway, even if we wanted to have them do so . . .
>
> There is an evident problem about the treatment of what I have called 'marginal cases' on this view, of course: infants, the feeble-minded, and the incapacitated are in varying degrees in the position of the animals in relation to us, are they not? True: but the situation is very different in several ways. For one thing, we generally have very little to gain from treating such people badly, and we often have much to gain from treating them well. For another, marginal humans are invariably members of families, or members of other groupings, which make them the object of love and interest on the part of other members of those groups. Even if there were an interest in treating a particular marginal person badly, there would be others who have an interest in their being treated well and who are themselves clearly members of the moral community on contractarian premises.

The principle underlying this view of morality is *egoism*: showing consideration for other people is really for one's own sake. By respecting the rules of morality one contributes to the maintenance of a society which is essential to one's welfare. And if persons free-ride they will be punished by loneliness, poverty – and maybe even confinement.

On this view there is a relevant difference between humans and animals. I am dependent on the cooperation of other people. If I treat other humans badly, they may treat me badly, whereas the animal community will not strike back if, for example, I use some of its members in painful experiments. From an egoistic point of view I need only to treat the animals well enough for them to be fit for my purposes.

This justification for giving humans moral priority over animals fits well into parts of the morality prevalent in our society, and logically it is coherent. Further, it serves to explain why legislation allegedly for the protection of animals usually protects those animals most which matter most to humans, for example dogs and cats. The main problem about this view is that most of us will find it difficult to maintain egoism with a clear conscience. As Narveson honestly spells out, on his view we do not have moral obligations to weak humans, unless they matter to some of the strong humans.

At this stage of the argument, most people will probably side with Bentham and say that if a human or animal suffers, then this matters *in itself* from a moral point of view. It follows that most people will not be willing to exclude animals from ethical consideration in the way that Narveson suggests.

What has been discussed until now is whether or not animals should have rights, not what kind of rights they should have – whether or not animals have *moral standing*. Bentham argues that they do, whereas Narveson claims that they don't. In what follows we shall assume that Bentham is right in thinking that animals have moral standing.

1.4. Four Views about Humanity's Duties to Animals

Assuming that animals do have moral standing, two new questions must be raised. What is the basis of our duties towards animals? And what duties do we have? There are no unanimous answers to these questions but here we shall present four competing views.

1.4.1. Utilitarianism

This view can be traced back at least to Bentham. In recent discussions about animal ethics it has been most forcefully defended by Singer who bases his view on a principle of equality (1989, pp. 74–79):

> I am urging that we extend to other species the basic principle of equality that most of us recognize should be extended to all members of our own species . . .
> Jeremy Bentham incorporated the essential basis of moral equality into his utilitarian system of ethics in the formula: 'Each to count for one and none for more than one.' In other words, the interests of every being affected by an action are to be taken into account and given the same weight as the like interests of any other being. A later utilitarian, Henry Sidgwick, put the point in this way: 'The good of any one individual is of no more importance, from the point of view (if I may say so) of the Universe, than the good of any other.' . . .
> The racist violates the principle of equality by giving greater weight to the interests of members of his own race, when there is a clash between their interests and the interests of those of another race. Similarly the speciesist allows the interests of his own species to override the greater interests of members of other species. The pattern is the same in each case.

For the utilitarian what matters are the interests of those who are being affected by what we do – not the race or the species of the creatures who have the interests. The strongest interests should prevail no matter who has them. This view has radical consequences when it comes to an ethical assessment of modern intensive livestock production.

Broiler chickens, stalled sows and other farm animals will often suffer and will lack the ability to do things which could contribute to their 'positive welfare'. The interests of these animals are set aside so that production can be efficient and that consumers can buy cheap meat and other animal products. However, in the rich part of the world these cheap products are not vital to human interests. If we paid 30 or 50% more and the extra money was used to improve the living conditions of the animals this would mean an immense increase in their welfare. In a country like Denmark where ordinary consumers spend less than 13% of their available income on food this would have only a marginal effect on income available for other purposes, and since income is generally high it would not significantly decrease the welfare of the affected humans. Therefore, according to the utilitarian view, we ought to make radical changes in the way farm animals are being treated.

However, it should be noted that from this view even less radical changes may be welcomed. A utilitarian speaks not only in terms of right and wrong but also in terms of better and worse. A small step towards more consideration of the interests of animals is better than no step. The discussion between those with a compromise-seeking attitude to the improvement of animal welfare and those with radical views is from the utilitarian point of view not a discussion of principle, but a discussion about which strategy will have the best effects on animal welfare.

Singer himself argues in favour of a rather radical attitude to the welfare of farm animals: that we should boycott animal products and become vegetarians. However, this is not because he thinks it is in principle wrong to kill an animal but because consumption of meat and other products from commercially reared animals leads to animal suffering (1979, pp. 152–153):

> As long as a sentient being is conscious, it has an interest in experiencing as much pleasure and as little pain as possible. Sentience suffices to place a being within the sphere of equal consideration of interests; but it does not mean that the being has a personal interest in continuing to live. For a non-self-conscious being, death is the cessation of experiences, in much the same way that birth is the beginning of experiences. Death cannot be contrary to a preference for continued life, any more than birth could be in accordance with a preference for commencing life . . . Given that an animal belongs to a species incapable of self-consciousness, it follows that it is not wrong to rear and kill it for food, provided that it lives a pleasant life and, after being killed, will be replaced by another animal which will lead a similarly pleasant life and would not have existed if the first animal had not been killed. This means that vegetarianism is not obligatory for those who can obtain meat from animals that they know to have been reared in this manner . . .
>
> I am sure that some will claim that in taking this view on the killing of some non-human animals I am myself guilty of 'speciesism' – that is, discrimination against beings because they are not members of our own species. My position is not speciesist, because it does not permit the killing of non-human beings on the ground that they are not members of our species, but on the ground that they lack the capacity to desire to go on living. The position applies equally to members of our own species who lack the relevant capacity.

Singer here says that it is all right to kill animals for meat as long as we make sure that they have a good life and are killed in a painless way. This view seems to be shared by many of those engaged in animal welfare science. It would be difficult to work on improving the quality of life of animals in livestock production and in animal research if one thought that the slaughtering of healthy animals constituted a major ethical wrong.

However, the argument may be questioned. Thus one may ask whether Singer really manages to draw a clear moral distinction between the killing of humans and of animals. A case may be made to the effect that Singer in the end will have to take a similar view on the killing of humans as of animals. If self-conscious humans are killed some of their forward-looking preferences will not be fulfilled, but frustration of these preferences may be outweighed by the satisfaction of preferences of persons by whom they are replaced.

A more consistent utilitarian line of argument would be to say that in principle it would be all right to kill a self-conscious human being if the killing were painless and if the person were replaced by another person who lives as good a life as the first and who would not have existed if the first person hadn't been destroyed. However, in real life the utilitarian may argue that the killing of humans and of animals have very different consequences. Thus the killing of a human usually has negative effects on survivors in a way that the killing of an animal does not. When a human is killed relatives will often grieve, and fear and anxiety may arise among the survivors. Another related difference concerns the indirect consequences on society if we do not hold human life in respect. Lack of respect for human life will undermine the foundations of society and will lead to the barbarism that we know all too well from history. Finally, killing of humans will normally not have the consequence that others come into existence instead, whereas with animals this is mostly the case. Thus with farm animals it is evident that we only have these animals because we can kill them. The same is true for laboratory animals – those destroyed are normally replaced.

One may be worried not only about how utilitarianism affects respect for human life. Conclusions on the killing of animals may also in some instances seem quite hideous (Lockwood, 1979, p. 168):

> Many families, especially ones with young children, find that dogs are an asset when they are still playful puppies (capable of keeping the children amused), but become an increasing liability as they grow into middle age, with an adult appetite but *sans* youthful allure. Moreover, there is always a problem of what to do with the animal when they go on holiday. It is often inconvenient or even impossible to take the dog with them, whereas friends tend to resent the imposition, and kennels are expensive and unreliable. Let us suppose that, inspired by Singer's article, people were to hit on the idea of having their pets painlessly put down at the start of each holiday (as some pet owners already do), acquiring new ones upon their return. Suppose, indeed, that a company grows up, 'Disposapup Ltd', which rears the animals, house-trains them, supplies them to any willing purchaser, takes them back, exterminates them and supplies replacements, on demand. It is clear, is it not, that there can, for Singer, be absolutely nothing directly wrong with such a practice. Every puppy has, we may assume, an extremely happy, albeit brief, life – and indeed, would not have existed at all but for the practice.

Lockwood himself says that though the example gives him pause he 'remains ultimately unconvinced'. Others, however, have argued that the utilitarian view fails because it does not respect the moral value of each individual (human or animal). This leads us to the second view to be discussed here.

1.4.2. The animal rights view

One of the most prominent adherents of the animal rights view is Regan who defends it (1984) in explicit opposition to utilitarianism:

> Unlike utilitarianism, the view in *principle* denies that we can justify good results by using evil means that violate an individual's rights – denies, for example, that it could be moral to kill my Aunt Bea to harvest beneficial consequences for others. That would be to sanction the disrespectful treatment of the individual in the name of the social good, something the rights view will not – categorically will not – ever allow . . .
>
> We are each of us the experiencing subject of a life, a conscious creature having an individual welfare that has importance to us whatever our usefulness to others. We want and prefer things, believe and feel things, recall and expect things. And all these dimensions of our life, including our pleasure and pain, our enjoyment and suffering, our satisfaction and frustration, our continued existence or our untimely death – all make a difference to the quality of our life as lived, as experienced, by us as individuals. As the same is true of those animals that concern us (the ones that are eaten and trapped, for example), they too must be viewed as the experiencing subjects of a life, with inherent value of their own . . .
>
> In the case of the use of animals in science, the rights view is categorically abolitionist. Lab animals are not our tasters; we are not their kings. Because these animals are treated routinely, systematically as if their value were reducible to their usefulness to others, they are routinely, systematically treated with lack of respect, and thus are their rights routinely, systematically violated. This is just as true when they are used in trivial, duplicative, unnecessary or unwise research as it is when they are used in studies that hold out real promise for human benefits . . .
>
> As for commercial animal agriculture, the rights view takes a similar abolitionist position. The fundamental moral wrong here is not that animals are kept in stressful close confinement or in isolation, or that their pain and suffering, their needs and preferences are ignored or discounted. All these *are* wrong, of course, but they are not the fundamental wrong. They are symptoms and effects of the deeper, systematic wrong that allows these animals to be viewed and treated as lacking independent value, as resources for us – as, indeed, a renewable resource.

The rights view differs from utilitarianism in cases where there is a conflict of interest. According to utilitarianism such conflicts should be decided by giving most weight to the strongest interests. The rights view on the other hand claims that it is never justified to sacrifice the interests of one individual to benefit another. This affects, for example, the discussion of whether it is wrong to kill animals. First, it may be argued that healthy animals do in a morally relevant sense have an interest in not being killed (Johnson, 1983, pp. 144–145):

> According to a common view, animals lack the concept of death, and so cannot mind death, any more than they mind not having a ticket to the opera. Rational creatures, however, can mind, and normally do, and this is the reason why it is wrong, *prima facie,* to kill them. Is such a view correct?
>
> You can have an interest in avoiding death if you are capable of conceiving death, and so of minding it; you can have an interest in your own continued existence if you are capable of conceiving it, and so of wanting it. But you can also have an indirect or derivative interest in life that feeds off your other

interests. If a cow likes to chew her cud, then it is, other things being equal, in her interest to be allowed to do so. She is benefited by having opportunities to satisfy her desires: the more the better. But does this not give the cow an interest in continued life? When to have a desire satisfied is to be benefited, isn't one benefited more, other things being equal, the more opportunities one has to satisfy it (perhaps – where this is relevant – up to some point of satisfaction)? This will be so even if one lacks the concept of a future, of personal identity over time, etc. Of course, if one does have such concepts, since one will then be able to *care* about the future, that will give one an additional interest in living. But the lack of such concepts does not mean that one has *no* interest in, or claim to, life: the derivative sort of interest in life remains. Insofar as life seems likely to satisfy one's desires, fulfils interests that one has, one has an interest in life.

The utilitarian and the adherent of the rights view may agree that in the sense here specified, animals have an interest in a continued life. However, the utilitarian claims that the interest of an animal in going on living may be outweighed by conflicting interests, i.e. the combined interests of the future animal which will replace it and human interests in animal production. Against this, the adherent of animal rights claims that it is unethical to sacrifice the interests of the first animal for the sake of others.

Another issue which gives rise to conflict between the two views is the use of animals for research. Thus animal experiments which are vital to the development of human medicine may on the utilitarian view be considered morally acceptable because benefits outweigh costs in animal suffering or discomfort. According to the animal rights view on the other hand it is not justified to conduct a harmful experiment on one individual only for the sake of the interests of others.

According to the rights view we should not only look upon animal (and human) welfare as something to be promoted *en bloc*. Rather it is our duty to protect the right of each individual animal (and human) not to be killed nor deprived of the means necessary to live a good life. Regan formulates this idea with reference to a famous eighteenth century slogan from Kant (Regan, 1984, p. 249):

> To harm . . . individuals *merely* in order to produce the best consequences for all involved *is* to do what is wrong – *is* to treat them unjustly – because it fails to respect their inherent value. To borrow part of a phrase from Kant, individuals who have inherent value must never be treated *merely as a means* to securing the best aggregate consequences.

The adherent of the rights view has, it seems, gained the moral high ground. However, there is a problem: how to handle cases where it is not possible to respect the rights of all individuals. The interests of two individuals (or groups) may not only be in conflict, but be mutually exclusive. For example it may be difficult to combine respect for the rights of mice and rats with the aim of securing human health and welfare. If these 'pests' are not 'controlled' they may pose a threat because they eat our food, and because they spread disease. It seems to be either them or us. What has the rights view to offer in such a case?

Regan's reply is that we are allowed to defend ourselves. However, this creates a problem for his abolitionist stance on animal experimentation. It is not implausible that some animal experiments (typically making use of rodents) may be as vital to human health as control of rodents. Thus, there is a problem for the rights view (pointed out by Singer among others) in drawing boundaries between cases where vital human interests allow us to kill or otherwise act against the interests of animals, and cases where respect for animal rights prevents us from pursuing our interests.

Despite the fact that the rights view may not in all cases give clear answers, there seems to be a genuine moral disagreement underlying the discussion between Singer and Regan. However, there are also points on which the two views agree. Thus they both think that it is important to consider the interests of all sentient creatures, and conversely that nothing but the interests of individual humans and animals matter. The latter point distinguishes these views from the third of the views to be discussed here.

1.4.3. The species-integrity view

According to this view it is not only individuals that ought to be the focus of our moral concerns. Rolston argues (1989, pp. 252–255) that we ought also to promote the value of species:

> Many will be uncomfortable with the view that we can have duties to a collection . . . Singer asserts, 'Species as such are not conscious entities and so do not have interests above and beyond the interests of the individual animals that are members of the species.' Regan maintains, 'The rights view is a view about the moral rights of individuals. Species are not individuals, and the rights view does not recognize the moral rights of species to anything, including survival.' . . .
>
> But duties to a species are not duties to a class or a category, not to an aggregation of sentient interests, but to a lifeline. An ethic about species needs to see how the species *is* a bigger event than individual interests or sentience. Making this clearer can support the conviction that a species *ought* to continue . . . Thinking this way, the life the individual has is something passing through the individual as much as something it intrinsically possesses. The individual is subordinate to the species, not the other way round. The genetic set, in which is coded the *telos,* is as evidently a 'property' of the species as of the individual . . .
>
> The species line is quite fundamental. It is more important to protect this integrity than to protect individuals. Defending a form of life, resisting death, regeneration that maintains a normative identity over time – all this is as true of species as of individuals. So what prevents duties arising at that level? The appropriate survival unit is the appropriate level of moral concern.

The species-integrity view as here expressed serves to explain the widely held view, that the extinction of a species is something to be deplored not only because of its consequences for the welfare of humans or animals but as something that is *in itself* bad. If the blue whale becomes extinct this will not be a problem for animal welfare – the whales do not suffer from being extinct. Many humans will regret the loss, but it seems to reverse the true order of things to say that loss of a species is bad because it is regretted by humans. It seems that we should regret the loss of a species because its existence is in itself morally valuable. This seems to imply that we have duties to species and not (only) to individual animals.

Also, the unease that many people feel about the development of transgenic animals may be explained by assuming that a species, as defined by its
genetic make-up, is something to be respected. A view of this sort has been
defended by Fox (1990, p. 32):

> The *telos* or 'beingness' of an animal is its intrinsic nature coupled with the
> environment in which it is able to develop and experience life. We can harm the
> *telos* in many ways, for example through environmental, genetic, surgical and
> pharmacological manipulation. To contend that we can enhance the natural
> *telos* of an animal – and thus by extension believe that we can improve upon
> nature – is *hubris*. Genetic engineering makes it possible to breach the genetic
> boundaries that normally separate the genetic material of totally unrelated
> species. This means that the *telos,* or inherent nature, of animals can be so
> drastically modified (for example by inserting elephant growth hormone genes
> into cattle) as to radically change the entire direction of evolution, and primarily
> toward human ends at that. Is that aspect of the animal's *telos* we refer to as the
> genome and the gene pool of each species not to be respected and not worthy
> of moral consideration?

Many people who are worried about genetic engineering will believe that
the question at the end of the quotation should be given a positive answer.
However, there are still problems about the view that we ought to respect
species defined in terms of genetic structures.

The first problem is the question of what is special about the genetic
structures which exist right now. Throughout evolution genetic structures have
changed continuously. There is no stage in evolution at which animal species
have reached their 'final' development. To say that the present genetic make-
up is special is arbitrary – like saying that art and literature have reached their
final points and should not change further.

The second problem with this view is that breeding for increased health –
for hens resistant to Marek's disease or pigs without malignant hyperthermia
– is usually considered a good thing. Although this may be seen as a remedy
of damages in the gene pool established during genetic selection of high
yielding domestic species, such breeding may eradicate genotypes disposed to
certain illnesses and secure the health of domestic stock. However, the demand
to respect species-integrity will also tell against selective breeding: like transgenesis selective breeding will result in significant genetic changes in species.
This tells against the idea of species-integrity.

Finally, the adherent of species-integrity faces the problem of explaining
how it benefits the animals. For example, there will be consequences concerning which animals come into existence and which don't. If we respect genetic
integrity we will be more reluctant to start programmes of selective breeding
and more disposed to maintain existing breeds. This will only affect which animals
benefit and which are being harmed not *whether* animals benefit or are harmed.
The net result in terms of harms and benefits may be the same or even negative.

It should be noted that the latter objections beg the question against an
adherent of the species-integrity view. They are only objections if what really
matters is animal welfare. However, this is just what the adherent of genetic
integrity wants to deny.

1.4.4. The agent-centred view

The theories we have discussed claim that we have duties to animals because of what happens to the animals. The first two focus on the suffering and rights of *individuals*, while the integrity view focuses on *species*. Many people, however, feel that what is important about our treatment of animals is what it does to *us* as moral agents. This is what we call the agent-centred view.

This view may involve little direct concern for animals at all. Thus Kant argued (1989, pp. 23–24) that we have duties to animals because otherwise we are more likely to act wrongfully to humans:

> Our duties towards animals are merely indirect duties towards humanity. Animal nature has analogies to human nature, and by doing our duties to animals in respect of manifestations of human nature, we indirectly do our duty to humanity. Thus, if a dog has served his master long and faithfully, his service, on the analogy of human service, deserves reward, and when the dog has grown too old to serve, his master ought to keep him until he dies. Such action helps to support us in our duties towards human beings . . . If then any acts of animals are analogous to human acts and spring from the same principles, we have duties towards the animals because thus we cultivate the corresponding duties towards human beings. If a man shoots his dog because the animal is no longer capable of service, he does not fail in his duty to the dog, for the dog cannot judge, but his act is inhuman and damages in himself that humanity which it is his duty to show towards mankind. If he is not to stifle his human feelings, he must practice kindness towards animals, for he who is cruel to animals becomes hard also in his dealing with men.

Other adherents of an agent-centred view do think, however, that animals fall within the scope of morality. A person who causes pointless suffering to animals will be described as 'cruel' and this will be thought to be a morally bad thing. In recent years, one aspect of moral character has been thought by several philosophers to be of special importance: our capacity to *care*. According to this agent-centred view, we should demonstrate care for others, and this may involve concern for their pain or suffering (Noddings, 1984, pp. 149–150):

> Pain crosses the line between the species over a wide range. When a creature writhes or groans or pants frantically, we feel a sympathetic twinge in response to its manifestation of pain. With respect to this feeling, this pain, there does seem to be a transfer that arouses in us the induced feeling, 'I must do something'. Or, of course, the 'I must' may present itself negatively in the form, 'I must not do this thing'. The desire to prevent or relieve pain is a natural element of caring, and we betray our ethical selves when we ignore it or concoct rationalizations to act in defiance of it.

So according to the 'ethics of care', what is wrong with causing suffering to animals is not the fact that suffering is increased (utilitarianism) or that it violates rights (the animals rights view) but that it demonstrates a flaw of character – a lack of care – in the person concerned.

Possessing the capacity to care is one of 'the virtues'. It is often called the virtue of compassion. Over the last three decades, many philosophers have advocated that, instead of basing moral theory on utility or rights (or integrity of species), we should instead develop an agent-centred theory of the virtues. So-called 'virtue ethics' requires us to act in accordance with the virtues: justly, generously, kindly and so on. The virtues, according to this view, should govern our treatment of animals.

Virtue ethics may not require the same things of us as other views. Consider on one hand use of rats in experiments, and on the other hand poisoning and trapping of rats in 'pest' control. Utilitarianism is likely to allow (perhaps even to require) both as long as care is taken to cause the animals as little suffering as possible. An agent-centred theory, such as virtue ethics, may forbid us to use animals in experiments for our own advantage, for this would be cruel, but that when rats cause us inconvenience it is prudent to trap or poison them. A radical version of the animal rights view, on the other hand, may forbid both. (Regan does, as emerged above, draw a distinction between animal experimentation and killing of animals in self-defence. However, he has problems defending this distinction, and here virtue ethics may be better able to draw this distinction in a consistent way.) What about the integrity of species view? That will probably allow both activities too, since rats are plentiful and their species is threatened by neither activity.

One advantage of virtue ethics and other agent-centred theories is that they can make room for moral distinctions which seem to play a role in common-sense ethics. For example, many people draw a distinction between pet animals and animals used for production, and again between those animals and 'pest' animals such as wild mice and rats. They say that a dog is man's friend and should be treated better than production animals. We do, however, also owe duties to the latter because we have taken them into our care. The relevant virtue here is 'stockmanship'. To rats, on the other hand, we do not owe any duties. Rather, the virtue of prudence tells us to get rid of these animals as efficiently as possible.

However, there are also problems with this view. One problem which in a sense is the same as the advantage just mentioned is that it is rather con-servative and makes it too easy to justify what we do. As long as we do things in accordance with traditional norms then we act in a virtuous manner − since the virtues seem to embody traditional ways of doing things. However, some-times it is possible to criticize traditional ways. Thus all the three other views are highly critical of traditional and common-sense views concerning human duties to animals.

Another problem with agent-centred theories such as virtue ethics is their vagueness. First, it is hard to determine whether certain activities are allowed by the theory or not. Why is experimentation cruel and 'pest' control not − especially if scientists do everything they can to reduce suffering and if those involved in 'pest' control do not care whether the animals suffer or not?

A related difficulty concerns conflict between virtues. Scientists who experiment on animals may be seeking a cure for a painful human disease. Imagine that one of them has a daughter who suffers from this disease, and is motivated by a powerful concern to relieve her suffering. Could this scientist not be described as benevolent? If so, what does virtue ethics require of the scientist? It is not clear that our views about who counts as a virtuous person are precise enough to decide. And in this case it is open to proponents of other views to claim that the virtuous person will be the person who maximizes utility, who does not violate rights, or who respects the integrity of species.

This last criticism amounts to saying that an agent-centred view is not really an alternative to the other views. Rather, it seems to presuppose an account of the moral status of animals like one of those given by the other views.

1.4.5. Hybrid views

The views outlined above give incompatible answers to the questions raised at the beginning of this section: What is the basis of our duties towards animals? And what duties do we have? This means that if one accepts, for example, utilitarianism one cannot, on pain of inconsistency, accept the animal rights view and the species-integrity view – although agent-centred views may be compatible with the others.

What is possible, however, is to hold a view that is distinct from each of those views but combines elements from at least two of them. For example, most of those who are attracted to the species-integrity view do also think that it is important to promote animal and human welfare. Thus they may hold a view according to which decisions have to make a trade-off between welfare and respect for genetic integrity.

Another hybrid view which is attractive to many people combines elements from utilitarianism and the animal rights view. One version of this would say that there are certain things that one may not do to animals, no matter how beneficial the consequences, for example causing the animals to experience intense suffering. As long as we abstain from these things we can, on this view, reason as a utilitarian would do. For example, killing of animals or causing them mild distress or inconvenience may be allowed if sufficiently good consequences follow.

The possibility of combining elements from the four main views does not by itself make it an easier task to formulate a full account of human duties to animals which is both plausible and logically consistent. For example, it is very difficult to combine in a consistent way the following two views, both of which most people seem to hold: (i) the utilitarian view of the killing of animals; (ii) the view that it is in principle never, or only in extraordinary circumstances, morally acceptable to kill an innocent human. Here the problem is that the principle underlying the utilitarian view of killing animals will also in some (maybe hypothetical) instances allow killing of, for example, mentally handicapped humans.

At this stage of the argument the question may be asked why one should engage in ethical thinking at all. Why not simply stick to gut reactions and forget justification?

1.5. What is the Point of Engaging in Ethical Thinking?

From our cultural background we have inherited elements from all the main views presented above. Normally, when we form opinions on ethical issues we draw on these views without clarifying the underlying ethical principles. Furthermore, public debates concerning animal issues take place without much ethical thinking being invoked. Two examples may illustrate this.

In the debate about animal research, antivivisectionists show gruesome pictures of animals being experimented on, appealing to our compassion for animals. Those in favour of research show pictures of crying children and seriously ill people, appealing to compassion for those who are ill. Rarely do those participating in the debate tell us which ethical principles underlie their view.

Another example is provided by campaigns against hunting of seals and whales. Appeals are made to fears concerning the environment, reverence for the animals, disgust towards cruel treatment of animals, etc. However, it is not made clear whether the campaigners are against other forms of hunting or other ways of using animals, for example in livestock production, and if they are not, what is the ethically relevant difference between hunting of sea animals and other ways of using animals.

Thus in many debates and campaigns concerning animals the 'arguments' presented are mainly emotional appeals focusing on narrow issues with no attempt to view these issues in a broader ethical context.

Also there is no reason to think that ethical arguments will have much effect in a public debate with strong emotions involved. Even the best moral arguments in favour of controlled whaling will probably not affect the strong antiwhaling sentiments found in some countries. Most likely those who present such arguments will simply be branded as morally corrupt and insensitive.

Why then take interest in ethical arguments rather than simply focus on the best means of promoting the cause that one happens to favour? Or, to put the same question in a slightly different way, why not instead of wasting intellectual resources on difficult philosophical issues rather take an interest in rhetoric, marketing and PR? There seem to be three good answers to this question.

The first answer is that not all people have a cause that they favour. A lot of people have sincere doubts about the extent to which we owe duties to animals. One can use rhetoric to try to convince others but it does not work as a means to convince oneself. Therefore, ethical thinking is needed by all those who want to have an opinion but do not know what to think. Of course, ethical arguments do not provide simple answers – often they generate further doubts. This leads to the second answer.

A value shared by most people who read books like this is intellectual integrity. We like to think of ourselves as people who form their opinions on the basis of evidence rather than superstition and prejudice. Of course, moral views cannot in the same way as scientific hypotheses be based on objective evidence. When we do moral thinking we are not concerned with finding facts about a mind-independent reality. Rather, our aim is to find out what our attitudes should be, if we think rationally and impartially about the matters at issue. That is, we want our attitudes to be *justified*. To uphold intellectual integrity we must therefore be able to justify our moral views.

The third answer is that even though moral arguments may not directly affect the general public they may have an indirect, long-term effect. Thus journalists interested in animal issues may be affected by moral arguments. Journalists often get their information by interviewing scientists or other resource persons. If the persons interviewed are able to engage in an ethical dialogue with the journalist, they will stand a good chance of being quoted and may affect the way the journalist approaches the whole issue. Also animal welfare regulation is not mainly decided by opinion polls. Rather, members of ethical councils and committees, civil servants and politicians who take a special interest in the issues are the key persons, and they will often be both willing and able to listen to ethical arguments. Even if one's views are not fully accepted, they will be taken more seriously if they are backed by ethical thinking which addresses the worries of the public.

Engaging in ethical thinking only seems to have two disadvantages. The first is that it takes time and energy. The other is that ethical arguments may turn out to have quite significant effects on one's ethical attitudes.

However, ethical thinking may reveal that these alleged disadvantages are really to be counted as advantages.

Acknowledgements

The authors want to thank Michael Appleby, Birgitta Forsman and Barry Hughes for helpful comments on an earlier version of this chapter.

CHAPTER 2

Understanding animal welfare

Ian J.H. Duncan (University of Guelph, Canada) and
David Fraser (University of British Columbia, Canada)

Abstract

Scientific study of animal welfare is pursued because of ethical concern over the quality of life of animals. Historically people have expressed this concern by exhorting others to treat animals in certain ways. However, disagreement over what is important for the quality of life of animals led to attempts to study and conceptualize animal welfare in more scientific ways.

Three broad approaches have emerged. (i) 'Feelings-based' approaches define animal welfare in terms of the subjective experiences of animals (feelings, emotions), and emphasize the reduction of negative feelings (suffering, pain, etc.) and/or promotion of positive ones (comfort, pleasure, etc.). Relevant research methods include measures of animals' preferences and motivations, plus behavioural and physiological indicators of emotional states. There is widespread agreement that subjective experiences such as suffering and contentment are important for an animal's welfare, but much work will be needed to produce scientifically based understanding of such experiences. (ii) 'Functioning-based' approaches define animal welfare in terms of the normal or satisfactory biological functioning of the animal. Many relevant (and sometimes conflicting) measures are used, based on health, longevity, reproductive success, and disturbances to behaviour and physiology. Although many of these variables are straightforward to quantify, there is much debate about the link between functioning-based measures and animal welfare. (iii) A third set of approaches call for animals to be raised in a manner that suits the 'nature' of the species or such that the animal performs its full repertoire of behaviour. Performance of the full behavioural repertoire has been widely criticized as a criterion for welfare, but more useful variants of this idea may yet be developed.

The different approaches, although based on different principles, often lead to similar conclusions. However, such agreement does not always occur, especially if genetic selection or artificial environments cause the natural behaviour and motivation of an animal to be maladaptive. In such cases, a broad base of information about the animal may help us reach a consensus about its welfare, but the assessment of an animal's quality of life can never be entirely objective because it involves a mixture of scientific knowledge and value judgements.

2.1. Introduction

'Animal welfare' is not a term that arose in science to express a scientific concept. Rather it arose in society to express ethical concerns regarding the treatment of animals. The 'welfare' of an animal refers to its quality of life, and this involves many different elements such as health, happiness, and longevity, to which different people attach different degrees of importance (Tannenbaum, 1991; Fraser, 1995). However, because science plays an important role in interpreting and implementing social concerns over the quality of animal life, animal welfare was adopted as a subject of scientific research and discussion. This adoption has led to a remarkably protracted debate on how to concept-ualize, in a scientific context, a concept that is fundamentally rooted in values.

One problem is that scientists have often tried to 'define' animal welfare as if it were a purely scientific concept. However, because our conception of animal welfare involves values as well as information, a conventional definition does little more than establish the general area of discourse (Duncan and Dawkins, 1983). To say what we mean by animal welfare requires not that we 'define' the term, as we might define a technical term like 'mass' or 'viscosity', but that we set out the underlying values (Tannenbaum, 1991; Sandøe and Simonsen, 1992; Fraser, 1993, 1995; Mason and Mendl, 1993; Stafleu *et al.*, 1996).

2.2. Welfare and Human Action

The earliest commentaries relevant to animal welfare simply prescribed how animals ought to be treated. For example:

> Six days you shall do your work, but on the seventh day you shall rest; that your ox and your ass may have rest, and the son of your bondmaid, and the alien, may be refreshed. (Exodus, 23: v12)
> You shall not muzzle an ox when it treads out the grain. (Deuteronomy, 25: v4)

Some of the most socially effective modern writing has taken much the same approach. For example, Ruth Harrison (1964, p. 178), in a critique which led to a major public enquiry into modern animal production practices, recommended:

1. The complete abolition of battery cages for laying hens.
2. The complete abolition of the intensive methods now used in veal production . . .
3. . . . specific legislation banning the rearing of animals on deficiency diets . . .
4. Permanent tethering should be banned.
5. Slats should be banned.
6. The keeping of animals in dim light or darkness should be banned.

Astrid Lindgren, whose writings played a key role in the development of animal welfare legislation in Sweden, urged:

> It might even be possible to guarantee that young animals, both bulls and heifers, get a little summertime happiness, at least a temporary reprieve from the floors of barns and the crowded spaces where the poor animals are stored until they

die. Let them see the sun just once, get away from the murderous roar of the fans. Let them get to breathe fresh air for once, instead of manure gas.

(Anonymous, 1989, p. 3)

Positions such as these, which exhort others to take certain actions, may be effective as long as there is a shared understanding about what is truly beneficial for the animal. However, this agreement may be lacking. For example, one veterinarian disagreed that animals are better off in more traditional agricultural systems:

My experience has been that more problems of animal welfare are to be found in the extensive – the open range – the old-fashioned methods and that by-and-large the standard of welfare among animals kept in the so called 'intensive' systems is higher. On balance I feel that the animal is better cared for; it is certainly much freer from disease and attack by its mates; it receives much better attention from the attendants, is sure of shelter and bedding and a reasonable amount of good food and water.

(Taylor, 1972, p. 428)

Disagreements of this type make us go back to first principles and examine more rigorously the values we hold about what constitutes a good or satisfactory life for animals. Three main schools of thought can be distinguished (see Fraser *et al.*, 1997, for further discussion).

2.3. Welfare and the Subjective Experience of Animals

2.3.1. Concepts

Animals can be objects of ethical concern for many different reasons. We may think it wrong, for example, to destroy an animal because it is rare and its death would reduce the genetic diversity of the planet, or because it is part of an ecological system that should be preserved, or because it is beautiful or interesting. However, these sorts of arguments can also be applied to other organisms such as plants.

Animal welfare refers to the particular kind of moral concern we have for animals ('higher' animals, at least) as a result of their capacity for subjective experience. With a few exceptions (e.g. Kennedy, 1992), most people appear to believe that animals experience affective states ('feelings', 'emotions'), and hence that animals can suffer if conditions are bad, and enjoy life if conditions are good. Suffering and happiness are important elements in ethical decisions about our treatment of fellow humans, and it seems natural to use the same criteria in evaluating our treatment of animals. Bentham (1789, p. 283), objecting to the then-common view that animals fall outside our sphere of moral concern because they do not use logic or language, proposed: 'The question is not, Can they reason? nor, Can they talk? but, Can they suffer?' In recent decades, most major critics of animal use have agreed that the capacity of animals to experience suffering and enjoyment is central to concern about their welfare (e.g. Midgley, 1983; Singer, 1990; Rollin, 1992).

Similarly, many scientists have emphasized the subjective feelings of animals as a key component in the scientific investigation of animal welfare (Dawkins, 1980, 1990; Baxter, 1983; Duncan and Dawkins, 1983; Duncan, 1987; Fraser, 1993). For example, Dawkins (1988, p. 209) stated, 'To be concerned about animal welfare is to be concerned with the subjective feelings of animals, particularly the unpleasant subjective feelings of suffering and pain.' Duncan (1993, 1996), noting that we speak of welfare only for organisms that are capable of experiencing subjective feelings, proposed that animal welfare should be defined only in terms of what the animal actually experiences:

> Neither health nor lack of stress nor fitness is necessary and/or sufficient to conclude that an animal has good welfare. Welfare is dependent on what animals feel.
>
> (Duncan, 1993, p. 12)

2.3.2. Research approaches

According to these 'feelings-based' approaches, welfare will be reduced by negative subjective states such as pain, fear, frustration, hunger and thirst, and will be improved by such positive states as comfort, contentment, and the pleasure of certain types of social interaction. The task for science, then, is to study and understand these subjective experiences of animals.

One research approach involves studying the preferences of an animal for different environments, and the strength of the animal's motivation to obtain or avoid certain features of the environment (see Chapter 11). Underlying such research is the assumption that animals will choose (and work to obtain) environments in which they experience more contentment and/or less pain, fear, and other negative states.

Performance of abnormal behaviour (see Chapter 9) is often interpreted as a symptom of some form of negative affective state. For example, various types of stereotyped behaviour have been interpreted as indicating hunger, frustration, boredom, or a desire to escape from unpleasant circumstances (Rushen *et al.*, 1993a; Wemelsfelder, 1993).

Vocal and other signals used by animals in communication may provide information about their subjective experiences. Using 'honest signalling theory', Weary and Fraser (1995a,b) outlined the conditions which should favour the evolution of signals that indicate pain, distress and other negative states.

Apart from evolved signals, other behavioural and physiological features may indicate subjective states. For example, Morton and Griffiths (1985) proposed a range of symptoms, including laboured respiration, reluctance to move, and abnormal salivation, thought to denote pain in laboratory animals.

In the future it may be possible to improve our understanding of subjective experiences by studying their physiological correlates in the nervous system. At present, most physiological measures used in animal welfare research (heart rate, secretion of 'stress' hormones) reflect more general types of arousal, but these may still be useful in comparing different levels of a given affective state. For example, Duncan *et al.* (1986) found that the heart rate of broiler chickens returned to normal more quickly if the chickens were captured by a mechanical device rather than by human handlers. Assuming that capture resulted in fear,

Duncan *et al.* (1986) interpreted the difference in heart rate as indicating a difference in fear. Similarly, increased levels of 'stress' hormones have been used to quantify the reactions of animals to situations believed to involve discomfort (Ladewig and Smidt, 1989) and pain (Shutt *et al.*, 1988; Mellor and Murray, 1989).

2.3.3. Commentary

The use of science to understand the subjective experiences of animals raises a long-standing debate. The idea that behaviour and physiology can help us understand the feelings and emotions of animals was common well into the twentieth century (e.g. Holmes, 1916; Cannon, 1929). Rollin (1990) argued that the widespread influence of Positivism in science caused this to change. Positivist thinkers held that scientific enquiry can extend only to processes that can be observed directly. In line with this view, many (but not all) behavioural scientists considered that understanding the subjective experiences of animals is not part of the behavioural sciences (Tinbergen, 1951; Lorenz, 1963). At the end of the twentieth century, the situation is changing rapidly. In fact, given the widespread discussion by scientists of cognition and affective experience of animals, Burghardt (1995) has proposed that the original 'four aims' of ethology (Tinbergen, 1963) now include a fifth: understanding the subjective experience of animals.

This is, however, a challenging enterprise. The feelings and emotions of animals, like the movement of subatomic particles, cannot be observed directly. Therefore, our understanding of these events is not simple, observational knowledge as we may have of the visible behaviour of animals or the movements of tennis balls. Rather, we have to postulate that these unobservable phenomena have certain properties, are affected by certain influences, and in turn have certain effects on other events that we can observe. For example, we may postulate that suckling piglets experience a particular kind of distress when separated from the mother, and that this distress causes the piglets to give certain characteristic vocalizations. Then we use the occurrence or intensity of these vocalizations to assess the degree of distress when piglets are separated in different ways, for example at the time of weaning (Weary and Fraser, 1995a). Compared to the simple, empirical study of processes that can be observed directly, developing an understanding of unobservable processes involves additional logical steps and assumptions, all of which are open to questioning and revision. Consequently, some scientists prefer to use more traditional measures based on the functioning of the body.

2.4. Welfare and the Biological Functioning of Animals

2.4.1. Concepts

Alternative approaches assess an animal's welfare based on whether its biological systems are functioning in a normal or satisfactory manner. According to these 'functioning-based' approaches, welfare will be reduced by disease, injury and malnutrition; good welfare will be indicated by high levels of growth

and reproduction, normal functioning of physiological and behavioural processes, and ultimately by high rates of longevity and biological fitness.

Fraser and Broom (1990) explain this position as follows:

> Animals have to contend with a complex environment and they have a variety
> of methods of attempting to cope with it. That environment includes physical
> conditions, social influences and any predators, parasites or pathogens which
> may attack the individual. The coping methods include physiological changes in
> the brain, adrenals and immune system and, linked to some of these, behavioural
> changes. Some factors which affect an animal may result in it having great
> difficulty in coping. It may fail to cope in that its fitness is reduced and either it
> dies, or it fails to grow or its ability to reproduce is reduced in some direct way.
> The welfare of an animal is its state as regards its attempts to cope with its
> environment.

Different commentators have adopted a functioning-based approach to
animal welfare for quite different reasons. Many consider that although the
animal's experiences of suffering, contentment, etc. are the defining traits of its
quality of life, such states are difficult to assess scientifically, whereas measures
based on biological functioning provide an adequate and convenient means of
obtaining relevant information. For example, Gonyou (1993a, p. 43) proposed:

> Although the animal's perception of its condition must serve as the basis for
> well-being, research in this area is only beginning. At the present time much can
> be accomplished by using more traditional approaches involving behavioural,
> physiological and pathological studies.

Other commentators adopt a functioning-based approach because they
attach little or no importance to how an animal feels. McGlone (1993, p. 28)
proposed:

> Recently, scientists have suggested that if an animal perceives that it feels poorly
> (as measured primarily by behaviour) then the animal is said to be in a poor state
> of welfare. I dismiss this view as simplistic and inappropriate. I suggest that an
> animal is in a poor state of welfare only when physiological systems are
> disturbed to the point that survival or reproduction are impaired.

A third group proposes that both the subjective experience and biological
functioning of animals are relevant to welfare but in a hierarchically ordered
manner. For example, Curtis (1987) conceptualized animal welfare by drawing
on the 'hierarchy of needs' proposed by the psychologist Abraham Maslow.
As summarized by Curtis (1987, p. 370):

> Our most prepotent needs are the physiologic ones, including those for adequate
> nutriture and a tolerable thermal environment. Once these needs have been
> satisfied, the safety needs emerge, including physical security and freedom from
> fear and anxiety. Most human beings develop other needs in approximately the
> following order: love, esteem, the need for self-actualization, the desire to know
> and understand, and the aesthetic needs.

On this basis, Curtis (1987, p. 370) proposed that animal welfare depends on
a similar hierarchy of needs: (i) physiologic needs, which are well understood
and reasonably well met in agricultural animals, (ii) safety needs, which are 'less
well understood and less well attended', and (iii) behavioural needs, which are

'not well understood'. In a similar vein, Hurnik and Lehman (1985, 1988) proposed that 'life-sustaining' needs are the most basic, followed by 'health-sustaining' needs, and finally 'comfort-sustaining' needs.

2.4.2. Research approaches

Research using biological functioning as an indicator of animal welfare involves a wide range of methods (see Fraser and Broom, 1990, and Chapters 8–10). Studies of veterinary epidemiology and pathology identify injuries and potential threats to health arising from how animals are kept. Studies of animal productivity quantify rates of growth and reproduction on the assumption that impaired welfare will reduce commercial productivity. Measures based on disturbed physiology or behaviour include changes in the endocrine system, suppression of immune competence, and performance of abnormal behaviour. Longer-term measures include longevity and reproductive success.

Many scientists who use a functioning-based approach to animal welfare have been greatly influenced by the concept of 'stress' as developed especially by Selye (1950) (see Chapter 10). Selye had noted that a variety of challenges to the animal (physical restraint, exposure to cold, injection of toxins) produce several characteristic changes in the body, including activation of the anterior pituitary and the adrenal cortex, and increased secretion of glucocorticoids such as cortisol. These changes were interpreted as indicating 'stress' in the animal. Animal welfare scientists seized on this idea, and have used glucocorticoid secretion and related processes in a wide range of studies of animal management and housing, generally assuming that increases in indicators of 'stress' imply reduced welfare (see reviews and critiques in Wood-Gush *et al.*, 1975; Dantzer and Mormède, 1983; Moberg, 1985b; Fraser and Broom, 1990; Rushen and de Passillé, 1992; Broom and Johnson, 1993; and Chapter 10).

Such measures, however, raise difficult issues about the boundary separating impaired welfare from routine adjustments in bodily processes (Barnett and Hemsworth, 1990; Mendl, 1991). Features such as heart rate and cortisol secretion vary routinely in response to many changes in the animal's environment and behaviour; consequently, we need some criterion to decide at what point such measures cease to be routine bodily adjustments and become relevant to assessing the animal's welfare. Moberg (1985b) proposed one such criterion. He noted that increases in the body's 'stress' responses, although not necessarily harmful or unpleasant in themselves, may eventually lead to some 'pre-pathological' state involving increased likelihood of harm to health and reproduction. Moberg recommended that these pre-pathological states (e.g. reduction of immune competence, suppression of endocrine responses needed for reproduction, and increased social aggression) be used as criteria for impaired welfare. As a more quantitative criterion, Barnett and Hemsworth (1990, p. 182) proposed: 'It is reasonable to suggest a risk to welfare when a sustained elevation of >40% in free corticosteroid concentrations . . . is evident.' Difficulties with such 'cut-off criteria' of animal welfare are discussed by Mendl (1991).

A different way of linking biological functioning to welfare was recommended by Hurnik (1993). Hurnik argued that the welfare of an animal is related to how well its 'needs' (for survival, health and comfort) are met. He noted that needs differ in importance to the animal, and that humans cannot easily assess the relative importance of the different needs. Hurnik proposed that the more adequately an animal's needs are met, the longer it may be expected to live. Hence, longevity should, in effect, integrate the satisfaction of the more important and less important needs, thus eliminating the errors that people might make in judging the relative importance of different factors. Limitations of this approach have been noted (Fraser, 1995). For example, McCay *et al.* (1939) found that laboratory rats lived considerably longer if severely restricted in their energy intake, compared to rats fed *ad libitum*. In this case, the fact that longer life was achieved at the cost of chronic under-nutrition (and presumably chronic hunger) casts doubt on the usefulness of longevity as a fully satisfactory indicator of welfare.

2.4.3. Commentary

For practical purposes, we expect changes in biological functioning to be easier to demonstrate scientifically than changes in what an animal experiences. It is easier, for example, to establish that an animal is injured or malnourished than that it is experiencing pain or hunger.

Conceptually, however, a functioning-based approach runs into difficulties because the link between biological functioning and the animal's welfare is not always apparent. Where there are clear differences in health (e.g. Ekesbo, 1966; Lindqvist, 1974; Tauson and Abrahammson, 1994), there is likely to be little disagreement that the animal's quality of life is affected. However, there is less agreement that high levels of other aspects of functioning (growth rate, reproduction) necessarily denote a better quality of life, and there is little consensus on the baseline that should be used in assessing such measures. For example, if a dairy cow is producing large quantities of milk, would a further increase really indicate better quality of life?

Finally, it is difficult to draw conclusions about animal welfare if different measures of biological functioning fail to agree. In veal calves, for example, Wiepkema *et al.* (1987) found that calves with a high incidence of a form of abnormal behaviour (stereotyped tongue-playing) had fewer ulcers of the abomasum. In broilers, sudden death syndrome is associated with birds that have a higher than average growth rate (Leeson *et al.*, 1995). As noted by Mendl and Deag (1995, p. 125), 'there are significant problems in amalgamating all the different types of measures . . . into a single "welfare" currency'.

2.5. Welfare and the 'Nature' of Animals

2.5.1. Concepts

A third view considers that to promote animal welfare we should raise animals in 'natural' environments and allow them to behave in 'natural' ways. The idea is reflected in the much quoted proposal that animals should have the 'freedom to perform most types of natural behaviour' (Webster *et al.*, 1986, p. 1) and in Lindgren's view that farmers should raise animals in sunshine and fresh air (see above). Rollin (1992, 1993) gave more formal expression to this idea. He proposed that each animal species has an inherent, genetically encoded 'nature' which he called its 'telos'. For example, it is in the nature of canaries to fly, of pigs to root, and of cattle to ruminate. Rollin (1993, p. 48) suggested that to promote the welfare of animals, we need to raise them in ways that respect their natures:

> It is likely that the emerging social ethic for animals . . . will demand from scientists data relevant to a much increased concept of welfare. Not only will welfare mean control of pain and suffering, it will also entail nurturing and fulfillment of the animals' natures, which I call telos.

Rollin was deliberately vague about how to identify or define the 'telos' of an animal, and he called upon ethologists to flesh out the concept through the study of behaviour (Rollin, 1992). Scientists who have thought along similar lines have sometimes proposed that animals should be kept in environments where they perform their full 'repertoire' of natural behaviour. For example, Kiley-Worthington (1989, p. 333) proposed:

> If we believe in evolution . . . then in order to avoid suffering, it is necessary over a period of time for the animal to perform all the behaviors in its repertoire, because it is all functional; otherwise it would not be there . . . Inevitably, then, if we take evolutionary arguments seriously, we already have a blueprint on how to optimize an animal's environment so that prolonged suffering is reduced or eliminated. It will be one in which the animal is able to perform all the behaviors in his repertoire.

2.5.2. Research approaches

Scientists applying this conception of animal welfare often study the behaviour of animals in a wild state, and compare this with similar animals living in captivity, apparently on the assumption that differences will denote deficencies in the captive environment. For example, Veasey et al. (1996) compared the behaviour of giraffes in four different zoo environments with that of free-living wild giraffes, but concluded that the observed behavioural differences did not allow clear conclusions about animal welfare.

Scientists have also attempted to design environments that allow animals to express their full behavioural repertoire. For example, Stolba and Wood-Gush (1984) studied domestic pigs in a partly wooded area and noted that the animals often rooted in the soil, rubbed against trees, and defecated in visually protected areas. Stolba and Wood-Gush then designed a multi-area pen where these and other forms of natural behaviour were possible. Other research has tried to identify environments that promote normal behavioural development. For example, Schouten (1986) compared piglets raised for the first weeks after birth in small or large pens, and found that the more confined animals failed to develop certain elements of normal social behaviour.

2.5.3. Commentary

The view that animals should perform their full 'repertoire' of behaviour was common in early animal welfare research, but Dawkins (1980) and others pointed out its shortcomings as a criterion for animal welfare. In particular, the behavioural repertoire of animals includes certain activities that are adaptations to cope with adverse circumstances. For example, rabbits hide from predators, attack intruders, and fluff their coats in the cold. By most criteria, however, the environments that bring out these behaviours tend to reduce well-being, not increase it. Poole (1996, p. 218), objecting to this approach to animal welfare research, suggested:

> Animals suffer severe and often fatal problems in nature, and their natural behaviour reflects their efforts to survive. To consider that wild behaviour is always indicative of well-being is therefore unrealistic; it most often represents a life and death struggle for survival.

The more general idea that we can improve animal welfare by respecting the 'nature' of animals is intuitively appealing and fits well with popular critiques that call for animals to be raised in more natural environments. However, the concept of an animal's 'nature' would need to be made more specific before it could give clear guidance in judging animal welfare; generalizations might lead us astray. For example, we might conclude that seagulls (*Larus* spp.) had evolved to live in such close association with the sea that this is an essential part of their 'nature'. However, within the past 30 years, the herring gull (*Larus argentatus*) and the lesser black-backed gull (*Larus fuscus*) have changed their habits in north-western Europe and now voluntarily live in very artificial environments created by human beings: they nest on buildings, roost on playing fields, and forage on garbage dumps. Gulls are so successful in this mode of living that such populations are expanding rapidly (Furness and Monaghan, 1987). Thus, it turns out that the sea is not an essential part of the 'nature' of these seagulls.

However, Rollin's concept of a genetically encoded 'telos' could be interpreted in ways that are more useful in welfare assessment. In the 'higher' animals at least, evolution favours not simply a repertoire of actions that are performed with a characteristic frequency, but a series of conditional rules whereby the animal uses certain types of behaviour in response to certain circumstances. If we construe 'telos' to mean these conditional rules, then the concept may be more useful in assessing quality of life (Fraser *et al.*, 1997). That pigs fail to wallow or huddle in a given type of housing may not indicate any deficiency in the environment, but if pigs are completely prevented from huddling when cold and wallowing when hot, then their natures are arguably not being respected and their welfare may be compromised.

2.6. Discussion

The three conceptions of animal welfare described above, although based on different basic principles, will often lead to similar conclusions. In general we expect the natural behaviour of animals to be adaptive; that is, natural behaviour should generally promote biological functioning in the sense of survival, health, and reproductive success. Likewise, pleasant and unpleasant subjective experiences are widely seen as adaptations that promote the same positive outcomes by motivating animals to perform beneficial actions and to avoid harm (Dawkins, 1980). As long as natural behaviour and subjective feelings do promote biological functioning, the different conceptions of animal welfare should lead to similar conclusions.

In fact, research does indicate that feelings-based and functioning-based interpretations often correspond. For example, domestic pigs (Baldwin and Ingram, 1967; Morrison et al., 1989) and chicks (Morrison and McMillan, 1985) will 'work' to turn on heaters, presumably to avoid feeling cold, and the temperatures they choose correspond well to their thermal requirements for optimum functioning. Similarly, epidemiological studies have shown that laying hens produce more eggs and have a lower mortality when space allowance is high and group size is low (Hughes, 1975). In preference tests, hens do choose small group sizes (Hughes, 1977) and 'work' to increase cage space (Lagadic, 1989) to approximately the same level at which improvements in egg production have been noted (Hughes, 1975).

Similarly, permitting animals to perform natural behaviour has often been shown to promote biological functioning. For example, confined pigs that are given an outlet for natural foraging behaviour are less likely to injure each other through tail-biting (Fraser et al., 1991); and allowing bucket-fed calves to suck by providing an artificial teat leads to greater secretion of digestive enzymes (de Passillé et al., 1993).

However, the three approaches do not always give rise to similar conclusions. Shortly before farrowing, sows seek isolated farrowing sites and create elaborate nests, thus providing their piglets with a warm, protected environment. This nest-building is part of their natural behaviour, and sows that are prevented from performing the behaviour may experience frustration. However, the functional outcome of the behaviour – a high rate of piglet survival – can be achieved as well or better by keeping the sow in a small enclosure which provides a high level of hygiene, warmth, supervision, and physical protection of the piglets. Here the natural behaviour (nest-building) is prevented, and a negative state (frustration) may be experienced, yet the functional outcome (piglet survival) can be very satisfactory. In such cases, the conclusions that we draw about the sow's welfare will depend on the relative importance that we attach to the different criteria, and no single, purely objective assessment is possible (Sandøe and Simonsen, 1992; Fraser, 1995).

The different criteria of animal welfare can disagree for a number of reasons. First, the environment in which the animal is kept may not correspond to the environment in which the species evolved and the individual developed. In the example just given, the farrowing sow's natural behaviour (nest-building) and feelings (frustration if the behaviour is prevented) would help the sow to reproduce successfully in a natural environment, but they may no longer be the best way to achieve the functional outcome in an artificial environment. Second, genetic changes to domestic animals may also result in disagreement among the different criteria for animal welfare. Modern strains of broiler chickens have been bred to consume so much food that they develop 'diseases of fast growth' such as skeletal problems and ascites (e.g. Duff and Hocking, 1986;

Thorp and Maxwell, 1993). In this case the motivation to eat, and presumably feelings of hunger, results in a level of food intake that is harmful to health and biological functioning.

How do we draw conclusions about animal welfare when such conflicts arise? A common recommendation is to use a large number of measures (Duncan and Dawkins, 1983; Fraser and Broom, 1990; Broom, 1996). For example, Dawkins (1983b, p. 23) suggests:

> Different measures of welfare do not always correlate. It is dangerous to put too much weight on any one . . . We should take a synthetic view involving all possible measures and in this way avoid the pitfalls involved in any one of them.

However, even with a broad base of information, science is limited in its ability to generate consensus. The relative importance that different people attach to different elements of animal welfare is, by the very nature of the issue, not a purely factual matter (Tannenbaum, 1991), nor can it be made a purely factual matter by any known type of scientific research (Fraser, 1995). As long as people disagree on what constitutes a good or satisfactory life for animals, there can be no single conception of animal welfare.

2.7. Conclusions

- Different conceptions of animal welfare used by scientists reflect different value positions on what constitutes a good or satisfactory quality of life for animals.
- 'Feelings-based' conceptions correspond to the widespread view that our treatment of animals should not cause undue suffering nor unduly deprive animals of comfort and contentment. Much work is needed to develop a scientific understanding of the subjective experiences of animals.
- 'Functioning-based' approaches correspond to the view that animals should be allowed to thrive and be healthy. This conception provides some widely accepted criteria for poor welfare, such as increased incidence of disease and injury. However, consensus is lacking on how less extreme alterations in biological functioning (reduced rates of growth and reproduction, increased indicators of 'stress') relate to the quality of life of animals.
- A third conception, which assesses the welfare of an animal by whether it can live according to its inherent 'nature', remains to be given a satisfactory biological interpretation. One common version of the idea – that animals should perform their entire behavioural repertoire – often fails to agree with other conceptions of welfare.
- When disagreements arise among the three conceptions of animal welfare, more complete information may help a consensus to form. However, science cannot provide a purely objective assessment because the conclusions we draw about an animal's welfare are based on value judgements as well as knowledge.

Acknowledgements

We thank Dan Weary, Ed Pajor, Barry Milligan, Allison Taylor and Tina Widowski for valuable discussion of these ideas. David Fraser was on the staff of the Centre for Food and Animal Research, Agriculture and Agri-Food Canada, during the preparation of this chapter.

PART II
Problems

This part of the book starts by considering the subject of natural and artificial environments, including variability in environments and in animals' responses to environments. Chapter 3 does this by concentrating on exploration, and emphasizes that animals are not just passive in their interactions with environments (as implied by some ideas about stimuli and responses) but also active, and that this can be a major cause of problems.

Problems for welfare are diverse, because welfare is not a simple scale, from bad to good: it has many different aspects. One way of expressing this diversity is the Five Freedoms: the UK's Farm Animal Welfare Council suggests that ideally animals should have freedom from hunger and thirst, freedom from discomfort, freedom from pain, injury and disease, freedom to express normal behaviour and freedom from fear and distress (Farm Animal Welfare Council, 1992). Such categories are neither definitive nor independent of each other, but provide a useful framework. The rest of Part II is largely based on the Five Freedoms but without a specific chapter on discomfort. Discomfort frequently occurs in association with other problems or as a lesser form of such problems and there have been few studies concentrating on this topic. A notable exception is the study on thermal discomfort by Mitchell mentioned in Chapter 12. It demonstrates the importance of defining and measuring problems before attempting to solve them.

CHAPTER *3*
Environmental challenge

Françoise Wemelsfelder (Scottish Agricultural College, UK)
and Lynda Birke (University of Warwick, UK)

Abstract

Environmental challenge is what life is all about. Artificial environments present different challenges to natural ones and this may cause problems for the animals; lack of challenge may also cause problems. This chapter provides discussion of models of exploration, and their implications for animal welfare. Information-acquisition and agency (the ability to create novelty) are examined; both are needed to explain the propensity of animals to interact with and to investigate their environment actively. Given this tendency, environmental challenge should be seen as an integral part of behavioural development and well-being. The absence of challenge in captive environments appears undesirable and may engender apathy and an enduring sense of boredom.

3.1. Introduction

Animals in the wild face unpredictable and challenging environments. Predators, food-shortage, weather, floods, illness – all threaten their health and survival. Whether, and how, animals deal with such challenges depends upon many attributes of the environment: places to hide or rest, availability of resources, the geography of the terrain and conspecifics – other adults or young. For captive or domesticated animals, moreover, they include relationships with human caretakers, as well as transient interactions with humans such as occur during transportation. Each aspect may help an animal deal with challenge, or may present challenge in its own right. In addition, animals may be challenged as a result of their own activities. Active individuals with large home ranges or territories face different challenges to animals that are sedentary. Animals in complex social groups must deal continuously with the intricacies of social interaction and communication. Challenges are thus intrinsic and natural, yet if too many occur, particularly within a short period of time, welfare is likely to be compromised.

By contrast, animals in captivity tend to live in highly predictable and structured environments, where they are challenged infrequently or not at all. One might expect this to be an improvement: the animal can relax and get on with its life. But what is life without some kind of challenge? Could it go too far the other way – might animals also suffer from a lack of environmental challenge? Is an animal's ability to deal with challenges in itself a necessary condition for good welfare? In this chapter we pursue these questions. We focus discussion on exploration, a notion which, in its most general sense, indicates the ability of animals to investigate and deal with novel aspects of the environment. Any environment presents an animal with novelty and potential information, which it will inspect and evaluate for further use. Furthermore, environments may offer opportunities for interaction and manipulation, for creating novelty rather than merely inspecting it. In this case, animals appear voluntarily to seek challenge. This ability we will designate as 'agency'.

These two aspects of exploration, 'information' and 'agency', will provide an outline for discussion in this chapter. Section 3.2 reviews theories which focus on exploration as information-acquisition; these indicate that a middle range of environmental novelty provides 'optimum' challenge in terms of welfare. Section 3.3 deals with studies bearing on the notion of agency; these suggest that environmental challenges may be conducive to welfare by enhancing behavioural competence and versatility. In conclusion, we propose that both aspects of exploration (information and agency) are needed to define adequately the concept of animal boredom.

3.2. Exploration as Acquisition of Information

The precise nature and function of exploration have always been difficult to define – patterns of exploration merge so easily into other kinds of behaviour, such as foraging, or play. One early theorist (Welker, 1961) claimed that:

> I find it virtually impossible to think of play and exploration as unique
> behavioural categories with characteristics distinct from other phenomena
> within the behavioural repertoire of mammals.

Yet if we observe a laboratory rat placed into an unfamiliar arena, or cattle or horses led out to new pasture, what we are likely to see is the animals moving around inspecting all kinds of stimuli in their new surroundings. There can be little doubt that a major function of exploratory behaviour is to provide animals with information about their environment. Despite the obvious importance of this function for survival in the wild, exploration has not been the focus of much research interest from ethologists. Even Hediger, in his seminal work 'Wild Animals in Captivity' (1950), while raising many issues relevant to the welfare of wild animals in a captive zoo environment, did not discuss exploratory behaviour. Most theories of exploration have been proposed by experimental psychologists in the context of learning and motivation. In this section, we will discuss and review these theories, in two categories: the older drive-reduction models and more recent cognitive models.

3.2.1. Drive-reduction models of exploration
In the 1950s to 1970s, several reviews were written in an attempt to define and explain exploratory behaviour in the light of the major psychological theories of motivation at the time, particularly those centred on drive reduction (Welker, 1961; McReynolds, 1962; Fowler, 1965). An especially influential work was Berlyne's 'Conflict, Arousal and Curiosity', published in 1960. In

this book, Berlyne identified several different types and categories of exploratory behaviour. These are still relevant today, providing a framework for study and discussion in recent studies of exploration (Russell, 1983; Wood-Gush and Vestergaard, 1989).

Berlyne's three types of exploratory behaviour are: (i) orientation towards a particular stimulus (through any of the sense organs); (ii) locomotor exploration (movement around an area for general investigation); (iii) investigation of a particular stimulus or object (mostly sniffing, licking, or manipulating the object). These three types of response frequently merge into larger patterns of exploration and may also intersperse with other behaviour such as foraging or play. Because locomotor exploration cannot easily be distinguished from locomotion directed at primary goals such as food or drink, Berlyne recommended that research should focus on the investigation of specific stimuli and objects. In this category, he distinguished two further sub-categories: inspective and inquisitive exploration. The former category, Berlyne suggested, describes exploration in response *to* a stimulus change, while the latter indicates exploration *for* a stimulus change. Inspective exploration is primarily passive, where the subject reacts to a perceived change and is affected by it, whereas inquisitive exploration appears more active, in that the subject creates change through its own actions. In Berlyne's words (1960, pp. 78–80):

> Exploratory behavior is by no means confined to the service of selective attention, all three forms of which – attention in performance, attention in learning, and attention in remembering – mean selection from elements that are actually present in the stimulus field. Exploratory responses are subject to no such limitation. Their principal function is, in fact, to afford access to environmental information that was previously not available. They do so by intensifying or clarifying stimulation from objects that are already represented in the stimulus field . . . or else by bringing receptors into contact with new stimulus objects . . . We shall call these inspective and inquisitive exploration respectively.

A critical question facing Berlyne and other early psychological theorists was how such exploratory behaviour is motivated. Does it occur largely in response to internal changes in the animal's physiology, as eating is motivated by a deficit in blood sugar? With regard to welfare, this is an important question. For, if it should be demonstrated that animals are internally motivated, i.e. have a need, to explore, then depriving them of the opportunity to do so means violating one of the basic freedoms. As we shall see, this is not easily done.

Simple (Lorenzian) drive-reduction models postulate that as the internal physiological deficit grows, drive increases and eventually 'overflows' into the performance of appetitive and consummatory behaviour. The intake of, say, food, then reduces the drive to eat, and the behaviour eventually ceases. In line with such a view, psychologists postulated that exploratory behaviour may arise either from a curiosity drive, or from a drive to reduce boredom. Berlyne was among those who argued for a curiosity drive, presumably evoked by exposure to novel or conspicuous stimuli. And indeed, numerous experiments have confirmed that incentives such as 'stimulus-change' (Kish, 1955), 'stimulus-complexity' (Dember et al., 1957), or 'stimulus-novelty' (Welker, 1956) reliably motivate animals to approach and explore an experimental arena. The notion of a curiosity drive is thus useful in that animals (or at least many species) clearly do appear to be curious about a great many things. On the other hand, it is problematic theoretically, in that contact with the novel stimulus is assumed both to elicit the drive and reduce it; without a clear physiological correlate of curiosity, this explanation appears circular.

An alternative view was that exploration occurs in response to a boredom drive, evoked by exposure to a prolonged lack of novel or interesting stimulation. Glanzer (1958, pp. 311–312) argued that a boredom drive arises from an intrinsic need to acquire and process information:

> The organism is viewed as an information processing system that requires certain amounts of information per unit time . . . An organism that has had a high flow of information directed in the past would have a high requirement or standard. An organism that has lived in an impoverished environment would have a low requirement or standard.

This conception accounts for the propensity of animals to go out and search for novel information, for example by patrolling and checking the boundaries of territories or home cages (Cowan, 1983). However, without an independent (physiological) measure of boredom, this concept, like that of curiosity, suffers from circularity: a state of boredom can be inferred only when exploration of a particular stimulus actually occurs, and thus has little explanatory value.

The strong and weak points of such motivational accounts of exploration are illustrated by recent experimental studies on exploration in piglets. Pigs seem interesting subjects for the study of exploratory behaviour, being opportunistic foragers highly motivated to gather information about a diversity of environmental features (Wood-Gush *et al.*, 1990). Accordingly, Wood-Gush and colleagues have repeatedly expressed their concern that modern intensive farming systems may appear highly monotonous to growing pigs, and give rise to chronic apathy and boredom (Newberry *et al.*, 1988; Wood-Gush and Vestergaard, 1989). The motivation of pigs to explore novel stimuli was investigated in two experimental studies. The first showed that piglets housed under relatively bare conditions spent more time examining a novel arena than animals living in a more complex environment and also spent longer examining a novel object presented in their home pen (Wood-Gush *et al.*, 1990). The second study provided evidence that piglets select an arena containing a novel object rather than one containing a familiar object (Wood-Gush and Vestergaard, 1991). The authors conclude (p. 603):

> These results clearly demonstrate that piglets 5–6 weeks of age are able to perform inquisitive exploration, i.e. carry out a response to initiate a change in their environment that has no primary reinforcement such as food, water, heat or illumination, but that will provide novelty. This type of curiosity indicates the presence of a motivational system with endogenous activating mechanisms, unlike inspective curiosity which is reactive.

They support their postulation of an endogenous motivation for exploration by arguing that both the greater persistence of the pigs to explore novelty in the first study, and the observed increase in locomotor play observed in the second study, should be interpreted as a rebound effect due to prolonged exposure to unstimulating environmental conditions. They suggest that in such conditions piglets redirect their investigation to inappropriate stimuli such as the ears and tails of litter mates. Rushen (1993) takes issue with this interpretation, proposing instead that, rather than providing evidence of an endogenous motivation to explore, the observed effects are related to the various stimulus-aspects of the test situation. The increase in play, he suggests, arises from the increase in available space offered by the test situation, while the more persistent interest in novelty shown by pigs in bare environments may be due to a reduced threshold to perceive novelty. Lastly, he suggests that redirected behaviours such as tail-biting may indicate nutritional deficiencies rather than boredom. Wood-Gush and Vestergaard (1993) retort that there is no evidence showing that frequency of play is dependent on space availability, that the barren-housed pigs did not show any signs of fear or other evidence of increased reactivity to novelty, and that their piglets were fed *ad libitum*. They maintain that inquisitive exploration is an internally motivated behaviour, and as such should be facilitated by the captive environment.

The different stances taken by these authors reflect the problem of circularity associated with drive-reduction models. Although the results clearly indicate the propensity of pigs to seek out environmental change, the problem is that this propensity shows itself only in the experimental test situation. An alternative account in terms of a more reactive, inspective form of exploration in response to the test situation can therefore easily be construed. Thus, providing experimental evidence that animals have an internally motivated need to explore is not at all straightforward. Certainly, many species will readily explore new environments or novel stimuli if given the chance. But does this indicate a need to explore, the hampering of which causes animals to suffer some form of distress? To investigate this question in more naturalistic conditions is hard, since it is extremely difficult to separate the need to explore from other needs, such as those of finding food, shelter or the company of conspecifics. However, given the all-pervading tendency of animals to investigate their surroundings, one cannot rule out a 'need to explore', nor the possibility that deprivation leads to an aversive state of boredom.

Novel stimuli elicit not only orienting or investigatory responses, they may also lead to withdrawal or avoidance. An unexpected loud noise, or the sudden appearance of an unfamiliar individual, may startle the animal into a fear response. This suggests that novelty *per se* is not always desirable. Some theorists working with drive models have suggested that only moderate discrepancy will promote exploration, and that for most animals there is an optimum degree of novelty. Hebb (1955) proposed a model in which he links exploration to an optimal level of arousal. Too little novelty would fail to arouse the animal's attention due to a lack of discrepancy with its previous experience, whereas too much would startle or frighten it into a fear- or stress-response. Again, however, the predictive validity of this model depends on the independent measurement of arousal. Several physiological correlates of stress-related arousal have been proposed (e.g. plasma corticosterone); however, a unitary and consistent measure of arousal, linking the concepts of boredom, curiosity and fear into a continuous scale, has not been established. Stress and arousal are now recognized as complex and multi-factorial phenomena, making the search for a single scale of arousal unlikely to succeed (Wiepkema and Koolhaas, 1993).

Drive-reduction models focused on 'optimal' levels of stimulation do have heuristic value, however, in that they alert us to the implications of general environmental stimulation for welfare. Lack of stimulation has been linked to the development of abnormally redirected and stereotyped patterns of behaviour (e.g. Stevenson, 1983), and this in turn has motivated animal keepers and scientists to design an array of devices and techniques for the enrichment of captive environments. These efforts have been successful in reducing the occurrence of abnormal behaviour, eliciting a variety of species-specific appetitive and investigatory patterns. For example, Chamove et al. (1982) showed that providing various primate species with woodchip floor coverings greatly increased the time they spent on the floor searching for food items. In contrast, researchers have become increasingly aware of the potentially arousing and stressful consequences of too much disturbance. The importance of stable and familiar relationships between farm animals and their caretakers, for example, has been well established (Hemsworth et al., 1994a). In zoos, the potentially stressful effect of the general public on the animals on display is the subject of increasing scrutiny. In addition to such efforts, it may be useful to try and identify what animals perceive to be an 'optimal range of stimulation', through preference tests and operant conditioning (Dawkins, 1990; Ladewig and Matthews, 1996).

Useful as such models may be practically, they remain problematic theoretically. Firstly, it is not easy to determine how different animals and species perceive and evaluate 'novelty'. An unfamiliar conspecific or inanimate novel object may excite and interest some animals but frighten others. Secondly, how animals evaluate novelty will vary with circumstance. The presence of conspecifics influences the way in which an individual – particularly of a social species – responds to a novel stimulus. Thus, what constitutes 'optimality' is notoriously difficult to determine: as Marian Dawkins (1990) notes, environmental preferences can be altered by previous experiences, and may not be stable over time. In general, models which present exploration in terms of some form of internal drive or need have difficulty in dealing with the specific stimulus-aspects which elicit and guide exploration. At the very least exploration should be seen as a resultant of an interaction between internal motivational states and external environmental factors (Toates, 1983). In this light, later theorists became interested in more cognitive accounts of exploration, postulating that animals have a fundamental need to acquire and process 'information' about the external environment.

3.2.2. Cognitive models of exploration

Cognitive models of behaviour regard the ability to gather and process information as fundamental: exploration is not merely another drive, it is a primary motivator in the quest for survival. Inglis has investigated information-gathering in animals in considerable detail (Inglis, 1975; Inglis and Freeman, 1976; Inglis and Ferguson, 1986) and proposes (1983) that information-gathering, and the concomitant reduction of uncertainty, are primary activities of animals living in a variable environment, with other behaviour subsidiary to it. He argues that, through systematic and persistent movement through an environment, animals acquire knowledge of the spatial and temporal relationships surrounding them. This in turn allows them to form expectancies, to detect novelty and to classify items into categories (e.g. food items). Inglis' model shares with drive-reduction models the prediction that extremes of stimulation are undesirable: too little information-processing activity will induce boredom, too much will lead to fear. But it adds another twist: Inglis (1983, p. 97) suggests that 'an animal prefers the greatest degree of discrepant input to occur when it is best able to assimilate that input'. In other words, it is the balance between stimulus input and the animal's ability to assimilate it that determines whether, for example, the animal explores or flees. 'Optimality' is thus seen as partly dependent on an animal's current behaviour and situation, a view which concurs with research on how animals value information (Stephens, 1989). As Inglis points out (1983, p. 104):

> An animal should only strive 'optimally' to reduce a specific need when the relevant deprivation state is sufficiently intense to gain attentional priority. Therefore 'optimal' behaviour should become 'less optimal' as the deprivation state is reduced, for the valence of the need-related expectancies will fall, thereby enabling other environmental cues successfully to compete for attentional priority.

An important feature of cognitive models such as these is that they allow for developmental and experiential change in the animal's perception of 'optimal input'; an aspect absent from drive-reduction models. A new-born animal soon begins to move independently, away from the nest and/or mother, to seek stimulation in its own right. It increasingly ventures into unfamiliar areas, gaining information as it goes. For altricial species, such map-building begins with mother/nest as reference points; for many precocial species, maps must be built from the first day of life. At the same time as building maps, young animals acquire systems of classification which form the basis for later evaluations of novelty. To mature animals, 'novelty' is relative to whatever they had to face before, and to how much they remember of that experience, so animals raised in captivity are likely to acquire systems of classification which are less intricate and varied than those of their wild conspecifics. These animals will have less expectancy, and perceive fewer major discrepancies with stored environmental information. However, if subsequently moved to a richer stimulus environment, an animal's expectancy increases and it will seek more input. 'Optimum' stimulus input may thus vary according to an animal's stage of development and its previous environmental history (Inglis and Freeman, 1976).

Such a conception of exploration has implications for animal welfare. Texts on animal welfare rarely discuss how developmental and environmental changes may affect and alter behavioural needs. Yet such changes occur, colouring an animal's perception of the environment and the challenges it presents. Glanzer's suggestion (1958, see quotation above) that animals growing up in a relatively impoverished environment require less input would imply that for such animals, boredom may be less of an issue; they simply expect less excitement than animals used to the vagaries of a diverse and changing environment. However, this argument can be turned on its head. It could equally be argued that animals from an impoverished background, because of poorly developed expectancy, are less well able to classify and evaluate perceived environmental stimuli. Unexpected or novel events will startle and arouse more, so that animals fail to exploit the novel information available. Laboratory animals, for example, may adjust poorly to experimental procedures which involve transport and handling, while for farm animals arrival at a slaughterhouse, with its crowded, noisy, unfamiliar conditions, may be particularly stressful. Thus, rather than living in quiescent adjustment to their surroundings, animals from an impoverished background may be overwhelmed by events, and fail to cope.

Cognitive models of exploration, then, seem to overcome some of the problems of earlier drive-reduction theories. The notion of 'information' incorporates the effect of both internal and external factors on exploratory behaviour. Such models allow for an animal's developmental and environmental history, and can account for much of the variation in exploration under different circumstances. However, cognitive models cannot account for some aspects of inquisitive exploration (Berlyne, 1960). The persistence and versatility with which animals explore and manipulate their environment cannot easily be explained in terms of incentive, homeostatic reward (the acquisition of information). 'Information' is not an object which can readily be 'found' at a certain location. Animals must interact actively with their environment and evaluate it, through orientation, searching and monitoring, for any information-processing to occur at all. Cognitive models turn this view around, regarding the active role of animals as a by-product of their information-processing capacity. However, this view leaves important aspects of exploration unconsidered; we will therefore turn to a strand of theorizing which focuses more on the animal-as-agent.

3.3. Exploration as Agency

The notion of agency, though not influential in studies of animal exploration, has been more so in human studies, especially those of exploration and play in children (Woodworth, 1958; White, 1959; Hutt, 1970; Hughes, 1983). These studies brought to light the propensity of children to direct their attention to an object or some other aspect of the environment and to engage in various kinds of interaction, seemingly just for the sake of it. A broom stick, for example, can be used as a horse, a weapon, a staff or a bench; each creating an opportunity for trying out new forms of behaviour and practising new skills. Such observations led Woodworth (1958) to propose his 'behavior-primacy' theory, that 'all behavior is directed primarily toward dealing with the environment'. A contemporary theorist, White (1959), subscribed to this theory and proposed the concept of 'competence' to interpret the voluntary character of child behaviour and development. In his paper 'Motivation reconsidered: the concept of competence', White (1959, p. 323) argued:

> The urge toward competence is inferred specifically from behavior that shows a lasting focalization and that has the characteristics of exploration and experimentation, a kind of variation within the focus . . . it is characteristic of this particular sort of activity that it is selective, directed and persistent, and that instrumental acts will be learned for the sole reward of engaging in it.

Such voluntary interaction, both Woodworth and White argued, falls outside the range of the homeostatic model. It does not, like homeostatic incentives, have a particular functional end-point; instead, the open-ended character of competence-related behaviours indicates that their performance should be seen as an end in itself. Versatile patterns of behaviour such as exploration and play reflect the organism's ability to create for itself novel opportunities of inter-action, and to take advantage of these and learn to deal with them. The non-directedness of inquisitive exploration and play is thus not random; it reflects a structured attempt at diversification and expansion of the behavioural repertoire. In this section we will review studies of animal exploration which have focused on various aspects of this ability.

Before we do so, it may be useful to consider the relationship between agency and a related notion, behavioural control. To exert control over envir-onmental challenges is important to an animal's welfare. Controllability and predictability play a central role in current theories of stress and animal welfare (Wiepkema and Koolhaas, 1993). These concepts have an information-based, cognitive connotation, reflecting the ability of animals to acquire and use in-formation for the anticipation and control of future events. The question is whether agency and competence are merely control-related behaviours, aimed at achieving optimal controllability, or whether they introduce an added element of interest and explanation.

Agency and competence are behavioural, not cognitive, concepts. They emphasize the organism's ability to enhance and expand its behaviour, not its knowledge, and are therefore not based on information-primacy theory. But why could such competence not be regarded as a form of knowledge, which the animal can use to predict and control its environment? Indeed, diversi-fication of behaviour (e.g. through play) will uncover new and useful forms of (proprioceptive) information, and thus qualifies as 'information-gathering'. But this misses the point. It fails to emphasize the innovative character of this type of behaviour; the fact that the animal, by expanding its repertoire, creates, rather than detects, new levels of expectancy and evaluation. Diversive explora-tion, in Hutt's terms (1970), is a response-oriented activity, not a stimulus-oriented one. The animal creates more uncertainty, rather than reducing it, and takes the risk of losing control rather than seeking it. It is this ability to which the concept of agency refers; it encompasses the notions of control and information-seeking, but cannot be reduced to it.

When the issue of competence was taken up in the animal literature, it was, unsurprisingly, from an evolutionary perspective. The first to consider the relationship between environment, individual competence and evolutionary fitness was Robert Fagen (1982), choosing behavioural flexibility as his key concept. In his paper 'Evolutionary issues in the development of behavioral flexibility', Fagen (1982, p. 365) defines flexibility as 'the capacity of an animal to alter its behavior or its ecology through behavioral means when faced by novel challenges so as to increase its chance of leaving surviving offspring or kin'. Fagen proposes that play and exploratory manipulation are crucially important behavioural mediators of this capacity; a supposition borne out by experiments indicating that voluntary interaction with the environment is prerequisite for normal development of behaviour and brain plasticity. Ferchmin *et al.* (1975), for example, housed a group of 'observer' rats in small wire-mesh cages inside a larger, stimulus-rich cage environment. These rats inhabited the same sensory environment as the rats actually living in contact with the stimuli available in the larger cage but they did not develop similar brain weight. Equally, rats taught to perform a complex operant motor task in an otherwise impoverished environment had smaller brains than animals in the enriched cage (Ferchmin and Eterovic, 1977). Apparently, neither complex sensory stimulation nor prolonged motor activity in and by themselves can match the effect on general brain development of free and unhampered interaction with the environment. The authors conclude 'it is not the amount, but the type of interaction which is important', and suggest that play may be of particular importance (Ferchmin and Eterovic, 1977).

Supporting evidence was found in studies with human children: here, too, spontaneous exploration and play were better facilitators of general learning ability than either perceptual or motor training *per se* (Sylva *et al.*, 1976; Smith and Dutton, 1979). The authors suggest that the versatility of explorative play stimulates a child's ability to integrate existing elements of behaviour into novel sequences. Likewise, Fagen (1982, p. 378) suggests with regard to animal play that 'Play experience produces flexible behavior by developing complex skills used in interacting with the physical and social environment.' He points out (1982, p. 366) that the experimental results reported 'reveal the need for ethological observations of the behaviors that animals actually perform under the conditions of the experiments (such observations have not yet systematically been made).'

Such observations were instigated by Michael Renner and his colleagues in a series of studies with white rats, which were raised in environmental conditions defined as either 'impoverished' or 'enriched'. The aim was to describe in detail the exploratory behaviour shown by both groups, under novel and potentially dangerous conditions. Renner and Rosenzweig (1986, p. 229) write:

> Exploration is a naturally occurring behavior that creates situations in which learning is likely to occur. The particular behaviors used by an animal in gathering information are important in determining what types or quantity of information it obtains from the world. Because exploratory behavior is not believed to be a stereotyped behavior or fixed action pattern, it seems plausible that the behavioral sequences employed in exploration are subject to change through experience, but this has not been established. Exploratory behavior as well as similar activities such as foraging expose an animal to some risk; this and other reasons make it reasonable to infer that rapidity and skill in gathering

information would have selection value. There is evidence to suggest that animals from enriched environments may process information differently than their impoverished littermates . . . but little is known of possible differences in the information-gathering strategies of animals with different histories.

Subsequent investigation did indeed demonstrate that rats with different environmental backgrounds employ different strategies in investigating a novel environment (Renner and Rosenzweig, 1986; Renner, 1987). The major difference appeared to reside in the quantity and quality of interaction with novel objects placed in the environment. Animals from enriched conditions tended to sniff, bite and climb objects more, used their paws more when investigating objects, and generally manipulated the objects more frequently. These results indicate, Renner suggests, that these animals are better able than animals from impoverished backgrounds to take advantage of the feedback available from the presented objects. He adds that this ability may well have functional significance under conditions of challenge.

Further testing confirmed this hypothesis, showing that 'enriched' adult male rats escaped more quickly from a simulated predatory attack than their 'impoverished' conspecifics (Renner, 1988). When both groups were given two hours' prior exposure to the arena in which the hidden escape route was located, this difference in escape time became even bigger. These results indicate that the more differentiated patterns of investigation shown by rats from enriched conditions reflect their greater ability to deal effectively with environmental challenges. Such patterns are stable over time, show relatively little individual variation and become more elaborate with age (Renner and Seltzer, 1991; Renner et al., 1992). Renner and Seltzer (1991, p. 338) conclude that:

> This consistency provides strong evidence that exploration is not . . . simply an expression of neural noise (i.e. a random element in behavior). Exploratory behavior, if adequately characterized by descriptive work such as reported here followed by experimental investigations of its structure and function, will almost certainly offer a window into the means by which each species adapts to the environment.

To sum up, exploratory behaviour, by providing contact with the environment, can be considered as an end in itself. If given the opportunity, animals try out various ways of interacting with an environment. The richer the environment, the more opportunities the animal has and the more versatile its behavioural repertoire becomes. This in turn creates more potential starting-points for interaction, giving the animal a more flexible disposition to deal with challenges. Thus, behavioural diversification, and the concomitant development of competence, appears a spontaneous, self-propagating process. It can only take place within the constraints of the species-specific repertoire, but its defining characteristic appears to be its voluntary nature.

This supposition leads to a final topic. The voluntary aspects of behaviour feature prominently in discussions of 'contrafreeloading': the observation that animals will work to 'earn' their food even when they can obtain it 'free'. At first sight, this phenomenon, too, suggests that animals will engage in interaction with the environment for its own sake (Neuringer, 1969). As such, it has direct and important implications for the welfare of animals in intensive housing systems (Duncan and Hughes, 1972). However, further experimental investigation revealed a simple explanation of contrafreeloading to be elusive. In a recent and comprehensive review, Inglis *et al.* (1997) put these results to close scrutiny. Adopting a naturalistic perspective, these authors take as a starting-point that animals in the wild are primed to deal with highly variable, unpredictable conditions. The tendency of animals to 'work for food' under artificial experimental conditions, they propose, may be taken as evidence of a need to gather, update and improve information about potential food sources.

This account is formulated along the terms of information primacy theory, yet is not incompatible with a more competence-oriented approach. The authors concede that competence, the ability to select an appropriate response to environmental change, is vital for testing the accuracy of acquired information. Thus the need to exert and maintain competence is an intrinsic part of their proposed explanation of contrafreeloading. However, consistent with their information primacy approach, the authors regard competence as an expectancy rather than a behavioural skill; an interpretation which we consider too limited (see above). We propose that contrafreeloading, while reflecting the need to gather and update information, also shows that animals 'prefer to work'; animals will voluntarily interact with their environment when given the chance. Agency, of course, implies the need for information. Competence and information-acquisition should therefore be seen as mutually inclusive notions, indicating that animals can and will seek to deal with environmental challenge.

Such a conception has important consequences for the understanding of animal welfare. A cognitive approach emphasizes the importance of information, of something useful to know, but an agency-based approach suggests the importance of meaning, of something useful to do. In this light, the notion of boredom does not merely point towards a chronic lack of sensory stimulation, but first and foremost indicates a chronic lack of opportunities for interaction (Wemelsfelder, 1993). Animals provided with complex sensory stimulation, but prevented from interacting with it, like the 'observer' rats (Ferchmin *et al.*, 1975), could thus still be bored. They can store and process perceived visual information about their surroundings, but are prevented from generating a meaningful response. Such a situation deprives animals of the very core on which their physical existence is based, namely the ability to act. This may lead, simultaneously or alternately, to apathy and high levels of anxiety (Rowan, 1988; Wood-Gush and Vestergaard, 1989). Environmental challenge thus appears important for welfare; its absence may render animals unable to cope.

This conclusion sheds doubt upon forms of environmental enrichment which are too artificial, too far removed from the animal's natural background, such as televisions. The animal may be fascinated at first, but eventually, due to lack of meaningful interaction, may lose interest or even become frustrated. In contrast, stimuli which simulate aspects of an animal's natural habitat may give rise to persistent and increasingly diverse and versatile forms of species-specific behaviour (Hutchins *et al.*, 1978; Newberry, 1995). Such stimuli need not be complex or technically advanced, but can be straightforward and easy to provide (e.g. straw or woodbark). Finally, opportunities for versatile interaction can in principle never be excessive. Given the voluntary nature of inquisitive exploration, the animal can choose to interact or not, whichever it decides. Opportunities for interaction do not, like stimulus-novelty, have a 'middle range optimum'; they should simply be there. However, in many natural and domestic conditions, inquisitive exploration and play are rarely experienced luxuries. In the wild, as soon as survival is under threat, play is strongly reduced (Barrett *et al.*, 1992); in intensive housing systems, environments mostly lack the substrates necessary to evoke it (Lawrence, 1987). But this is not to say that agency and competence are luxuries in terms of welfare. Agency is a fundamental principle of behavioural organization and may well be central to the animal's ability to experience a state of well-being.

3.4. Conclusions

- There is ample evidence that exploration is something many animals will do, even when their basic needs are met. Depriving animals of the opportunity to explore or to seek other environmental challenges may be stressful. However, this hypothesis is not easy to test experimentally. Different approaches have different implications for welfare, as indicated in the following points.
- Older drive-reduction models of exploration regard it as subordinate to more basic motivations and as less relevant to welfare. In more recent models this view is rejected.
- Recent cognitive models of exploration consider information-gathering the most important motivation of animals, dominated by other motivations only in acute need. Such a conception provides a strong case for animals to live in varied, complex sensory surroundings. Yet cognitive models, in their emphasis on information and knowledge, are vulnerable to the surmise that animals born and raised in deprived conditions do not miss what they do not know.
- Agency-based models of exploration focus on the voluntary, interactive aspects of exploration. That animals actively seek challenge indicates that behavioural competence and versatility are motivators in their own right. In this context, the need of animals to be provided with rich, species-specific environmental conditions seems persuasive. Environmental challenge should be seen as an integral part of behavioural development and well-being; in its absence, animals may succumb to apathy and boredom.

Acknowledgements

We would like to thank Björn Forkman and the editors of this book for helpful comments and discussion.

CHAPTER 4
Hunger and thirst

Ilias Kyriazakis (Scottish Agricultural College, UK) and
C. John Savory (Roslin Institute, UK)

Abstract

New definitions of hunger and thirst are offered, arising from the notion that animals have specific requirements for nutrients (including water) to carry out their physiological functions. There are circumstances in which animals are malnourished or undernourished or both; 'water undernutrition' is termed here water restriction. Conditions resulting in these states are discussed, paying specific emphasis to the more subtle ones, such as failure to allow the individual – as opposed to the average – animal to meet all its nutrient requirements. The welfare problems arising from malnutrition, undernutrition and water restriction are categorized as (i) abnormal or disturbed behaviours, (ii) stress-related physiological problems and (iii) illness; these categories are not mutually exclusive. Behavioural problems arise when malnourished and undernourished confined animals are unable to express 'normal' foraging behaviour: redirected foraging behaviour as a result of malnutrition and food-related stereotypies as a result of undernutrition. Assessment of animals' welfare in relation to nutrition is thus based on physiological as well as behavioural evidence. The overall framework proposed here is sufficiently general to deal with alternative approaches (such as 'subjective experiences') to the assessment of animal welfare.

4.1. Introduction

It is perhaps not accidental that in most existing codes of recommendations for the welfare of animals (Farm Animal Welfare Council, 1992; Animal Welfare Advisory Committee, 1994) 'freedom from hunger and thirst' features as the first requirement that has to be satisfied. This prioritization probably reflects their importance, because 'hunger and thirst are the two most basic, primitive and unremitting of all motivating forces' (Webster, 1995). Complete failure to eat or drink leads to relatively rapid death (especially in the case of water deprivation) while failure to satisfy the requirement for any essential nutrient leads to illness, deterioration and eventual death.

These are extreme examples. At the other end of the spectrum, mild deprivation of nutrients and water has little effect on health, vigour or welfare (e.g. the water intake of experimental animals can be reduced to 70–80% of *ad libitum* without any adverse physiological effects (Forbes, 1995)). Furthermore *ad libitum* feeding of animals (e.g. the breeding stock of many farm animals selected for fast growth and consequently increased adult body size) can lead to increased incidence of disease and reduction in the animal's reproductive performance. These examples raise the following questions: what constitutes hunger and/or thirst, and when is freedom from hunger and thirst being denied and, most importantly, welfare compromised?

This chapter offers definitions of hunger and thirst and ways of measuring them; once clear definitions are offered, the conditions that lead to them are detailed. The ways in which these conditions affect welfare are discussed.

4.2. Hunger: Definitions and Measurements

4.2.1. Definitions

There is much confusion in the physiological and psychological literature over the term 'hunger' and its equivalents, 'feeding motivation' and 'eating tendency'. The most frequently used definition (e.g. Le Magnen, 1985) '[the state of the animal] in which it is stimulated to eat', implies that when an animal is not feeding, it is in 'a passive state of no hunger'. Such definitions do not take into account the nutritional properties of the food (i.e. food is treated as having a unitary value), the physiological state of the animal, nor the external factors which could influence (or prevent) feeding. Perhaps because of this limitation some recent Codes of Animal Welfare (e.g. New Zealand) have extended freedom from hunger and thirst, to freedom from thirst, hunger and *malnutrition* (Animal Welfare Advisory Committee, 1994), but this extension can only increase confusion. Added confusion could arise because 'freedom from hunger and thirst' is a *non sequitur*. Animals need to be hungry or thirsty in order to eat or drink.

It might be more useful if feeding behaviour is viewed within the context of what the animal is trying to achieve. Animals have nutrient requirements to carry out specific bodily functions (e.g. to grow and reproduce), and at the same time 'possess the desire' to meet these requirements (the latter being an extension of the Aristotelian concept of 'telos', that all animals desire or strive to reach the functional end for which they were designed):

> In the Aristotelian and evolutionary sense an immature animal seeks resources such as food and water from its environment because it desires to grow. This desire is to grow towards the mature size in the shortest time that is consistent with reproductive success and thus to ensure the preservation of the animal's genetic material.

> (Kyriazakis, 1994, p. 85)

This presupposes a set of nutritional and environmental conditions (ideal or non-limiting), which will allow the animal to meet its requirements. If nutritional conditions are limiting by being inappropriately balanced in relation to the animal's requirements, then it is *malnourished*; if they are limiting by being insufficient it is *undernourished*. It is also possible to have combinations of the two situations, with an animal receiving too few nutrients in total and these nutrients also being incorrectly balanced. The latter is most frequently the case for animals kept extensively in harsh environments. Similarly, environmental restrictions (physical or social) may result in undernutrition and/or malnutrition; for example, when an animal in a very hot or competitive environment is given a non-limiting food. The terms 'undernutrition' and 'malnutrition' are preferred in this chapter to 'hunger', because they describe this aspect of feeding behaviour more appropriately. The conditions which lead to these two situations are considered separately and discussed below.

4.2.2. Measurements

Measurements of hunger can be divided into three categories. The first includes measurements of food intake, rate of eating and the time spent in food-directed activity. These are the most frequently taken and direct measurements, but until recently involved techniques that were far from perfect (mainly observations, Le Magnen, 1985). However, recent advances in electronics have allowed for continuous automated recordings of all three variables, with consistent accuracy.

The second category encompasses the operant methodology for measuring 'hunger', where animals make specific responses such as pressing a lever or pushing a door open to obtain food (Petherick and Rutter, 1990; Day *et al.*, 1995). By varying the amount of work required to obtain food, one can assess the importance of the food to the animal (Dellmeier, 1989). The disadvantage of this widely used method is that the requirement to work is an artificial condition 'which modifies the spontaneous microstructure of feeding behaviour' (Le Magnen, 1985). Nevertheless, this method is useful in distinguishing between the cessation of feeding and continuing feeding motivation, for example in situations where animals have stopped feeding because the physical capacity of their gastrointestinal tract has been reached, but nutrient requirements have not been satisfied (Day *et al.*, 1995).

The third category includes methods where animals are willing to undergo an aversive stimulus to obtain food (e.g. an electric shock) (Cabanac and Johnson, 1983). These are the least frequently used perhaps because of problems in interpreting results and also the ethical problems of obtaining dose/response effects over an adequately broad range. The disturbance caused to the animal by the aversive stimulus may induce considerable changes to its general, as well as to its feeding, behaviour.

4.3. Sources of Malnutrition

Malnutrition can arise when an animal is given access to a food which is inappropriately balanced (deficient in one or more nutrients) in relation to its requirements. There are cases where farm animals are intentionally exposed to malnutrition to meet specific husbandry or production requirements. Veal calves are sometimes fed on a liquid diet deficient in iron to produce 'pale meat' (van Putten, 1982) and newly weaned pigs are given a low protein food to reduce the diarrhoea which frequently accompanies the abrupt change from milk to a solid diet (Miller and Stokes, 1994). However, the most common cases of malnutrition are probably those arising from the failure to meet the specific requirements of the individual animal given access to a single food.

The nutrient requirements of an individual reflect its genotype, sex, stage of growth or reproduction and previous nutritional history (reviewed by Kyriazakis, 1994). These individual requirements can be both demonstrated and satisfied when animals are given a choice between two or more appropriate foods (Kyriazakis, 1994; Sclafani, 1995; Tolkamp et al., 1996). Nevertheless, under commercial farming or laboratory conditions animals generally receive a single food designed to meet the requirements of the 'average' individual for a given stage of production (e.g. between two weights, or at a certain stage of lactation). Inevitably many if not all individuals will, at some point experience a discrepancy between the nutritional content of the single food and their requirements for specific nutrients.

Animals could attempt to meet requirements for the deficient nutrient(s) by increasing intake of the imbalanced food. Pigs and sheep on a low protein food increase their intake to compensate for the protein deficiency (Leng, 1990; Kyriazakis et al., 1991), as do chickens on a vitamin A deficient food (Ogunmodede, 1981). Sometimes, however, the magnitude of the (specific) nutrient deficit is large or there are environmental or physical constraints and the animal fails to compensate fully, perhaps because of adverse effects caused by increasing the amounts of other non-limiting nutrients.

One solution would be to provide a food that is non-limiting in all nutrients, which exceeds every individual's requirements. Although possible with certain nutrients, and indeed the preferred method of providing certain trace-elements and vitamins, this is unrealistic for many of the major nutrients (e.g. protein) because of the increased costs and environmental pollution (increased rates of excretion of nutrients in excess of requirements).

4.4. Sources of Undernutrition

There are several circumstances where animals are exposed to conditions of undernutrition, including (i) directly or intentionally imposed undernutrition, which is most frequently the outcome of certain (farming) practices; and (ii) indirectly imposed undernutrition, where food is freely available, but the animal is unable to consume sufficient.

4.4.1. Directly (or intentionally) imposed undernutrition

Directly imposed undernutrition can be the outcome of *quantitative* food restriction, when animals are given insufficient amounts of food, or *qualitative* food restriction, when animals are given access to a bulky food where intake is limited by volume. Quantitative food restriction is frequently imposed on the breeding stock of farm animals, to prevent excessive fatness during reproduction, to improve reproductive performance, to reduce the incidence of skeletal and metabolic diseases, and to reduce food costs. The extent of restriction can be severe: breeding sows and boars are given approximately 60% of the amount they would consume on a concentrate food offered *ad libitum*

(Lawrence *et al.*, 1993), and broiler breeders are offered 'roughly a quarter to a half as much food as unrestricted birds, depending on age and on whether birds of the same age or weight are compared' (Savory *et al.*, 1993). Lawrence *et al.* (1993) suggested that of all intensively kept farm animals broiler breeders are exposed to highest levels of quantitative food restriction. Until recently (Riley, 1989) growing pigs were also subjected to quantitative food restriction to reduce unwanted fatness, but recent genetic improvements, that have resulted in leaner pigs, have reduced the need for the practice. A special case of quantitative food restriction is complete food withdrawal for up to 12 days to induce a moult in laying hens (Brake *et al.*, 1982), used in the USA but illegal in the UK.

Because of serious behavioural and welfare problems associated with quantitative food restriction (see below), some have advocated the use of qualitative food restriction as an alternative feeding method for monogastric breeding stock (Robert *et al.*, 1993; Zuidhof *et al.*, 1995). Ruminant livestock are often faced with such a restriction when given poor quality roughage. Offering a concentrated food diluted with a source of 'bulk' (such as sugar beet pulp or oat hulls) to monogastric animals, greatly increases the time they spend eating (Zuidhof *et al.*, 1995). However, the animal still consumes insufficient nutrients, i.e. it is undernourished, because its food intake is limited through the 'gut-filling' properties of the bulky food (Kyriazakis and Emmans, 1995).

4.4.2. Indirectly (unintentionally) imposed undernutrition

Indirectly imposed undernutrition occurs when ruminant animals forage in areas where their food (herbage) is unevenly distributed, or is difficult to harvest (because bite size is small). In these cases factors limiting food intake are the amount of time which the animal can spend grazing each day and the number of bites it can take (Illius and Gordon, 1991). Animals under such conditions often fail to consume sufficient food and move into negative energy balance (Oldham *et al.*, 1993).

Restrictions imposed on feeding behaviour by other group members are common. Most farm animals prefer to feed together (Young and Lawrence, 1994). Where the primary food source limits access to one or more individuals, this can result in certain individuals being prevented from feeding freely by others. In many cases animals respond to social restriction by changing how and when they feed (Nielsen *et al.*, 1995; Tolkamp *et al.*, 1996) but as group size becomes larger the risk of some individuals suffering from food restriction increases.

Lastly, environmental conditions can restrict food intake and lead to undernutrition. The most important is the effect of increased ambient temperature in reducing food intake (Verstegen and Close, 1994). This is caused by reduced ability to dissipate the heat production associated with food intake. For highly-producing animals even small increases in ambient temperature can lead to significant reductions in food intake and production (Charles, 1989). Environmental temperature affects not only the total amount of food eaten, but also when and how the animals feed. During hot Australian summers sheep tended to graze during the night, with an increase in grazing activity near dawn (Brown and Lynch, 1972).

4.5. Thirst: Definitions and Measurements

4.5.1. Definitions

In their monograph entitled 'Thirst', Rolls and Rolls (1982) suggested that:

> [It] is a subjective sensation aroused by lack of water . . . It can strictly only be studied directly in man, according to this definition. However, animals including man, when deprived of water, are in a state of drive in which they will search for and ingest water, and 'thirst' can be used in a different way to that described above as a name for this state of drive.

However, substituting the term thirst with 'drive for ingesting water' or perhaps 'drinking tendency', when it is applied to animals, does not appear any more helpful. This is because the decision to perform, and the extent of, a 'drive' or a 'tendency' will be the outcome of the interactions between internal factors (such as physiological state and diet) and external factors (such as environmental temperature, ease of access to a water source and water quality). If on the other hand, water is treated as a single nutrient (perhaps the most important, because its lack leads to rapid death (Forbes, 1995)), then animals can be seen – by analogy with hunger – as being either 'water undernourished' or preferably 'water restricted'. This definition, which we shall use in this chapter, implies that the only function of water intake is to meet physiological requirements. These physiological functions have been described by Brooks and Carpenter (1990, p. 116) as:

> (i) the adjustment of body temperature, (ii) the maintenance of mineral-homeostasis, (iii) the excretion of the end products of digestion, (iv) the excretion of antinutritional factors ingested in the diets, (v) the excretion of drugs and drug residues, (vi) the achievement of satiety (gut fill) and (vii) the satisfaction of behavioural drives.

To those we can add the function of 'lubrication' for wetting food in the mouth and stomach(s) (Forbes, 1995). Functions (vi) and (vii) are not considered by many as physiological functions and this is the view we shall take.

The above view excludes instances where water consumption exceeds physiological requirements. This type of consumption has been termed 'secondary drinking' (Rolls and Rolls, 1982), 'adjunctive drinking' (Rushen, 1985b) or 'luxury drinking' (Fraser *et al.*, 1990). Examples include hunger-induced drinking (Yang *et al.*, 1981) and 'scheduled-induced polydipsia' (Falk, 1961), where animals (most often rats), reduced to about 80% of normal body weight and given small amounts of foods at regular intervals, develop excessive drinking. These instances however, constitute abnormal (extreme) types of behaviour, induced only under certain experimental or husbandry conditions (Rolls and Rolls, 1982), and will not be considered further, although their significance will be re-addressed briefly in the 'Problems' section of this chapter.

4.5.2. Measurements

Methodologies identical to the ones used to measure hunger can be applied to measure thirst: (i) measurements of water intake, rate of drinking and amount of time spent on drinker-directed activity, (ii) operant methods and (iii) aversion methods. The measurements taken by the first method probably reflect requirement for water intake, whereas the latter two reflect motivation to obtain water. An additional difficulty associated with the first methodology is that under certain conditions (e.g. sows in tether stalls (Fraser *et al.*, 1990)) animals play excessively with the water supply system (e.g. nipple drinker); this can severely impair the ability to measure water intake. This excessive wastage of water and inaccuracy of water meters has often been considered responsible for introducing important errors in assessing the true water requirements of animals, and contributes to the large variation in water intake among similar animals in different studies (Forbes, 1995).

4.6. Sources of Water Restriction

Water restrictions fall into two categories: (i) intentionally imposed limitations on how much and when the animal may drink; and (ii) unintentional restriction as a result of physical, environmental and social factors. The first arises from systems or practices for intensively kept animals (mainly pigs or poultry), whereas the second is common to both intensively and extensively kept animals. Extensively kept animals (especially ruminants) in semi-arid or arid environments and high environmental temperatures are clearly water restricted but will not be considered here.

4.6.1. Intentional water restriction

There are systems of production, mainly for pigs and poultry, where the water supply is either restricted to certain periods of the day or mixed with the food (liquid or wet feeding systems). Pigs may also be allowed to opt for a preferred water to food ratio by operating a water valve in their feeding trough (Brooks and Carpenter, 1990). The advantages of these systems are that delivery of both water and food can be automated; some researchers have reported increases in productivity with this practice (Danish National Committee for Pig Breeding and Production, 1986). Water restriction programmes are often employed for broiler breeders and sows as a means of reducing the overdrinking and wet droppings that result from the severe food restriction programmes often imposed on this kind of animal.

These systems of production and practices fail to recognize many of the physiological functions that water can serve and their additive nature which can lead to an increase in requirements (Brooks and Carpenter, 1990). These systems can prove particularly risky when employed in conjunction with high environmental temperatures, where the animal has to regulate its body temperature, or where foods high in protein and/or minerals are offered (see below). The justification for such systems on the grounds of both productivity and welfare seems limited.

4.6.2. Unintentional water restriction

The most common unintentional restriction to intensively kept animals results from the failure of the water supply (e.g. blocked or burst pipes). There are, however, more subtle features of the delivery system which could impose a variable degree of restriction. For example, water delivery rate can significantly restrict intake and performance of weaned (3–6 weeks of age, Barber *et al.*, 1989) and growing pigs (10–14 weeks of age, Nienaber and Hahn, 1984). Although pigs on a lower water delivery rate spent longer drinking, their intake was lower than for those on high water delivery rates. Inappropriate design of drinkers can similarly restrict the water intake of goats kept at high temperatures (Brooks and Carpenter, 1990). Social competition or ease of access to drinkers can result in water restriction, in particular for ruminants which take only a few large drinks per day, mostly associated with meals (Forbes *et al.*, 1991).

Water quality (e.g. cleanliness and existence of mineral and toxic substances) also plays a role in the water intake of animals, especially pigs and poultry (NAC, 1974), which rely heavily on water supply (being fed on dry foods). Pigs prefer uncontaminated water (Brooks and Carpenter, 1990) while chickens reduced their water intake to about 75% of normal when it was adulterated with quinine (Yeomans and Savory, 1989). It is well established that water with a high mineral content or containing toxic substances reduces the water intakes of farm animals.

As with intentional water restriction, the importance of the above factors is exaggerated in conditions of high temperatures or when animals are given access to certain foods. High dietary protein content (where animals have to excrete through urine the products of deamination), mineral content (particularly sodium and potassium (Wahlstrom *et al.*, 1970)), and water holding capacity (which traps water in the gastrointestinal tract (Kyriazakis and Emmans, 1995)) also aggravate effects of water restriction.

Extensively kept ruminants under temperate conditions are generally assumed to meet their water requirements through the water content of their food (Lynch *et al.*, 1972). This is probably true when their diet consists of high water content grass and root crops. However, if the availability of green grass declines and/or the physiological state of the animal changes (e.g. during lactation) then these animals may become water restricted.

4.7. Welfare Problems

4.7.1. Categorization

In the wild or under free-ranging conditions an undernourished and/or malnourished animal will ordinarily direct most of its behaviour towards finding and consuming food items (foraging behaviour) until either it satisfies its nutrient requirements, or some constraint is imposed (e.g. time available for foraging). Sheep under extensive conditions are known to walk up to 20–25 km per day whilst foraging between nutrient-poor food patches (Squires and Wilson, 1971), while sows under free-ranging conditions (Edinburgh Pig Park) and offered only a small amount of concentrate food, spent over 50% of their time foraging (Stolba and Wood-Gush, 1989). For animals in conditions where their nutrient requirements are not met and the expression of their foraging behaviour is restricted (i.e. intensively kept farm animals, laboratory animals), it is accepted that this foraging activity will be directed towards alternative available stimuli (Lawrence *et al.*, 1993).

The continuing failure of an animal to meet its nutrient (including water) requirements, despite directing its behaviour towards finding food or water, can be seen as a (chronic) stressor. If, in addition, the animal's failure is severe then body reserves (fat, protein and major minerals in the bones) may be utilized for some of its physiological functions. Growing pigs are known to lose body fat and gain small amounts of protein under severe conditions of nutrient restriction (Kyriazakis and Emmans, 1992), while lactating mammals given restricted amounts of food utilize body reserves to produce milk (Oldham *et al.*, 1993). If prolonged, such a 'negative nutrient balance' will lead to deterioration, illness and eventual death.

Welfare problems arising from malnutrition, undernutrition and water restriction thus fall into three categories: (i) behavioural problems related to the expression of foraging behaviour in confinement; (ii) stress problems related to failure to meet nutrient requirements; and (iii) problems associated with 'illness', arising from prolonged periods of severe nutrient restriction. The latter (clinical manifestations of illness) will not be considered here, because they belong more appropriately to Chapter 9. The three categories above are not mutually exclusive because, for example, malnourished or undernourished animals might have behavioural problems, whilst at the same time being physiologically stressed (see below).

4.7.2. Behavioural problems

Confined animals whose nutrient requirements are not met will direct their foraging activity towards the most appropriate available stimuli. In some instances it is directed towards suitable foraging substrates (such as straw bedding), but in many cases the physical constraints are such that it is actually directed towards the pens or cages, or even towards conspecifics. In the latter cases redirected foraging activity can lead to specific behavioural problems such as tail-biting in growing pigs (Fraser, 1987), 'wool-stripping' in sheep kept indoors (Cooper *et al.*, 1994), or food related stereotypies (Rushen, 1985b). Because these behaviours are widely considered 'abnormal', may indicate reduced welfare and are of public concern, they will be considered here.

Redirected foraging behaviour as a result of malnutrition

Malnourished, intensively kept animals offered *ad libitum* access to an imbalanced food have been reported to show increased general activity, exploratory, chewing and rooting behaviours. These behaviours have been interpreted as manifestations of their foraging behaviour. For example, growing pigs offered *ad libitum* food deficient in protein increased their general activity, walking, and rooting of straw, relative to pigs given food excessive in protein or pigs offered a choice between the two foods (Jensen *et al.*, 1993). Similar observations have been made on pigs offered diets deficient in minerals (Fraser, 1987). Ruminants kept indoors on food low in roughage, but otherwise 'balanced' in all nutrients, show increased levels of general activity compared to those given a high roughage food (Spensley *et al.*, 1993).

It is during foraging that animals encounter substrates with nutritional value. Behaviour towards these substrates would be sustained because of its incentive value. Fraser (1987, p. 917) attempted thus to explain the persistence of tail-biting in pigs, by viewing blood as a substrate providing a nutrient (salt), as follows:

> Once the chewing of tails has caused a bleeding wound, then an attraction to blood could add a further impetus for the behaviour to continue or escalate. At this stage, a lack of salt in the diet will increase the animal's attraction to blood . . . Other dietary problems, such as low levels of fibre or protein might also contribute.

In other words tail-biting can start accidentally, as a result of increased foraging activity by malnourished individuals, but persists because of the reinforcing properties of blood ingestion. A similar hypothesis has been advanced to account for the initiation and persistence of feather-pecking in *ad libitum* fed hens (Blokhuis, 1989). Support for this view is provided by the fact that supplementation of the diet with nutrients such as salt (Fraser, 1987) or folic acid (Robert *et al.*, 1991) reduces activity in *ad libitum* fed growing pigs, and in the latter case reduced nibbling of pen-mates in growing pigs restricted to 95% of their *ad libitum* intake.

Food related stereotypies (as a result of undernutrition)

One of the first clear and conclusive observations which related stereotypies (behaviours regularly repeated in a similar way and lacking obvious function; see Chapter 9) and other 'abnormal' behaviours to food restriction, were those of Rushen (1985b, p. 1064) on tethered sows. He observed that:

> Rubbing the snout against bars, manipulating the drinker, bar-biting and head-weaving were clearly adjunctive behaviours, associated with the feeding period. These could be classified as either terminal responses (bar-biting, rubbing, and head-weaving) that occurred immediately prior to the delivery of food, or interim responses that occurred immediately after food delivery. Interim responses involved either long duration drinking combined with rooting, rapid short duration drinking, or rapid rubbing. The last two behaviours tended to occur in stereotyped sequences. Vacuum-chewing and playing with the chain however, appeared to occur with equal frequency before and after feeding.

The observations were subsequently confirmed (by comparing sows on different degrees of food restriction) by Appleby and Lawrence (1987). Similar behaviour, related to the delivery of food in food-restricted situations, has been reported in many species under restricted feeding regimes, in conditions where foraging is limited. Examples include stereotyped spot-pecking in pigeons (Palya and Zacny, 1980), pecking at the feeder and floor litter in broiler breeders (Kostal *et al.*, 1992), tongue-rolling in small cats (Shepherdson *et al.*, 1993), pacing, running in and out of the nest box and head-nodding in mink

(Mason, 1993) and wool-stripping, wool-chewing and slat-biting in sheep (Cooper *et al.*, 1994).

It is now widely believed that such stereotypies represent the expression of foraging behaviour, modified by the physical constraints of the environment (Lawrence *et al.*, 1993). In some animals (e.g. mink and small cats) these behaviours are mostly performed before feeding and are more or less abolished once food is delivered (Mason, 1993), whereas in others (e.g. pigs and poultry) they occur at low levels before feeding and actually increase following food consumption (Terlouw *et al.*, 1991). In addition, some of these behaviours are locomotory (e.g. pacing), whereas others are clearly oral (e.g. pecking and tongue-rolling).

Terlouw *et al.* (1991, p. 988) were the first to argue that the above differences in food-related stereotypies could be explained by species-specific differences in the temporal sequences of foraging behaviour.

> In carnivores, in which [foraging] behaviour tends to precede the meal, stereotypies are largely found before feeding . . . In omnivores, such as the pig, in which [foraging behaviour] sequences may be interspersed over long periods of time, one might expect [foraging] behaviour to be stimulated by the ingestion of food, and result in stereotypy following a meal.

This idea has obvious attractions, but would have to be thoroughly tested before it could be used to predict the food-related stereotypic behaviour of animals in various husbandry conditions (Mason and Mendl, 1997).

These types of behaviours are substantially reduced if suitable substrates are provided to which more 'natural' foraging behaviour of food restricted animals can be directed (Shepherdson *et al.*, 1993; Spoolder *et al.*, 1995). A similarly reduced incidence is observed when the bulkiness of the food increases but the amount of nutrients remains unaltered (Robert *et al.*, 1993; Savory *et al.*, 1996). Nevertheless, general activity levels continue to reflect the degree of food restriction and remain high.

4.7.3. Stress-related physiological problems

Temporary or sudden restriction of food and/or water to an animal that has been previously able to meet its nutrient requirements could be regarded as an acute stressor. Rats and pigs respond to extinction sessions of operant responding for food rewards by an increase in their plasma cortisol concentrations (Dantzer *et al.*, 1980) which may reflect the 'general adaptation syndrome' (Chapter 10). Whether animals malnourished or undernourished for prolonged periods are similarly (chronically) stressed is less well established, for it has been proposed that 'it is reasonable to suggest a risk to welfare when a sustained elevation of >40% in free corticosteroid concentrations is evident' (Barnett and Hemsworth, 1990).

Published evidence on 'chronic stress' induced by malnutrition, undernutrition and water restriction appears equivocal. Hocking *et al.* (1993) and Savory *et al.* (1996) found that both quantitative and qualitative undernutrition of broiler breeders resulted in a 2- to 5-fold increase of plasma corticosterone. In contrast, Terlouw *et al.* (1991) and Maxwell *et al.* (1992) did not observe any changes in corticosteroid levels of long-term undernourished sows and broiler breeders respectively. These discrepancies may depend on the length of the imposed undernutrition (the longer the undernutrition, the less likely are high corticosteroid levels), the time of day, and the fact that apparent adaptation of plasma cortisol does not always imply normality. Chronic undernutrition of tethered sows was not accompanied by increased cortisol but rather an increased cortisol response to an acute stressor and to adrenocorticotropin hormone challenge (von Borell and Ladewig, 1989). This suggests that the animals were suffering from sensitivity of the pituitary–adrenal axis, which has been considered a symptom of chronic stress in animals (Dallman and Jones, 1973).

A further characteristic of chronic or repeated stress is that it can lead to immunosuppression (see Chapter 10). Although it is difficult to distinguish between the direct and indirect effects of malnutrition and undernutrition on the immune system, there is evidence mainly from broiler breeders, that chronic undernutrition could affect the plasma heterophil to lymphocyte ratio, and the frequencies of basophil and monocyte blood cells (Hocking *et al.*, 1993; Zuidhof *et al.*, 1995; Savory *et al.*, 1996). These findings support the view that undernourished animals are subjected to chronic stress.

A further consideration is whether malnutrition and undernutrition cause different degrees of chronic stress in confined animals deprived of the possibility of looking for food items, compared to extensively kept or wild animals which seek but eventually fail to obtain sufficient food. This is an intriguing and difficult question, especially in view of the possibility that some 'abnormal' behaviours may have stress-reducing properties and so allow animals to 'cope' with the malnutrition or undernutrition (Savory *et al.*, 1992).

4.8. Discussion

We have stated explicitly that an animal kept under 'appropriate' conditions will consume food and water sufficient to meet its nutritional requirements. By doing so it maintains its fitness and can carry out the most natural and ultimate of its functions: reproduction. The paradox of animals (e.g. breeding broiler chickens and sows) given *ad libitum* access to balanced diets, consuming so much that reproductive performance is impaired and (metabolic) diseases are increased, should not be seen as contradictory. These cases reflect the outcome of 'artificial' genetic selection, not for a fit and healthy reproducing adult but for other traits. Broilers are selected for rapid growth of lean tissue at slaughter (at 6 weeks of age). This results in heavy adults with bone and joint problems which are 'outgrowing their strength' (Webster, 1995). A similar apparently paradoxical case is that of zoo animals overeating and becoming obese when fed *ad libitum*. This reflects the unnatural environment in which they are kept, which denies them free movement and exercise, and most importantly food which does not resemble their natural diet (Leus and Morgan, 1993).

Our view also implies that intakes of food and water serve only to meet the animal's requirements. This is not a universally held view, for it has been suggested that animals derive 'a positive source of pleasure' through the actions of feeding and drinking (Webster, 1995). Supporters of this view contrast the long time spent foraging by many animals on a relatively low quality, fibrous food source, against the rather short time they take to consume the restricted amount of concentrated food offered to them whilst they are confined. They propose that this reduced 'oral stimulation' is the cause of oral stereotypies. This suggestion, however, is not sufficient to account for the non-oral food-related stereotypies, and the species difference in the temporal sequencing of the stereotypies (in relation to food delivery). The framework we have proposed earlier appears to be more general and sufficient to account for the variations in food-related stereotypies.

Our view does not preclude the possibility that animals derive pleasure (i.e. reinforcement) from the action of drinking or eating, especially when they have been deprived of a particular nutrient and subsequently gain access to food high in this nutrient (e.g. protein deprived rats encountering a protein rich food, Deutsch *et al.*, 1989). We suggest that this sensation is specific, relates to the state of the animal and is induced by the specific nutrient deprivation. It may be analogous to the pleasure humans derive from drinking water after deprivation (Rolls and Rolls, 1982).

Although not stated explicitly, the assessment of welfare in relation to malnutrition, undernutrition and water restriction must rest on whether animals' biological systems are functioning normally (on the basis of physiological and behavioural evidence). Welfare problems arising from these three states fall into three distinct but not mutually exclusive categories: abnormal or disturbed behaviour, stress-related physiological problems and illness. There is of course an alternative view which asserts that welfare must be assessed in terms of the actual 'subjective experiences' that arise from the negative states of malnutrition, undernutrition and water restriction (Chapter 2). The overall framework we have proposed is sufficiently general to deal with either approach to the assessment of animal welfare.

4.9. Conclusions

- Animals have requirements for nutrients (including water) to carry out their physiological functions, and at the same time possess a desire to meet these requirements. Animals can be malnourished, undernourished or both; in the case of 'water undernutrition' animals can be water restricted.
- There is a range of conditions which lead both extensively and intensively kept animals to these three states, including subtle ones that arise from failure to allow the individual animal (as opposed to the average animal) to meet its nutrient requirements.
- The welfare problems that arise from malnutrition, undernutrition and water restriction can be categorized as abnormal or disturbed behaviours, stress-related physiological problems and illness.

- Abnormal and disturbed behaviours arise when malnourished and under-nourished confined animals are unable to express normal foraging behaviour, but instead direct it towards elements of their environment (including conspecifics). Welfare problems can be resolved either by removing the causes or by allowing the animal to find more appropriate expressions of its foraging behaviour.

Acknowledgements

We are grateful to Dr Jon Day and Professor Mike Forbes for their useful comments on the manuscript.

CHAPTER 5
Pain and injury

Paul A. Flecknell (University of Newcastle, UK) and
Vince Molony (University of Edinburgh, UK)

Abstract

Pain and injury in animals occur under a variety of circumstances – for example following accidental injury, as a result of methods of housing or husbandry, following surgical procedures or as a result of disease processes. The problems associated with pain are exacerbated by our current poor ability to assess the magnitude of the degree of pain experienced by individual animals. Further factors are the economic and other constraints on the use of analgesic drugs. Increased recognition of the significance of pain should lead to changes in our methods of care and use of animals and a reduction in the magnitude of this problem.

5.1. Introduction

Pain in animals is of obvious welfare concern if it is assumed that animals perceive pain in a similar manner to humans. Injury, arising from accidental trauma or as an almost inevitable consequence of some husbandry systems, is also recognized as a major animal welfare problem. Injury is of concern both because of the consequent pain which is likely to arise from traumatized tissues, and also because of its incapacitating effect on the animal. This incapacity can lead to other problems such as hunger, thirst and inability to find shelter. In this chapter the capacity of injury to cause pain will be considered. Other consequences are dealt with elsewhere in the book.

The assumption that animal pain is similar to that in humans is based on comparative anatomy, physiology and behaviour and has been extensively discussed elsewhere (National Research Council, 1992; Short and van Poznak, 1992). Pain in humans has both sensory and emotional components, and although the exact nature of the emotional component in animals must remain uncertain, the aversive nature of animal pain has been generally accepted. A broad summary of the views of many veterinarians and bioscientists was provided by Duncan and Molony (1986):

> We suggest that intact animals are capable of an experience which they avoid, given the opportunity, and which can dominate their physiology and behaviour in a similar way to the experience of pain in man.

This approach to animal pain avoids stating that the experience of pain is similar in animals and humans but points out the similar effects of the experience.

If animal pain is considered to be an aversive experience, this attitude should have led to concern to prevent or alleviate pain. Regrettably, simple solutions to this group of welfare problems have not been forthcoming. To appreciate the reasons for this lack of progress, it is necessary to examine some of our underlying assumptions concerning animal pain and to review the development of methods for preventing and alleviating pain.

5.2. Recognition of Animal Pain

Society's attitudes to animal pain are shaped largely by anthropomorphic views of animal consciousness. This uncritical view of animal pain often includes the expectation that when animals experience similar emotions to humans, they should behave in similar ways. This approach results in ready recognition of some responses to acute severe pain – for example a pet dog's reaction to having its tail trapped in a door – but pain in other circumstances may go unnoticed. Humans frequently show clear, prolonged behavioural changes in response to post-surgical pain, and our ability to communicate verbally reinforces these signals to our companions. Animal behaviour following surgery, or some other presumably painful condition, is often only subtly altered. As pointed out by Yoxall (1978, p. 423):

> Acute pain, such as that manifested by an animal with a broken bone, can readily be identified by eliciting manifestations of distress from the animal on palpation of the affected area. Sometimes the presence of pain may be inferred from clear clinical signs, such as lameness, dysphagia, dysuria and so on. In other cases, however, in which the presence of pain does not cause any functional impairment to the animal's normal activities, the manifestation of pain may be much less apparent, and only be demonstrated by the presence of behavioural changes. A dog with a prolapsed intervertebral disc, for example, may show no signs directly referable to the lesion, but may just remain sitting in an attitude which one can only describe anthropomorphically as indicative of misery and dejection. Equally, a dog in pain after a traffic or other traumatic accident, or following a painful surgical procedure, or with a painful tumour, may manifest the presence of pain by simply appearing less lively than usual.

A failure to show obvious pain-related behaviour leads to an assumption that significant pain cannot be present. A failure to recognize pain may account not only for attitudes in society in general, but also the attitudes of those most capable of producing solutions to the problem – veterinary surgeons, research scientists and others who directly work with animals. Early attempts at recognizing pain often returned to anthropomorphic criteria:

> It behoves the veterinary clinician, in his attempt to alleviate suffering in animals, to maintain a high index of suspicion for the presence of pain in dealing with conditions which are known to be painful when they occur in man. There is no doubt that the use of analgesics can significantly reduce morbidity in small animals suffering from a wide variety of conditions. One's own experience of pain in different circumstances is a useful guide in this context.

(Yoxall, 1978, p. 424)

Yoxall's statement that analgesic use can reduce morbidity in small animals has still not been fully evaluated by controlled clinical trials. A number of studies do offer support, for example reports of a reduction in body weight loss following surgery in rats when analgesics were administered (Liles and Flecknell, 1993) and improved pulmonary function following analgesic use after thoracotomy in dogs (Flecknell *et al.*, 1991).

Anthropomorphic criteria are also used in US government guidelines to research workers:

> Unless the contrary is established, investigators should consider that procedures which cause pain and distress in human beings may cause pain or distress in other animals.

> (IRAC, 1985, p. 82)

Although this sets out an apparently humane approach, uncritical anthropomorphism may actually have hindered our progress in alleviating animal pain. As mentioned earlier, the assumption that conditions that cause pain in humans also cause pain in animals almost inevitably leads to the assumption that the behaviour of animals in these circumstances should mirror that of humans. Yoxall (1978, p. 423) was aware of this problem and cautioned:

> Animals are unable to communicate abstract concepts such as this, so it is up to us to try to learn to recognise subtle behavioural changes which may indicate that an animal is suffering from some noxious sensation, which we may anthropomorphically label 'pain'.

The major developments in our attempts to recognize animal pain occurred during the early 1980s. The growing concern of the research community to reduce any pain and distress associated with the use of animals in experimental procedures was reviewed by Flecknell (1984). This paper dealt extensively with the available analgesics and their potential use in animals, but only briefly with the issue of pain recognition. A more extensive treatment of this latter topic was provided by Morton and Griffiths (1985), in what has arguably been the most influential paper on animal pain assessment: 'Guidelines on the recognition of pain, distress and discomfort in experimental animals and an hypothesis for assessment.' The authors stated (p. 431):

> It is intended that this article should be of help, not only to newcomers inexperienced in the recognition of pain, but also possibly to those relatively experienced workers who may be called upon to evaluate the pain involved in a new model or an individual animal. The clinical signs and observations detailed in this paper have been based on the experience of animal technicians, animal nurses, research scientists and veterinary surgeons who have looked after experimental animals for a number of years. Some of the signs referred to will appear conflicting and this may reflect the types of physiological abnormality that exist in a broad spectrum of progressive debilitation in an animal.

In the interval between publication of Morton and Griffiths' paper and reports of application of their scheme, the paper was criticized because of the non-specific nature of the signs used in the scoring system. However, the authors had not suggested that the signs were specific. They stated (p. 433) that:

> The assessment scheme may be used under the following circumstances: for the animal user, technician or nurse to assess if treatment is required urgently; to evaluate the effectiveness of any treatment given or any experimental variable; to predict the level of pain likely to be incurred during an experimental procedure and to retrospectively assess the accuracy of that prediction; to reach an agreed score at which an experiment may be terminated; and to retrospectively assess the amount of suffering incurred by a procedure and its acceptability.

In other words, the signs involved indicate departures from normality, and pain could be one possible cause. Regrettably, very few attempts have been made to validate this approach to pain scoring. One study that examined the predictive value of the scoring system highlighted the need to tailor the assessment carefully (Beynen *et al.*, 1987) and pointed out the considerable between-observer variation that can occur when applying such schemes.

Further development of recognition of pain by clinical and laboratory evaluation was provided by the Association of Veterinary Teachers and Research Workers (1986, revised 1989) and subsequently by other groups (LASA, 1990; National Research Council, 1992; FELASA, 1994). All of these working party reports focused on experimental animals, reflecting not only the concern to alleviate pain, but also the requirement of legislation such as the Animals (Scientific Procedures) Act, 1986, in the UK, to assess the 'severity' of experiments.

In farm animals, attention had largely been focused on housing, husbandry and humane slaughter techniques; however, an EU-funded workshop brought together current opinion on the problem of pain in these species (Duncan and Molony, 1986). Although this workshop summarized a substantial body of literature, it also highlighted how few studies had been undertaken which directly addressed the problem of assessing pain in farm animals. Subsequently, reports from a number of research groups have appeared, focused primarily on the consequences of routine husbandry practices such as de-beaking, docking and castration (Mellor and Murray, 1989; Wood *et al.*, 1991; Gentle, 1992; Kent *et al.*, 1995). These studies highlighted the need for objective means of assessing pain, because without such a means of assessment it is not possible to determine which of two alternative techniques is to be preferred because it causes less pain. This same issue was reviewed by Flecknell (1994) who also pointed out that establishing methods of pain assessment was essential when selecting appropriate analgesics and establishing effective dosage regimens for pain alleviation.

Numerous attempts have been made to assess post-surgical pain in both companion and experimental animals (Reid and Nolan, 1991; Thompson and Johnson, 1991; Liles and Flecknell, 1993; Popilskis *et al.*, 1993; Nolan and Reid, 1993). In many instances the resulting data are difficult to interpret because of a failure to include appropriate controls. Where clinical signs were used to develop a pain-scoring system, the assumption was made that the signs indicated pain. Administration of an effective analgesic should therefore reduce the severity of these signs and hence the overall pain score. Without appropriate controls, the criteria used for scoring cannot be validated. Inclusion of an untreated control group, however, poses ethical concerns. Although these concerns are valid, they can be overcome to some extent by establishing criteria, before commencing a study, in which the investigators will intervene and administer analgesia. If a scoring system really is assessing the degree of pain, then this should present no problems, and the level of pain experienced either by untreated controls, or by animals receiving an ineffective analgesic therapy, can be limited.

Further difficulties associated with the use of pain-scoring systems in animals include the poor between-observer agreement for many scoring criteria (Beynen *et al.*, 1987) and the subjective nature of many assessments. Establishment of well validated pain-assessment techniques may therefore be difficult without the use of detailed behavioural analysis (Wood *et al.*, 1991; Liles, 1994).

5.3. Occurrence of Pain

5.3.1. Wild animals

Leaving aside the obstacles posed by our inability to assess pain accurately, it is possible to identify circumstances in which it is likely that pain might occur. In wild animals, the occurrence of pain might be thought to be an inevitable component of their life and not a problem of concern to humans. We do not, however, leave wild animals to live out their lives free from human interference and our interventions may result in them experiencing unnecessary pain. Obvious examples include hunting and trapping, both being activities which have provoked considerable public debate over the methods used, either when hunting for sport or commercially. Hunting of foxes, otters, stags and badgers, culling of seal pups and trapping of animals using leg-hold traps have all been criticized and in some cases legislation introduced to control the activity. Less attention has been directed towards fishing: either sports angling, in which hooking the fish may cause pain, or commercial fishing, in which fish may experience distress when suffocating after being caught. Objective scientific studies are needed to assess the welfare of animals in these circumstances, in order to determine whether they should correctly be identified as causing problems.

Wild animals, particularly rodents, may also suffer pain when killed as part of pest control programmes. Considerable efforts have been directed towards developing rodenticides which should cause less pain and distress, and discouraging or banning the use of less acceptable compounds such as strychnine.

5.3.2. Farm animals

Pain in farm animals may arise for a variety of reasons, many of which are associated with intensive husbandry systems. Leg injuries and fight wounds are seen in pigs (Webster, 1995), lameness and mastitis in cattle and lameness and myiasis in sheep. A number of routine animal husbandry practices such as tail-docking and castration may be carried out without anaesthesia and can be assumed to cause pain, but it is only relatively recently that serious attempts have been made to evaluate the severity and significance of this pain (Mellor and Murray, 1989; Wood *et al.*, 1991; Kent *et al.*, 1995). In addition to these instances of disease or traumatic injury, pain may also arise at parturition in cattle from the production of over-sized calves, or following Caesarean section if this is required for successful delivery of the calf. Although all of these potential causes of pain require consideration, Webster (1995, p. 156) concluded that pain in poultry might constitute 'the single most severe, systematic example of man's inhumanity to another sentient animal'. Based on a 25% incident rate of leg weakness and impaired locomotion in heavy strains of chicken by the time of slaughter (Kestin *et al.*, 1992), Webster concluded (p. 156) that 'Approximately one quarter of the heavy strains of broiler chickens and turkey are in chronic pain for approximately one third of their lives.'

Finally, as mentioned earlier, transport and slaughter of all species of food animal have the potential to cause pain.

5.3.3. Companion animals

Pain in companion animals can occur as a consequence of accidental trauma or elective surgery, such as ovarohysterectomy in dogs and cats. Taylor (1985) pointed out that pain could occur not only in these circumstances, but also in association with acute abdominal conditions, degenerative joint disease, tumours, periodontal disease and skin disease. This appears to be the first attempt explicitly to direct attention to such a broad range of clinical conditions in which pain could be present, and in which pain alleviation should be considered. Earlier, Yoxall (1978) had observed:

> It is surprising, for instance, how much a dog's 'quality of life', observed by the owner, may be improved by the administration of a simple analgesic if the dog is suffering from a tumour, which although painless on palpation, may be causing considerable chronic pain.

This appears to be the first publication that suggested that neoplasms could cause chronic pain in animals and that this could be a welfare problem, although the occurrence of obvious pain in association with specific tumours such as osteosarcoma had been emphasized as a diagnostic criterion. As with many other possible sources of pain, only anecdotal evidence has so far been published, and there appears to be a complete absence of controlled studies investigating the potential occurrence of cancer pain in animals.

It is also worth noting that pain may well occur as a result of inbreeding for the selection of certain breed characteristics, with inadvertent selection of undesirable traits such as hip dysplasia in dogs.

5.3.4. Laboratory animals

In laboratory animals pain can occur as a direct result of experimental procedures, or as a consequence of the method of housing and husbandry used in the laboratory. For example, sore hocks in rabbits and pododermatitis in guinea pigs can arise from the use of poorly designed grid floors, and are conditions that may produce chronic pain. As with companion animals, pain may occur as a result of neoplasia, arising either spontaneously in animals on long-term studies, or following deliberate induction of tumours in cancer research. The welfare problems associated with neoplasia have rarely been addressed, but recently guidelines have been developed to address this issue (UKCCCR, 1988).

Another area of special concern are studies in which chronic painful conditions are deliberately induced. Examples include chronic arthritis (Colpaert, 1987), neuroma production and a number of deafferentation models (Rossitch, 1991). Although these studies cause significant problems in respect to animal pain, they also indicate the progress that can be made in characterizing signs of pain and understanding the pathophysiology of the condition. In studies of arthritis in mice, Williams and colleagues (1993) used a series of functional parameters including strength of grip and gait analysis to follow the progress of this presumed painful condition. They concluded (p. 179): 'These experiments revealed that functional abnormalities of joints and of gait could predate, by weeks, the appearance of the first clinical symptoms of arthritis in mice.' Thus, although such studies pose significant ethical difficulties, they also indicate how the problem may be reduced by refinement of animal models. In this instance, early completion of studies could reduce the duration of arthritic pain, and possibly its severity.

5.4. Failure to Alleviate Pain

Although our inability to recognize the presence and assess the severity of animal pain may be a major factor in dealing with this significant welfare problem, it might have been expected that the widespread adoption of anthropomorphic criteria for pain recognition should have led to extensive use of analgesics. This has not been the case. In a survey of analgesic usage by small animal veterinarians in the UK, Townsend (1987, p. 25) concluded that:

> Less than half the respondents regularly used appropriate analgesia in a variety of situations in which dogs may be considered to be in severe pain . . . When information concerning repeat administration was included this figure fell to less than one third of the respondents.

More recently, a survey of Canadian veterinarians reported that only 49% could be classified as analgesic users (Dohoo and Dohoo, 1996).

A number of factors may contribute to the apparent underuse of analgesics to treat pain. A review of the veterinary literature of the 1960s and 1970s indicates a lack of emphasis on the need to alleviate pain. Although virtually all of the currently available analgesics were provided for use in humans at that time, they were not widely used in animals. Lumb and Wynn Jones in their text 'Veterinary Anaesthesia' (1973) emphasized the use of opioids (morphine-like drugs) as components of pre-anaesthetic medication, but did not consider post-operative pain. In the chapter dealing with post-operative care, the emphasis was on preventing anaesthesia-related problems.

The only mention of opioids (narcotics) was as follows (p. 607):

> When pre anaesthetic sedation has not been used, animals may thrash and
> struggle, bruising themselves severely and even breaking teeth during the
> recovery period. Coursing breeds such as greyhounds, Russian wolf hounds and
> Afghans are particularly prone to this phenomenon. Judicious use of
> tranquillisers or narcotics in small doses will quiet animals in this condition.

The authors clearly had a concern for the welfare of their patients but completely failed to address the problem of post-operative pain, viewing the value
of opioids primarily as sedatives. Given the close relationship between anaesthesia and surgery, this lack of emphasis might have been understandable
if there had been extensive discussion of pain relief in surgery texts; however,
this was not the case. The increasing concern to alleviate pain is shown,
however, by the greater emphasis given to the topic in the most recent edition
of this text. The editors affirm (Thurmon *et al.*, 1996, p. 40) that 'The prevention and control of pain is central to the practice of anaesthesia' and go on
to encourage use of analgesics by stating (p. 52) that:

> The commonly stated reasons for withholding analgesics (e.g. to avoid opioid
> induced respiratory depression or because pain relief would result in increased
> activity leading to self injury) are seldom valid.

Although this latter claim is widely supported by clinical opinion, no studies
specifically aimed at addressing this issue have been published.

A similar increase in concern about animal pain is shown in recent editions
of standard veterinary surgery texts. In the first edition of 'Textbook of Small
Animal Surgery' (Slatter, 1985) post-operative pain was relegated to a short
paragraph, whereas in the second edition of this text (Slatter, 1993) there is
much more extensive coverage of the topic.

Many older veterinary texts emphasized the potentially hazardous effects
of opioids and this is a concern which still persists. In their survey of factors
which influenced analgesic use by Canadian veterinarians, Dohoo and Dohoo
(1996) state that:

> Veterinarians were split roughly equally between analgesic users and non
> analgesic users. The two main factors influencing this dichotomy in patient
> management include the veterinarian's perception of the degree of pain felt post
> operatively, and maximum concern expressed regarding the risks associated with
> the use of potent opioid agonists in the post operative period.

Virtually identical concerns were expressed in human anaesthetic practice in
the 1960s and 1970s. These were well summarized by Utting (1984, p. 182):

> In a book on quality of care it can and should be said dogmatically that the
> standard of post operative pain relief in the UK, and probably everywhere else,
> is abysmal. This is well attested and documented.

Taylor (1985, p. 5), in addition to highlighting the need to assess pain,
pointed out that:

> Two further factors probably add to the underuse of analgesics in veterinary
> work. First, all the original strong analgesic opiates are subject to controlled

drugs regulations, necessitating tedious paperwork each time they are used. Secondly, the opiates have a considerable reputation for causing respiratory depression. Neither of these factors should prevent the clinical use of analgesics.

It is probably also relevant to point out that the relatively high cost of many analgesic agents may also be a factor in limiting their use.

In addition to the legal controls on the use of opioids, other legislation has impacts on the ability of veterinary surgeons to prevent or alleviate pain. In their investigations into the effects of castration in piglets, McGlone and Hellman (1988, p. 3049, emphasis added) stated:

> We conclude that castration is painful for 2 wk old and 7 wk old pigs. The 2 wk old pig seems behaviourally less affected by castration than does the 7 wk old pig. Local anaesthetic prevented pain induced behaviour changes for 2 wk old but not for 7 wk old pigs. *At present the FDA does not permit use of these anaesthetics in food producing animals.*

Legislation restricting the use of analgesics in food animals has become an important issue in Europe in the 1990s. European Union and local legislation resulted in a substantial reduction in the number of pharmaceutical products available for use in food producing animals. Although repeated reassurances have been issued in the UK by the Veterinary Medicines Directorate, there can be little doubt that absence of products licensed for use in food animals restricts the treatment of painful conditions. One particular concern relating to the use of analgesics in farm animals arises when injured animals are to be slaughtered with the intention that they are subsequently used for human consumption. If such 'casualty slaughter' animals, which may be in severe pain, are not immediately humanely destroyed, they may not be given analgesic and sedative treatment because of regulatory restrictions combined with the economic pressures to obtain some financial return from the animal.

The lack of emphasis on pain relief in veterinary texts should not lead to an assumption that the veterinary profession is unconcerned with pain. Analgesics are used extensively in particular clinical situations, notably the treatment of colic in horses.

Despite lack of information in standard texts, some members of the veterinary profession were attempting to provide information. Davis and Donnelly (1968, p. 1161), describing the use of experimental pain measurement to evaluate analgesics in cats, stated:

> The use of most of the common analgesic drugs has been considered to be contraindicated in cats because of toxicity or untoward side effects observed in this species. This view has been held by generations of veterinarians despite the fact that few fundamental studies of the pharmacology of these drugs have been performed in the cat . . .
>
> We believe that the results of this investigation justify the clinical trial of morphine and d-propoxyphene, alone or in combination with chlorpromazine, in the management of pain in the feline patient.

Over twenty years elapsed before more extensive evaluations of any analgesics in the cat were published (Lees and Taylor, 1991). Despite the lack of well controlled studies to evaluate the analgesic efficacy of such agents, anaesthetists teaching in veterinary schools continued to recommend the use of analgesics throughout the 1970s and 1980s, yet these recommendations seemed to have relatively little impact in veterinary practice. One other reason for failing to alleviate pain may also be of significance:

> It is as well, however, for the enthusiastic clinician to remember that pain is a natural protective response, which indicates that damage to the tissues is occurring. It is important to diagnose and treat the underlying cause of the pain, and to minimise treatment of pain in circumstances in which, by its presence, pain is reducing the likelihood of further damage occurring.
>
> (Yoxall, 1978, p. 435)

Over-concern with the protective nature of pain is still voiced as a reason for failing to administer analgesics. A similar concern pervaded clinical practice in humans but such concerns have been successfully set aside. In veterinary practice, it remains an obstacle to be overcome.

5.5. Additional Concerns

A number of the conditions identified as likely to cause pain may result in chronic pain rather than short, acute pain. The discovery of endorphins and descending regulatory pathways could imply that animals in chronic pain would experience other sources of pain less intensely. This appears not to be the case, and it has been demonstrated that animals in chronic pain may be hyperalgesic to certain types of noxious stimuli (Millan, 1987).

The finding that chronic pain could increase the perception of acute painful stimuli has significant welfare implications. Other sources of chronic pain were identified by Gentle (1992, p. 241), commenting on his own studies of the consequences of de-beaking in poultry:

> The acute pain from beak trimming is indeed short lived and some of the birds are not in pain for 24h after amputation. Following this pain-free period the birds may experience chronic pain for long periods of time.

This work, together with the reports of high incidence of lameness in birds, highlights the pressing need for us to review the impact of breeding programmes and husbandry procedures in poultry. In common with other painful conditions identified in farm animals, however, the problem of pain is related not simply to a failure to recognize pain or to treat it, but to economic factors that preclude effective action to prevent or alleviate pain.

5.6. Conclusions

- As with all the other groups of animals that society uses, the growing body of scientific evidence that a problem of pain does exist sets us on the path of finding effective solutions.
- In companion animals the use of analgesics remains variable, in spite of recent studies to evaluate the alleviation of post-surgical pain (Thompson and Johnson, 1991; Pascoe, 1993; Popilskis *et al.*, 1993).

- Nevertheless the range and use of analgesics is increasing: in the UK butor-phanol, buprenorphine, flunixin, carprofen, ketoprofen and meloxicam have all recently become available for veterinary use, suggesting that drugs for pain relief in companion animals are now seen as a commercially viable field.
- Greatest progress has been made in the area of pain in laboratory animals, reflecting both the introduction of legislation in Europe and the targeting of this field by animal welfarists.
- A requirement to use experimental animals to gain knowledge of benefit to science, to humans and to other animals remains. In spite of alternative and refined techniques, and increased use of analgesia, some of this use of animals results in pain.
- It should, however, be put into the context of our overall use of animals. In the UK about 3 million experimental animals are used each year, whereas 500 million are reared for food. Festing (1992, p. 65) has put it succinctly:

  > The average person in this country will consume in a 75 year lifespan approximately 600 chickens, 20 sheep, 22 pigs and 4 cows. They will use in research four mice, one rat and one two-hundredth of a dog. In other words, you can have all the benefits of medical research for a whole lifetime for approximately four mice and one rat.

- In farm animals the welfare issues caused by pain now receive serious attention. Analgesics are being marketed not merely for traumatic pain but also for other painful conditions, such as those with an inflammatory component like pneumonia.
- There has been a move towards husbandry systems, such as rearing un-castrated bulls and pigs, that avoid the need for surgical procedures in conscious animals.
- These are encouraging trends, though the same economic pressures that restrict the solution of many husbandry and transport problems inevitably prolong the problem of pain.

CHAPTER 6
Fear and distress

R. Bryan Jones (Roslin Institute, UK)

Abstract

Fear is one of the primary emotions that governs the way animals respond
to their social and physical environment. Ideally, fear is adaptive but the
restrictions imposed by many farming systems often interfere with the animal's
ability to respond in an adaptive fashion. Fear is now widely regarded as an
undesirable state of suffering and as a powerful and damaging stressor. Indeed,
it is one of the major problems facing the poultry industry; both acute and
chronic fear can dramatically reduce the animal's welfare and performance. In
chickens, for example, inappropriate fear responses can cause injury, pain or
death. Furthermore, fearful birds are less able to cope with challenges, are
difficult to manage, and show poorer growth, food conversion efficiency and
egg production. High fear levels could also compromise the use of more
extensive housing systems. It is imperative that we reduce fear but first we must
define it and measure it. Although fear is a complex concept, covering at least
five different processes or states, we can now measure it in operational terms.
Encouragingly, strong correlations between many tests of fear suggest that
they are measuring the same underlying characteristic, perhaps fearfulness, and
not just stimulus-specific responses. Potentially promising ways of reducing
underlying fearfulness include environmental enrichment, human stimulation,
and genetic selection. These remedial measures are briefly discussed in terms
of practical problems, ethical concerns and unanswered questions.

6.1. Introduction

Fear is one of the primary emotions that govern an animal's life. Although it
is often adaptive in ideal circumstances the 'sudden, unpredictable, intense,
prolonged or inescapable elicitation of fear can severely harm the mental and
physical wellbeing, growth and reproductive performance of laboratory, zoo
and farm animals' (Jones and Waddington, 1992, p. 1021).

Almost 75 years ago, Schjelderup-Ebbe (1922, p. 225) concluded that 'a
grave seriousness lies over the chicken yard and hens exhibit much anger and
fear'. The advent of intensive farming has meant that the chicken's environment has changed dramatically while the modern chicken also differs significantly from the barnyard fowl of 1922. Although I do not intend to debate the
advantages and disadvantages of intensive systems and of selective breeding,
I will examine some of their connotations for fear and distress.

Firstly, because many modern intensive farming systems provide chickens with a relàtively invariant and uneventful existence a misguided tendency to underestimate or even deny the occurrence and potential impact of fear has often accompanied their evolution. It has even been claimed that housing chickens in battery cages provided freedom from fear (Anonymous, 1992). However, it will never be possible, or even necessarily desirable, to totally eradicate fear and frightening stimuli from even the most sheltered farm environment. Neither must we lose sight of the fact that more extensive systems also have their attendant problems. For example, low-flying aircraft often cause intense fear and this problem is much more pronounced in flocks kept on free range (P. Cooper, personal communication). During its lifetime, a chicken could encounter a wide variety of alarming events. Their nature and incidence will vary according to the bird's genetic background, the precise nature of its housing and husbandry, and the quality of stockmanship. Generally though, exposure to novelty *per se* and contact with human beings are the commonest and potentially most frightening events; others include social disturbance, certain husbandry procedures, and all aspects of transportation and pre-slaughter processing.

Secondly, although many intensive systems offer benefits such as increased protection from disease, predation and climatic extremes, keeping animals in environments which minimize external stimulation and reduce the opportunities for decision making and control may engender monotony, physical debilitation, cognitive impairment, depression and the development of behavioural vices (Kendrick, 1992; Mench, 1992; Jones, 1996). Furthermore, animals kept under low levels of sensory input are more likely to overreact to novel events; consequently they may find it difficult to cope with subsequent changes in the environment and to acquire new knowledge (Kendrick, 1992; Jones, 1996). The value of avoiding under- as well as over-stimulation is now widely recognized and controlled exposure to mild or moderate fear and stress is thought to be beneficial (Jones, 1996; Zulkifli and Siegel, 1995). As Zulkifli and Siegel (1995, p. 71) point out, 'the challenge is to assess the degree of stress and provide an appropriate optimum stress environment'; they add cautionary notes concerning the lack of consensus over determinants of stress and the difficulties in constructing a universal scale due to the considerable genetic variability in stress responsiveness.

Thirdly, it has been argued not only that selective breeding for improved growth and reproductive performance implies selection for adaptability to an intensive environment but also that current high levels of productivity reflect adaptation. However, good productivity and health alone are not necessarily indicators of good welfare (Mench, 1992). Indeed, poor agreement was reported between measures of productivity and of physiological responsiveness to a known stressor (Zulkifli *et al.*, 1995). 'In large part, this is due to the way in which these measures are defined and manipulated within the commercial production environment' (Mench, 1992, p. 108). The deleterious effects of stress occur at the level of the individual animal whereas productivity is often measured at the level of the unit. Thus, 'individual animals may be in a comparatively poor state of welfare even though productivity', e.g. number of eggs per house, 'within the unit is high' (Mench, 1992, p. 108). Furthermore, farming practice has probably changed too rapidly and frequently for the chicken's biology and behaviour to have evolved in a suitable fashion and at the same pace (Faure, 1980). Domestication has undoubtedly reduced fear but chickens can still be easily frightened by environmental change and by exposure to people.

Not only can fear cause serious problems for the farm animal and for the farmer but its assessment and understanding pose problems for the scientist. This chapter attempts to define fear and its components and to discuss its assessment. The precise implications of high levels of fear for the welfare, management and performance of poultry are described. Various ways of alleviating fear are discussed in terms of their potential advantages and their associated problems. Although the chapter focuses primarily on the domestic fowl, important work on other species is also mentioned. Furthermore, many of the principles underlying the development and reduction of fear are relevant to farm, zoo and laboratory animals.

6.2. What Constitutes Fear?

The complexity and controversy surrounding the fear concept are illustrated by its numerous definitions. Some examples include: a state of alarm or dread, an unpleasant or painful emotion elicited by danger, an expectation of pain, a behaviour system which has evolved to ensure survival, a hypothetical state of the brain and neuroendocrine system, and a defensive motivational state (Jones, 1987a; 1996). However, many of these definitions focus on the protective aspects of fear and they are not mutually exclusive. Fear is normally listed among the emotions, like love, anger and hate, and I regard it as an emotional (psychophysiological) response to perceived danger. Indeed, fear is one of the primary emotions determining how humans and other animals respond to their physical and social environment. Ideally fear is an adaptive state with fear behaviour serving to protect the animal from injury (Jones, 1987a, 1996).

Our understanding has been further complicated because fear embraces at least five different phenomena or processes (Jones, 1996): (i) The first stage necessarily involves exposure to frightening stimulation; (ii) This may activate the brain and neuroendocrine system and thereby generate a flexible, internal fear state; (iii) The animal may then show one or more of a number of fear responses, such as cautious investigation, fight, flight or immobility. These may be altered and integrated according to changes in the perceived potency of the threatening stimulus and in the consequent intensity of the internal fear state; (iv) The level of underlying fearfulness (inherent and/or acquired propensity to be easily frightened) is crucial because fearful animals are more likely to show exaggerated fear responses than are their less fearful counterparts, regardless of the nature of the threatening stimulus. Boissy (1995) concluded that 'fearfulness has to be considered as a component of personality' (p. 183) and that it is:

> a basic feature of the temperament of each individual, one that predisposes
> it to respond similarly to a variety of potentially alarming challenges, but is

nevertheless continually modulated during development by the interaction of
genetic traits of reactivity with environmental factors, particularly in the juvenile
period. (p. 165)

Such interaction may explain much of the inter-individual variability observed
in adaptive responses; and (v) although there is no direct evidence, chickens
might experience a state of anxiety (a feeling of apprehension stemming from
the anticipation of an imagined threat). For example, some birds seem to
spend most of their time hiding and rarely mingle with the rest of the flock.

6.3. Assessment of Fear

Neither the fear state nor fearfulness can be measured directly in any species,
including man. Much debate has centred on whether or not fear varies over a
unitary scale. According to Archer (1979, p. 57), 'this would correspond to
asking in everyday speech "How frightened are you? Just a little, or scared out
of your wits?"' Like Hinde (1974), but unlike Gray (1971), Archer (1979,
p. 57) regarded 'such a unitary representation as too great an oversimplifica-
tion to be useful for precise analysis' and proposed that fear should not be
regarded as a unitary variable because correlations between different measures
of fear were weak, at least in laboratory rodents and human beings. He also
argued that putative fear responses must be considered specific not only to the
particular test stimulus but also to the species, age and sex of the subject.
Similarly, Murphy (1978, p. 430) concluded that 'the use of the words fear or
fearful to imply any trait of temperament or personality in any group should
be avoided'. If valid, these proposals would severely constrain attempts to reduce fear in practical situations, because the manipulation of narrow stimulus-
specific responses would be of little value in modifying general adaptability and
responsiveness to challenge. However, the limited numbers of tests and measures and the small sample sizes examined in the studies on which Archer's
(1979) criticism was based were unlikely to have yielded significant correlations,
and one cannot realistically expect correlations close to unity when measuring a complex, behaviourally disruptive phenomenon like fear (Gray, 1979;
Tachibana, 1982).

Duncan (1981a, p. 456) has claimed that 'Although a phenomenon such
as fear is really a hypothetical intervening variable, it is still possible to define
it operationally and measure it in the same way as hunger or thirst can be
measured'. Thus, fear can be assessed functionally in terms of the animals'
attempts to avoid danger. Because fear competes with and inhibits all other
behaviour systems we can infer how frightened an animal is by monitoring its
responses in test situations intuitively regarded as more or less frightening
(Jones, 1987b; 1996). Some of the behavioural methods commonly used to
measure fear in poultry, such as open-field, emergence, approach/avoidance,
and tonic immobility tests, are described elsewhere (Jones, 1987b; 1996).
Many researchers have also recorded physiological measures of alarm or
stress, such as heart rate and the concentrations of plasma catecholamines and
corticosterone. These indices are most useful when measured in conjunction

with behavioural observation; behavioural and physiological information should be regarded as complementary rather than alternative measures of fear.

Encouragingly, strong intra-individual associations have been found across scores in several tests of fear in chickens and Japanese quail (Jones *et al.*, 1991; Jones and Waddington, 1992), and in mammalian species, such as goats, sheep, cattle and service dogs (Fordyce *et al.*, 1982; Goddard and Beilharz, 1984; Lyons *et al.*, 1988; Romeyer and Bouissou, 1992). These positive correlations strongly suggest that the tests were measuring the same intervening variable, perhaps underlying fearfulness, and not just stimulus-specific responses. If so, this measurable, underlying characteristic or personality trait offers exciting opportunities for manipulating non-specific responsiveness to threat.

6.4. Impact of Fear

Fear represents a major problem facing the animal farming industry. Its many harmful effects on the welfare, management, performance and profitability of poultry are outlined in Box 6.1 and discussed below.

6.4.1. Welfare problems

Ruth Harrison's seminal and timely book 'Animal Machines' (Harrison, 1964) resulted not only in growing public awareness of the conditions of intensive farming but also in a vociferous concern for the welfare of farm animals. The Brambell Committee, which was consequently established to enquire into the welfare of intensively farmed animals, concluded that:

> There are sound anatomical and physiological grounds for accepting that domestic mammals and birds experience the same kind of sensations that we do [and that] animals can experience emotions such as rage, fear, and apprehension.
>
> (Brambell Committee, 1965, pp. 9,10)

Box 6.1. Some undesirable consequences of inappropriate fear responses, chronic fear states, and heightened fearfulness with particular reference to poultry.

Wasted energy
Injuries (scratches, cuts, bone fractures), pain and death
Feather-pecking, feather damage
Behavioural inhibition, social withdrawal, reduced ability to adapt to change and to new resources
Difficulties in handling and management
Delayed maturation
Decreased reproductive performance and egg production
Reduced growth and food conversion efficiency
Abnormalities of the egg shell, compromised hatchability
Downgrading of eggs and carcasses
Serious financial losses

Interestingly, it had already been proposed that a response preparing us for flight and defence was incompatible with the life of civilized man (Charvat et al., 1964).

Although fear and stress are adaptive in ideal circumstances, the questions of degree and context are crucial. In reality, the restrictions imposed by many farming systems can interfere with the animal's ability to respond in an appropriate and adaptive fashion to changes in its environment. For example, caged hens cannot run away from threatening stimuli, while chickens kept on a free-range area lacking in shelter are unable to hide from an aerial predator. There is 'growing support for the view that fear not only represents a state of suffering but that it is also a powerful, potentially damaging stressor' (Jones, 1996). The UK's Farm Animal Welfare Council (1993, p. 4) has consistently recommended that there should be 'freedom from fear and distress'.

Both acute and chronic fear states can seriously harm the animal's well-being, particularly if they are intense (Jones, 1996). Firstly, for example:

> Chickens often run into obstacles or pile on top of and trample each other when they panic . . . Birds at the bottom of the heap may suffocate and others might suffer bruising, broken bones, cuts and scratches.
>
> (Jones, 1996)

Such injuries represent a major welfare problem because they can lead to chronic pain, infection, physical debilitation, and perhaps social withdrawal. Damage to the plumage, caused by fear-related behaviour, such as clawing, trampling and perhaps feather-pecking (see below), can also result in increased susceptibility to claw-inflicted injury and in greater heat loss. Feather loss or damage is also perceived by the public to indicate reduced well-being. Secondly, if the animal is unable to escape from a frightening stimulus or to find an alternative coping strategy, or if it learns that none is available, it might give up and enter the dangerous realms of hopelessness, learned helplessness and behavioural depression (Job, 1987). These states may lead to psychosomatic symptoms or even death, at least in man and other mammals (Jones, 1987a).

Feather-pecking and feather damage may be associated with the chickens' level of underlying fearfulness, although the existence and direction of any causal relationship is unclear. Feather loss was more pronounced in hens characterized as fearful, regardless of whether they were housed individually or in groups (Craig and Swanson, 1994). Furthermore, birds likely to feather-peck also showed greater fear than did their low pecking counterparts (Vestergaard et al., 1993). However, comparisons of birds from genetic lines coincidentally showing high or low propensities to feather-peck indicated that this putative relationship was not straightforward and that differences in social motivation might also be influential (Jones et al., 1995).

Fear is such a powerful emotion that it can inhibit behaviour patterns generated by all other motivational systems (Jones, 1987a, 1996). Furthermore,

> Animals under constant stress do not learn well simply because they are unable to attend selectively to the changes in their environment that the learning task requires.
>
> (Kendrick, 1992, p. 226)

Thus, a frightened bird would be less likely to express exploratory, feeding, social and sexual behaviours. Such inhibition of generally beneficial behaviours and processes could dramatically reduce the animal's ability to adapt to changes in its physical environment, to learn new tasks, to utilize new resources and to interact successfully with its companions. For example, fearful broiler cockerels were less sexually active than calm ones and their fertility was compromised (Shabalina, 1984).

6.4.2. Management problems

> The dominant reaction of the progenitors of domestic poultry species to human beings is a fearful one which may have been attenuated but is unlikely to have been eliminated by the domestication process.
>
> (Duncan, 1990, p. 121)

Suarez and Gallup (1982) have even suggested that naïve chickens not only find human contact alarming but perceive people as predators rather than as benevolent caretakers. Visual or physical contact with people can undoubtedly elicit withdrawal, panic and violent escape reactions in chickens, often with associated injury, as well as acute stressor effects, such as cardiac acceleration and adrenocortical activation (Jones, 1996). Indeed, irregular handling and exposure to harsh caretakers were identified as stressors capable of severely limiting the performance of broiler breeders (Rosales, 1994), while inter-flock aggression was greater in strains of hens showing high fear of humans (Komai and Guhl, 1960). Animals predisposed to be easily and intensely frightened are also much more difficult to handle and manage than their less fearful counterparts. This could exacerbate the problems encountered during routine examination, translocation, depopulation, artificial insemination, etc. As well as 'the deleterious effects on the bird, their intractability could place a greater demand on the stockpersons' time as well as increasing the risk of their injury and/or disaffection' (Jones, 1996).

High or persistent fear of humans is undesirable from both the chickens' and the farmers' viewpoints. However, human contact could become even more traumatic as increasing automation reduces opportunities for birds to become accustomed to people. Some degree of contact between chickens and humans is inevitable regardless of the production system but this is not something to be avoided. Rather, we should find ways of improving the human–chicken relationship to maximize mutual benefits (see 6.5.2.).

Because novelty is potentially alarming, elevated fearfulness can cause problems when chickens are translocated from one environment to another. For example:

> The novel cage environment might pose a welfare problem for floor-reared chicks when they are transferred to it during late adolescence, [and] chicks reared in floor pens appeared to be more fearful initially and to engage in more agonistic activity [than those from cages].
>
> (Craig and Swanson, 1994, p. 929)

The growing tendency to adopt more extensive and putatively welfare-friendly systems could also be hampered by high levels of underlying fearfulness. The progenitors of the domestic fowl prefer habitats that provide good cover and Grigor (1993) suggested that modern day chickens may feel vulnerable and susceptible to attack by predators in open areas. Free-range environments are likely to incorporate numerous potentially alarming elements, such as novel places and things, lack of shelter, and the risk of predation. Not surprisingly therefore, many birds appear reluctant to leave the poultry house and to move out into a free-range area when given the opportunity; indeed only small proportions of the flocks were normally observed outside (Grigor, 1993). Interestingly, birds frequently using the free-range area were found to be less fearful than those which never ventured out of the poultry house (Grigor, 1993) although it remains to be determined whether this is cause or effect. Attempts to ensure greater usage of free range would probably benefit from application of the following approaches. Firstly, and in line with informed practice, its attractiveness could be increased by incorporating 'reassuring' features, such as shelter, feeding sites and familiar stimuli. Secondly, because some birds were consistently observed outside (Grigor, 1993), selective breeding for increased willingness to enter the free-range environment might offer a speedy solution. Thirdly, it may be worth determining if the birds would follow an imprinted robotic chicken out of the shed and onto free range.

6.4.3. Fear, performance and economic consequences

Despite the growing concern for the welfare implications of fear, its impact on production has received greater attention.

Exposure to frightening and otherwise stressful stimulation disrupted egg laying and resulted in numerous abnormalities of the egg shell, such as thinness, cracks, equatorial bulges, accretions and chalky deposits (Hughes *et al.*, 1986; Mills and Faure, 1990). Furthermore, 'birds which consistently laid eggs with abnormal shells were more fearful than "normal" layers' (Jones, 1996). Shell abnormalities can pose substantial problems for egg producers. Table eggs with abnormal shells may be downgraded or rejected, with the associated economic loss, because they fail to match the consumers' conception of the ideal egg. Thin shells and other abnormalities can also compromise hatchability. Thus, significant 'losses may also be caused in breeding flocks because seriously affected eggs are not usually sent to the hatchery' (Hughes *et al.*, 1986, p. 326).

The persistent or frequent expression of certain fear responses, such as panic or violent escape, is physically demanding, wasteful of energy and can result in serious injuries to the birds or their companions (see 6.4.1). These injuries may, in turn, cause downgrading of carcasses at slaughter with consequent falls in profitability.

It is thought that fearful birds take longer to reach sexual maturity and show poorer egg production than do less fearful hens. Convincing evidence for this sort of negative association was obtained when it was shown that 'fear of an approaching human was inversely related to egg production' in hens housed in battery cages in both laboratory (Hemsworth and Barnett, 1989) and commercial (Barnett *et al.*, 1992) situations. Fear of humans accounted for between 20 and 63% of the variance in egg production and mortality in the latter study which extended across 14 commercial farms. In economic terms, an assumption that fear of humans accounted for a conservative 20% of the variation in egg production in the latter study indicates a significant source of lost income (J.L. Barnett, personal communication). If losses were similar in the UK, fear of humans could cost the egg industry several million pounds a year. This estimate could be substantially higher if production losses caused by other frightening events, such as low-flying aircraft (see below), thunder, failure of services, reflected light, vermin, etc., were determined and included.

'Fear of humans may also be an important factor limiting the productivity of commercial broiler chickens' (Hemsworth et al., 1994b, p. 102). For example, avoidance of an approaching human varied hugely across 22 commercial farms and food conversion efficiency (FCE) was significantly lower at those farms at which the birds showed greater fear of people (Hemsworth et al., 1994b; Jones, 1996); indeed, the level of fear of humans accounted for 28% of the variance in food conversion at the farms. This relationship probably reflected variations in the quality of stockmanship; a variable which is known to be closely linked with both emotional state and productivity in several farm animal species (Hemsworth et al., 1993). Based on the above variance and on the range of 1.79 to 2.10 in FCE observed across the 22 farms, it was calculated that an improvement of 0.09 units in FCE would be available to the farm with the worst record (Hemsworth et al., 1994b). Given current costs, even a conservative improvement of 0.045 units in FCE would translate to a saving of AUS$8,400 per farm (Hemsworth, personal communication).

The financial importance of fear is further illustrated by the fact that the Ministry of Defence made compensatory payments to poultry farmers of approximately £700,000 in 1995 to cover fear-related losses caused by low-flying military aircraft (P. Cooper, personal communication). This figure does not include those additional production losses associated with overflights by civil aircraft or by hot-air balloons.

Fear and growth are also negatively related in chicks of both broiler and layer strains. Panic and hysteria have often been associated with reduced growth rates (Mills and Faure, 1990) and exposure to frightening procedures, such as beak-trimming, electric shock and blood withdrawal, depressed weight gain in chicks (McFarlane et al., 1989; Jones, 1996). Similarly, 'Commercial pigs may be highly fearful of humans [and] high levels of fear of humans by pigs may markedly reduce their growth and reproductive performance' (Hemsworth et al., 1993, p. 39). Remedial measures intended to reduce fearfulness in chickens, such as regular handling and environmental enrichment, have also resulted in increased FCE and growth (Jones, 1996).

There is convincing evidence that underlying fearfulness and product quality are negatively associated in a range of farm animals. Stress-induced reduction in meat quality was more pronounced in Japanese quail of a genetic line showing high rather than low levels of fear (Mills, personal communication), the incidence of pale soft exudative meat was increased in pigs that were nervous and difficult to handle (Grandin, 1991), and cattle characterized as fearful showed a greater incidence of bruising as well as reduced meat tenderness (Fordyce et al., 1988).

These negative relationships between fearfulness and performance may reflect chronic activation of the hypothalamo–pituitary–adrenocortical (HPA) axis or a series of acute responses. Persistent elevation of circulating levels of the stress hormone corticosterone (cortisol in certain mammals) causes many undesirable effects in chickens, including reduced energy retention, growth, egg production and immunocompetence (Jones, 1996). It is important to note firstly that fearful chickens showed greater adrenocortical responses to stressful stimuli and secondly that the artificial elevation of plasma corticosterone levels predisposed hens to react more fearfully to alarming stimulation (Jones et al., 1988; Beuving et al., 1989; Jones, 1996). Naturally increased pituitary–adrenocortical activity may also be associated with elevated fear in ducklings, rabbits and pigs (Jones et al., 1988; Jones, 1996) and with increased panic, anxiety and depression in human beings (Goldstein et al., 1987). It is thus conceivable that a progressively harmful positive feedback could develop. For example, not only might fearful chickens be frightened more easily, frequently and intensely than less fearful ones but the relatively greater activation of their HPA systems might, in turn, perpetuate or exaggerate fearfulness.

Whatever the mechanisms, a powerful warning note was sounded by the suggestion that:

> Larger negative correlation coefficients are likely to be found, for susceptible strains, between measures of fearfulness and productivity as periods of confinement in barren, high-density cage environments increase.

> (Craig et al., 1983, p. 272)

6.5. Alleviation of Fear

The question of whether we should adapt the environment to suit the animal or change the animal to suit the environment is frequently posed. On the one hand we know that:

> Environmental factors have profound and drastic effects upon the immature organism, and one can literally change an animal's behavioral and physiological capabilities through the appropriate manipulation of environmental dynamics.

> (Denenberg, 1962, p. 110)

On the other hand, given the great genetic diversity within populations, selective breeding probably represents the quickest, most reliable method of reducing fear and other welfare problems. In reality, an integrated approach is likely to be the most effective. Currently, the most promising ways of reducing fear and increasing adaptability include environmental enrichment, regular handling or related methods of promoting habituation to people, and selective breeding. Each is briefly discussed below and is covered in considerably greater detail elsewhere (Jones, 1996).

6.5.1. Environmental enrichment

Environmental enrichment involves introducing novel and putatively interesting stimuli into the home environment and thereby increasing its complexity and stimulus value. This procedure reliably reduced fear of novel places, things and food in numerous species, including the domestic fowl (Jones and Waddington, 1992; Jones, 1996). Furthermore, it reduced mortality, aggressiveness and cannibalism, and improved performance in chickens (Jones, 1996). Because animals seek novelty, e.g. chicks preferentially approach novel video images (Jones *et al.*, 1996), enrichment may also be beneficial in this respect.

However, several potential problems have to be overcome before the commercial poultry environment can be effectively enriched. The selected enrichment devices must be safe, affordable and practicable, not too easily soiled, lost or destroyed, accessible to all members of the flock, and retain the birds' interest and thereby prevent the need for frequent change. Ideally, we should determine what sorts of stimuli the chickens find attractive and interesting. Some of the many questions include: are there unlearned preferences, are movement and change important, is physical interaction with the enrichment stimuli essential, and at what rates of introduction and stages of the bird's development would enrichment be most beneficial? Identifying the factors which govern a chicken's perception of a safe and interesting world would greatly facilitate the development of effective environmental enrichment.

6.5.2. Regular handling

Picking an animal up and/or stroking it regularly is a powerful, rapid and reliable method of reducing fear of people (Hemsworth *et al.*, 1993; Jones, 1993; 1996). Although handling does not necessarily reduce chickens' fear of non-human stimuli, other desirable effects of this procedure include reduced aggressiveness, increased resistance to infection, and improved performance (Jones, 1996). However, despite its potential benefits, regular handling of large flocks is not a practicable option for the poultry farmer. Encouragingly though, the effects of handling generalized from one handler to other people regardless of differences in their gender, physical appearance or clothing (Jones, 1994; 1996). It was also recently shown that fear of humans was reduced simply by letting chicks see people regularly, and that this effect was common to broiler chicks and those of flighty and docile laying strains (Jones, 1993; 1995; 1996). Furthermore, exposing hens to close visual contact with humans daily (in addition to that involved in routine husbandry) from 19 to 36 weeks of age reduced their fear of people and increased hen-day egg production (Barnett *et al.*, 1994b). Stockpersons' attitudes and behaviour, which are known to modulate animals' fear of human beings (Hemsworth *et al.*, 1993), are also important. Indeed:

> One likely outcome of future research is the development of staff training and selection procedures which augment the productivity and welfare of farm animals by improving the attitudinal and behavioural profiles of stockpersons towards farm animals.
>
> (Hemsworth *et al.*, 1993, p. 44)

The apparent flexibility, ease of induction and pervasiveness of the 'human contact effect' clearly have important practical implications.

6.5.3. Selective breeding

The animal's genetic background strongly affects its ability to adapt to environmental changes and challenges. Craig and Swanson (1994, p. 933) concluded that:

> A solution to reducing or preventing harmful behaviours would be to use stocks that either do not show these behaviours or exhibit them at such low levels or so infrequently as to be of trivial importance.

Mench (1992, p. 120) had also argued that 'Genetic selection may prove to be a powerful tool for decreasing the incidence of behaviors associated with welfare problems.' Although decreased fear has accompanied domestication there is still considerable variability both within and between populations of poultry. Genetic selection programmes for reduced fear or for a dampened adrenocortical stress response to specific stressors have been established in turkeys (Brown and Nestor, 1974), chickens (Faure, 1980; Gross and Siegel, 1985) and Japanese quail (Satterlee and Johnson, 1988; Mills and Faure, 1991).

> Simple criteria for evaluating poultry husbandry using behavior–genetic analyses are not available and additional research is needed.
>
> (Siegel, 1993, p. 5)

Encouragingly, genetic selection of Japanese quail either for short tonic immobility (TI) fear reactions (Mills and Faure, 1991) or for a reduced plasma corticosterone response to mechanical restraint (Satterlee and Johnson, 1988) has alleviated the birds' underlying fearfulness as well as their physiological stress responsiveness to a wide range of potentially traumatic situations (Jones *et al.*, 1991; 1992; 1994a,b; Jones 1996; Jones and Satterlee, 1996). Parallels between the results of the two independent selection programmes suggest that they may have influenced the same underlying variable, perhaps fearfulness. Indeed, several behavioural measures of fear (e.g. TI, open-field responses, avoidance, struggling during restraint) differed markedly between the selected and control lines and may represent valuable selection criteria for breeding programmes intended to alleviate underlying fearfulness and non-specific stress responsiveness. Such behavioural tests have many advantages; they can be carried out on young chicks and are quick, simple, inexpensive and non-invasive. Studies of genetic lines like those described above should be extended to include other important traits, such as aggressiveness, immuno-competence, productivity and product quality.

Two possible objections must be considered before we accept and exploit genetic selection as a welfare-friendly tool. Firstly, selection sometimes modifies more than one trait. Therefore, we must ensure that there are no associated undesirable effects. Secondly, the ethics of genetic manipulation has raised widespread concern. However, I consider genetic selection for reduced fearfulness to be ethically sound because it is likely to increase the animal's ability to interact successfully with its physical and social environment and thereby to improve its welfare as well as its management and performance.

6.6. Conclusions

- Fear is an undesirable state of suffering and a powerful stressor which can seriously harm an animal's welfare, management, performance and profitability.
- It is imperative that we reduce fear, from the animals', the public's and the farmers' viewpoints.
- Fear is a complex concept and its assessment is controversial. Therefore, interpretational and methodological problems associated with our understanding and assessment of fear have often had to be addressed. Fear is now generally assessed in functional terms; strong correlations between many tests suggest that they are measuring the same underlying characteristic, perhaps fearfulness (propensity to be easily frightened).
- The manipulation of narrow stimulus-specific responses would be of little practical value. Our ability to measure and modify underlying fearfulness represents a crucial advance.
- Fearfulness can be reduced by environmental enrichment, human stimulation and genetic selection; but several questions need to be addressed before recommendations can be made concerning these remedial measures.
- The answers to these questions may identify the most appropriate approach, in terms of selective breeding, environmental enrichment, and human–animal interactions, in order to achieve the optimal levels of sensory stimulation, fear and stress.

CHAPTER 7
Behavioural restriction

J. Carol Petherick (Queensland Department of
Primary Industries, Australia) and Jeff Rushen
(Agriculture and Agri-Food Canada)

Abstract

Animals in human care are generally kept in conditions which prevent them
performing many of the behaviours they would normally use to attain their
functional goals. A central question in the study of animal welfare is whether
or not animals should be allowed to carry out most or all of their normal
behaviour patterns; there is a widespread belief that behavioural restriction or
deprivation will cause animals to suffer. One influential paper (Baxter, 1983)
has suggested that animals may not need to perform certain behaviours provided the functional consequences of those behaviours are met. Other workers
(Hughes and Duncan, 1988) have provided evidence to suggest that animals
may, indeed, need to perform the behaviour itself in order to ensure good welfare. It has been suggested that welfare is more likely to be jeopardized when
behaviours that are largely internally motivated are prevented or restricted,
when motivation remains high if the behaviour cannot be performed and when
it is the performance of the behaviour itself which reduces motivation. Nest-
building in poultry is given as an example, with details of its physiological basis.
However, it is recognized that it is not easy to distinguish between internal and
external motivation and that many behaviours are probably motivated in both
ways. Dust-bathing behaviour is given as an example. It is apparent that we
need to understand more fully the motivation for the performance of behaviours, and in particular what initiates and turns them off, before we can assess
the effects of their restriction or deprivation. Three methods by which it may
be possible to assess the impact of behavioural restriction on welfare are
discussed. These are the measurement of the demand (the 'price' that animals
are prepared to pay) for behaviours, the physiological consequences of behavioural deprivation and the occurrence of abnormal behaviours which arise from
behavioural restriction.

7.1. Introduction

A central question in the study of animal welfare is whether it is sufficient to
ensure that an animal's functional requirements for good health, protection
from environmental extremes and adequate nutrition are met, or whether it
is also necessary to allow animals to perform some or most of their normal
behaviour patterns. In most instances, animals in the care of humans, such as

laboratory animals, wild animals in captivity and farm livestock cannot perform many of the behaviours they would normally use to attain their functional goals: behaviours that are regularly seen in less restrictive environments. The majority of the work on behavioural restriction and deprivation has been carried out with farm animals, so most of our examples relate to them. However, the principles apply equally to any species kept in a restricted environment.

The implicit philosophy behind such animal management has been that if the animal's functional requirements are met then the often energetically expensive behaviour need not occur. However, for many animal welfare groups, such behavioural deprivation or restriction is one of the main faults of intensive animal husbandry (Dawkins, 1988) and there is a widespread belief that animals which are restricted or prevented from performing their full repertoire of behavioural patterns will suffer in the same way that they suffer if their physical requirements, such as for food and water, are not met. Furthermore, many captive animals will perform apparently 'irrelevant' behaviours, which are directed to an inappropriate object. Often this behaviour will be performed even when the normal functional consequences of the behaviour have already been achieved. For example, domestic hens and pigs engage in extensive nest-building behaviour even when provided with a preconstructed nest (Hughes *et al.*, 1989; Arey *et al.*, 1991) and young ruminants, separated from their mothers, perform non-nutritive sucking of pen mates, parts of the pen and non-functional teats even after drinking milk (de Wilt, 1985; de Passillé *et al.*, 1993). Understanding the causes of such apparently abnormal behaviour, and its relationship with behavioural deprivation, has become a major part of applied ethology.

7.2. Theoretical Background

7.2.1. Behavioural 'needs'

A central concept in discussions of behavioural deprivation and animal welfare has been the concept of a behavioural or ethological 'need' – a term often used to imply that frustration will result if a behaviour is prevented by the environment in which the animal is kept. Much of the scientific discussion that has occurred over animal welfare has involved trying to define more precisely what 'behavioural needs' might be. However, in this context, the word 'need' is used in two slightly different ways. Animals need food and water in the sense that without them they die. Dawkins (1983a) refers to these types of needs as ultimate, because if they are not met reproductive failure and death will result. These needs can be distinguished from another type of need which can be referred to as a proximate need. Failure to meet these needs may not result in death or loss of reproductive success, but it may cause the animals to suffer nevertheless. If they do exist, 'behavioural needs' are most likely to be proximate needs.

Baxter (1983) illustrates the difference between ultimate needs and proximate needs in his discussion of how the behaviour of farm animals can contribute to their welfare and productivity. For example, nest-building by pre-natal sows may function to provide climatic and mechanical protection for the new-born piglets. Therefore the ultimate needs of the sow could be achieved simply by providing a suitable environment for the piglets, and it may not be necessary for the sows to perform any particular behaviour patterns to achieve this. However, Baxter considers that welfare is very much concerned with the subjective experiences of animals and whilst ultimate needs may be met by the functional consequences of the behaviour, the proximate needs which ensure good welfare may not be met. Thus questions about how behavioural deprivation affects animal welfare are concerned with what motivates the animal to perform the behaviour.

7.2.2. Aspects of motivation important for animal welfare

To decide whether inability to perform a particular behaviour pattern reduces the welfare of the animal we need to understand the motivation behind the behaviour, especially what factors cause an animal to start performing the behaviour and what causes it to stop. One particularly important question is whether these factors are internal (i.e. arising from changes within the animal itself) or external (i.e. arising from changes in the animal's environment). Generally, welfare problems are more likely to arise when internal sources of motivation for the behaviour are present. However, it may not be an easy task to separate internal and external factors. As Hughes and Duncan (1988, p. 1700) state:

> It is impossible to divide the factors that govern the expression of behaviour strictly into internal and external ones, because all motivational systems are ultimately both internally and externally controlled . . . Nevertheless, when the proximate factors governing the expression of particular behaviour patterns are considered, it is clear that some are triggered primarily from within, some from without and others by complex interactions between the two.

A second issue concerns whether the factors that reduce the motivation to perform behaviour require the performance of the behaviour itself or the attainment of certain consequences of the behaviour. To deal with this issue, it is necessary to discuss some different models of motivation.

7.2.3. Motivation to perform behaviour or to attain consequences?

One widely held view is that animals are motivated to obtain certain consequences of behaviour, and that it is the consequences of the behaviour that turn the behaviour off. Models of motivation along these lines often assume that animals have some ideal state or 'set-point', and that when there is some discrepancy between this set-point and their actual state, then behaviour occurs with the aim of reducing this discrepancy. For example, Baxter (1983, p. 216) discusses such a model of the motivation of nest-building by sows:

> Welfare requirements are for behavioural control systems to remain at, or appropriately return to, their set points. [In sow nesting] the central issue is the nature and origin of the loop feeding back into the behavioural system to reduce motivation . . . From my studies of sow nesting behaviour, I speculated . . . that nesting motivation was reduced when the sow could lie down and her udder,

highly sensitive and distended with milk at this time, remained comfortable . . .
If a sow's welfare requirement was to be able to perform nesting behaviour,
it could only be accommodated by providing her with bedding material and a
large amount of space. If, however, her requirement is for udder comfort prior
to parturition, then this could be accommodated in many ways, one of which
would be to provide a soft resilient substrate for the sow to lie on.

While the above way of looking at motivation may seem to be common
sense, considerable research in animal behaviour has shown that the motivational systems are not as straightforward as this. Konrad Lorenz produced a
particularly influential model of behavioural motivation (Lorenz, 1981), which
suggested that animals are motivated to perform particular behaviour patterns
and not just to achieve particular functional goals. For example, an animal that
has consumed sufficient food to meet nutritional requirements may still need
to perform appetitive food-searching behaviours, simply for the sake of performing the behaviour itself. Furthermore, Lorenz suggested that the tendency
to perform these behaviour patterns increases with the time since their last
performance as a result of an accumulation of internal 'nervous energy'. At
normal levels of motivation, the behaviour will be elicited only by stimuli that
are close to the optimal. As time passes and the internal motivation increases,
the behaviour will begin to be elicited by a wider range of sub-optimal stimuli.
Eventually, the motivation is so high that the animal performs the behaviour
in the absence of any eliciting stimuli. If this scheme were true, it would have
major implications for the housing of animals, especially for the necessity of
allowing them to perform various behaviour patterns. Using Lorenz's motivational concepts, early critics of intensive animal husbandry took the occurrence
of vacuum behaviour by farm animals as evidence that performance of
behaviour itself might be necessary to reduce the underlying motivation.

In fact, the Lorenzian model of motivation had been attacked many times,
mainly on the postulated source of nervous energy. Recently, however,
Lorenz's ideas have been sympathetically re-evaluated. Toates (1986) and
Toates and Jensen (1990) argue that it is possible to dismiss the dubious
'nervous energy' mechanism while accepting that certain parts of Lorenz's
model do correspond with some aspects of animal behaviour. Two pieces of
evidence might be valuable in indicating a behavioural need. These are: (i) that
the motivation to perform a behaviour increases with the time since its last
performance and animals will begin to perform the behaviour when the level
of motivation reaches a sufficient intensity; and (ii) that it is the performance
of the behaviour itself, rather than the functional consequences, that reduces
the motivation.

To decide how much behavioural deprivation reduces an animal's welfare
it is necessary to determine whether the animal is highly motivated during the
period of deprivation. The most common method for assessing the level of
motivation during deprivation has been to observe how animals behave after a
period of deprivation. In many cases, preventing an animal from performing a
behaviour will cause it to perform the behaviour with increased intensity once
they have the opportunity – the 'rebound effect'. Such a rebound is often interpreted as evidence of internal motivation that continues to increase while the

animal is unable to perform the necessary behaviour. However, McFarland (1989) suggested an alternative explanation. When a stimulus is constantly present, or is repeatedly presented, the animals may habituate to it and not notice its subsequent absence. However, when the stimulus is removed for a long period of time, the animals will lose this habituation; a process known as 'dishabituation'. On re-presentation of the stimulus, they may show an exaggerated behavioural response because of reduced habituation to the external stimulus. In this case there would be no suffering during deprivation as there would have been no increase in motivation during the period of deprivation itself.

7.2.4. Motivation and welfare

The model of motivation proposed by Lorenz and that favoured by Baxter would seem at odds, but we should avoid thinking of these schemes as alternatives. It is likely that both motivation to perform behaviour and motivation to obtain certain consequences may be operating in different motivational systems or even to varying degrees within the same system. We should also avoid the temptation to think of all motivational systems as similar.

In an influential paper, Hughes and Duncan (1988) defended the notion of 'behavioural need' arguing that the problem of behavioural deprivation was a central issue for animal welfare, and that the concept should not be rejected simply because it was framed in terms of an inadequate model of motivation. They cited the classic work of Breland and Breland (1961) as further evidence that under modern conditions of domestication, animals show a tendency to perform appetitive behaviour patterns when they are no longer necessary for the completion of the consummatory act. Pigs were trained to pick up large wooden tokens and deposit them in a 'bank' several metres away in order to obtain a food reward:

> The pigs became conditioned rapidly but after a few weeks became progressively slower as they spent more and more time dropping the tokens and rooting them. Increasing the food deprivation made the problem worse. This could be interpreted as evidence of a rooting 'need' in pigs, with rooting behaviour becoming fixed to that stimulus, the token, which is most closely associated with the appetitive behaviour. Breland and Breland (1961) described trying to condition raccoons, *Procyon lotor*, to place 'coins' in a 'bank' and how they spent so much time rubbing and 'washing' the coins that the operant response was almost completely blocked. This rubbing and washing response appears to be a normal part of the appetitive phase of feeding behaviour. The findings suggest that these animals had a marked tendency to perform different appetitive elements of feeding behaviour, and that the more strongly the primary behaviour was motivated, the more obvious and fixated these secondary and fragmented behaviour patterns became.
>
> (Hughes and Duncan, 1988, p. 1698)

In trying to reconcile Baxter's model with Lorenzian processes, and to produce a more complex model of motivation, Hughes and Duncan (1988, p. 1703–1704) presented a schematic model (illustrated in Fig. 7.1):

> in which the functional consequences have a negative feedback effect, acting both on the motivation and through the animal's perception of external stimuli.

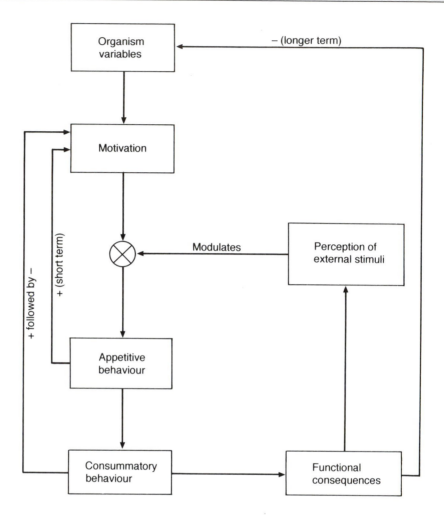

Fig. 7.1. Model of motivation presented by Hughes and Duncan (1988).

In the Hughes/Duncan model . . . the behaviour itself can have a positive feedback effect on motivation. There is evidence that this happens during feeding behaviour with hunger increasing during the early stages of the meal and only decreasing later . . .

The existence of a positive feedback loop such as this between behaviour and motivation also has the great advantage of helping to explain many of Breland and Breland's (1961) findings . . . In our model, motivation is eventually switched off by the functional consequences acting through organism variables (such as physiological changes) . . . Thus, an animal performing behaviour that does not have the appropriate functional consequences, or that does not have them soon enough, may get into a closed loop from which it cannot escape. Inappropriate behaviour, such as feather pecking in fowls, bar biting in pigs, navel sucking in calves and weaving in horses, *Equus caballus*, is thus repetitive, stereotyped and persistent, because it has become divorced from its functional consequences . . .

For any behaviour pattern which is largely governed by internal factors, motivation levels will sooner or later increase above threshold. This will trigger appetitive behaviour, but in some intensive environments it will be impossible to proceed to the consummatory sequence. The appetitive behaviour will continue, sometimes in an abbreviated or incomplete form, and this will have the effect of raising motivation further. Welfare considerations will arise in situations where motivation reaches high levels but the consummatory behaviour cannot be performed, and may also arise when the interaction of the appetitive behaviour with the environment does not provide the appropriate functional consequences . . .

Such a conclusion does of course challenge Baxter's (1983) view, that 'the performance of normal behaviour is not itself a requirement' for welfare. We believe that in certain cases it may be.

7.3. Examples of Motivational Analysis

In the previous section we have dealt with some of the more general issues involved in behavioural deprivation. Now we consider some specific instances.

7.3.1. Dust-bathing in poultry

Dust-bathing behaviour is frequently carried out by gallinaceous birds and, when carried out on an appropriate substrate, the well-defined series of behavioural patterns results in substrate particles being incorporated into the feathers and held in close contact with the body. However, in most modern housing conditions, domestic hens are prevented from performing this behaviour. Do the birds suffer as a result of this deprivation?

A number of studies of this behaviour pattern have led workers to hypothesize that this is a behaviour that is strongly internally motivated and, thus, fulfils one of the conditions of behavioural needs. Under normal light/dark cycles, both quail and fowl show a pattern of dust-bathing consistent with the behaviour being controlled at least partially by an endogenous circadian rhythm (Statkiewicz and Schein, 1980; Vestergaard, 1982; Hogan *et al.*, 1991). Furthermore, studies investigating the effects of dust deprivation (Vestergaard, 1982; Hogan *et al.*, 1991) have found increased dust-bathing activity when dust is returned, suggesting some rebound. Hogan *et al.* (1991) found that these deprivation effects appeared as soon as dust-bathing developed in chicks' behavioural repertoire and that the effects did not change over a 4-week period. These authors interpreted their results in terms of a Lorenzian hydraulic model (Lorenz, 1981), with a build-up of an internal factor in the absence of dust-bathing and a subsequent reduction of the factor by the act of dust-bathing itself.

In 1993 Hogan and van Boxel modified the model to incorporate a recovery process and a gating mechanism, along the lines suggested by Daan *et al.* (1984) to explain the timing of human sleep. The gating process of the model of Daan *et al.* (1984) determines thresholds for sleep and waking which vary according to a circadian rhythm, whilst the recovery process causes a regulating variable to decrease during sleep and increase while awake. In simple

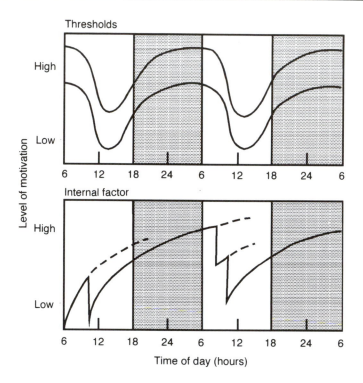

Fig. 7.2. A motivational model for dust-bathing. The internal factor for dust-bathing is assumed to increase in a negative exponential manner as a function of time, and to decrease during dust-bathing. Dust-bathing can occur when the level of the internal factor reaches the upper threshold and is inhibited when the level drops to the lower threshold. The threshold levels vary according to the time of day (circadian factor). External stimuli such as the light/heat stimulus or various types of dust are assumed to change threshold values and not the internal factor itself (Hogan and van Boxel, 1993).

terms the recovery process is responsible for the degree of sleepiness and a person is more likely to go to sleep in the evening, when the threshold for sleep to occur is lower, than during the day, when the threshold is higher. In a similar way waking is determined by a threshold which varies in parallel to the sleeping one. Thus, the final model for dust-bathing, proposed by Hogan and van Boxel (1993), is a Lorenzian process gated by a circadian pacemaker (Fig. 7.2).

Such a model explains the effects on dust-bathing of a light/heat stimulus which does not change the total amount of dust-bathing but changes the time when the dust-bathing occurs (Hogan and van Boxel, 1993). Thus, presentation of the heat/light does not change the level of the internal motivation, but rather results in an immediate lowering of the threshold. Removal of the heat/light stimulus results in an immediate raising of the threshold.

Consistent with the Lorenzian model, the authors interpreted the increased dust-bathing after the period of deprivation as resulting from an accumulation of motivation during the deprivation period, and hence as potentially indicative of suffering. However, it is possible that dishabituation was responsible for the apparent rebound.

To decide between these alternative explanations, Nicol and Guilford (1991) proposed that exploratory behaviour may provide the key to determining whether motivation rises during a period of deprivation, before external stimuli are re-presented. The advantage of using this technique is that it is not necessary to present the stimulus in order to observe a behavioural response.

For their tests Nicol and Guilford deprived hens of food and litter and measured their use of a circular tunnel attached to the test pen. Hens deprived of food for 3 hours spent significantly more time in the tunnel than non-deprived birds, although no food was provided in either the tunnel or the test pen. To test motivation during litter deprivation, Nicol and Guilford kept hens either on wire or on peat for 6 weeks prior to testing. During the test, half of each of these groups of birds were given peat in the pen ('Control'), while the other half were not ('Experimental'). They found that the deprived Experimental birds spent significantly more time in the tunnel than the non-deprived Experimental birds.

Nicol and Guilford pointed out that although their study had indicated an increase in motivation to obtain litter during deprivation, their results do not show which internal causal factors are responsible for the change in motivational state because hens use litter in a variety of ways (e.g. for dust-bathing, nesting and foraging). Identification of the precise internal cause of the behaviour may come when the physiological basis has been identified, and it is to this that we now turn.

7.3.2. The physiological basis of nest-building in poultry

For animal welfare, understanding the causal basis of nesting behaviour by hens is particularly important. In modern battery cages, hens are not provided with any special place for laying their eggs even though it is clear that hens are highly selective in terms of where they lay. Because of this, it has been claimed that the frustration of natural nesting motivation is one of the main behavioural problems for hens in battery cages, and that the welfare of the hens is compromised as a result (Appleby et al., 1992). Consequently it is important to understand the motivation of this behaviour and how much it is controlled by internal factors that are likely to be present in all environments. The classic work of David Wood-Gush into the physiology of pre-laying behaviour of domestic hens is one of the earliest and still one of the best studies of the physiological basis of behaviour in farm animals.

Shortly before laying an egg, hens engage in a typical sequence of behaviours, the end result of which is the construction of a suitable nest. Appleby et al. (1992) describe three phases of this nesting behaviour. The first phase is essentially a searching phase with the hen seeking possible nest sites. In battery cages, this often takes the form of a restless pacing around the cage. The stereotyped and repetitive nature of this behaviour strengthens the impression that the hen is frustrated at this point. The second phase consists of the choice of a suitable nest site from the alternatives available. In this phase the hen examines closely the alternative sites. Once a suitable site has been chosen, the hen then constructs a hollow, by manipulating the substrate with beak and feet, and sits on the nest in preparation for laying. Interestingly, providing the hen with a preformed nest does not prevent these behaviours occurring (Hughes *et al.*, 1989), suggesting that it may be triggered by internal factors. In his experiments, Wood-Gush (1963) provided hens with a trap nest and based the measures of nesting behaviour on the second phase, that is, the time taken to inspect the nest, and the entry of the hen into the trap-nest.

Nesting behaviour usually starts 1–2 hours before oviposition. The close association in time between the occurrence of nesting behaviour and the laying of the egg initially suggested a direct causal link: nesting behaviour seemed to be initiated by the presence of a mature egg in the oviduct. However, in a series of well-designed experiments, Wood-Gush (1963) eliminated this possibility. First, observations showed that hens which laid soft-shelled eggs prematurely engaged in nesting behaviour at the time expected had they had a hard-shelled egg, despite the absence of an egg in the oviduct. In fact, even complete removal of the oviduct did not prevent normal nesting occurring at the time expected, clearly showing that stimulation from the oviduct is not necessary to initiate nesting behaviour. However, some of Wood-Gush's results suggest that the act of laying the egg may play a role in terminating nesting behaviour: removal of the oviduct, with the result that no egg was laid, resulted in a considerably increased time spent on the nest. This illustrates an important point: the factors that initiate a sequence of behaviours or motivational system may be very different from those that terminate it.

These results also show how the factors that control the motivational system underlying a behaviour may be quite different from the factors that underlie the functional basis of the behaviour. The functional goal of nest building is clearly to provide a suitable environment for the eggs. However, it is clear from the above experiments that nesting behaviour will occur whether or not the hen actually lays an egg.

If stimulation from an egg in the oviduct does not initiate nesting, why are nesting behaviour and egg laying so closely associated in time? It seems that events during ovulation which initiate egg formation also control the onset of nesting behaviour. Ovulation occurs about 24 hours before egg laying and involves a well-known series of endocrine changes, notably the release of oestrogens and progesterone from the follicle after ovulation. First, Wood-Gush and Gilbert (1964) demonstrated the importance of an intact ovarian follicle for nesting behaviour. The follicles of hens were removed surgically and this largely prevented nesting behaviour from occurring, even though the hens successfully laid eggs. Wood-Gush and Gilbert (1973) then showed that injection of oestradiol and progesterone stimulated hens to inspect nests and to enter a nest (Fig. 7.3). However, this behavioural effect did not immediately follow injection but rather occurred 24 hours later, which is the normal period from ovulation to the beginning of nesting.

Although the main emphasis of the study was on documenting the role of progesterone, the amount of nest examination seen when the hens received just oestrogen was much higher than that by normal hens on non-laying days.

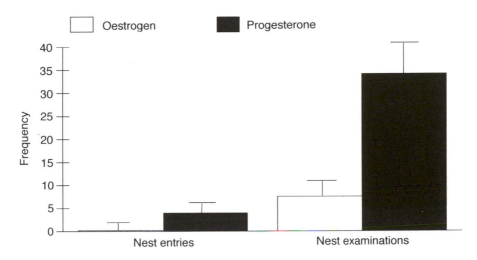

Fig. 7.3. Mean (± se) frequency of nest entries and nest examinations by hens injected either with oestrogen alone (open bars) or with a mixture of oestrogen and progesterone (filled bars). The figure is drawn from Table 1 of Wood-Gush and Gilbert (1973).

This suggested that oestrogen alone may also play a role in initiating some components of nesting behaviour. This was not the case for nest entry which rarely occurred when the birds were given oestrogen alone. This again suggests that the different components of nesting behaviour may have different causal bases, and shows the mistake in talking of 'nesting motivation' as a unitary motivational state.

Together these results suggest that pre-laying nesting motivation is initiated by internal factors, specifically the release of progesterone from the follicle, and is likely to be present regardless of the environment in which the bird is housed.

7.4. Assessing the Impact on Animal Welfare

The question remains: even if we have determined that the performance of a behaviour is motivated by 'internal' factors, how can we know whether deprivation of that behaviour will reduce the welfare of the animals? We will consider three possible methods to answer this question: measurement of the 'demand' for the behaviour, assessment of the physiological consequences of behavioural deprivation, and observations of abnormal behaviour that may occur as a result of deprivation.

7.4.1. Behavioural demand

Dawkins (1983a) introduced the application of this methodology, developed by economists, to assess the importance that an animal attaches to the performance of particular behaviours. When people have less to spend, their purchasing priorities may change. If they stop buying something when the price increases, their demand for that commodity is said to be 'elastic'. But if they consider that something is so important that they continue to buy it, although it may mean going without other things, the demand is said to be 'inelastic'. Demand elasticity can be quantified by measuring the slope of the function relating quantity purchased to price (Lea, 1978). This function is typically of the form $Y=aX+b$, where Y is the log of the quantity and X is the log of the price. The absolute value of the typically negative slope, a, is the elasticity coefficient and b is a constant. Curves with a small elasticity coefficient are described as inelastic while those with a larger coefficient, for example approaching or greater than 1.0, are elastic.

Lea (1978) proposed that an analogue for price, in behavioural terms, is the amount of effort required to obtain a particular commodity or stimulus, and the quantity of the commodity obtained is the equivalent of the amount purchased. In Dawkins' words (1983a, p. 1199):

> Here is the key to discovering which of the proximate needs an animal might possess are sufficiently strong to be likely to give rise to suffering if unsatisfied. Necessities showing inelastic demand . . . will be those commodities which the animal has the strongest proximate needs for. Luxuries showing elastic demand . . . would have some levels of causal factors present (some level of proximate need) but lower than those of necessities. The resilience associated with any given behaviour could be measured either by manipulating a variable which affected most or all of the behaviours in its repertoire, such as cutting time or energy budgets or restricting the total number of key pecks an animal was allowed to make. Or it could be measured by manipulating a variable which affected only one behaviour, such as the handling time of one food item or the number of pecks required for one type of commodity but not others . . . The economic approach is thus a way of ranking proximate needs into those which are important and those which are less important to the animal. If we can agree that denial of some proximate needs (e.g. hunger) denote suffering, then the animal's own ranking system will enable us to characterize the other into necessities (as much, if not more suffering) and luxuries (less suffering or none at all).

One way of measuring the amount of effort is to require an animal to perform an operant response, such as pressing a lever, to obtain the commodity and then increase the number of required operant responses for each access to the item. Matthews and Ladewig (1994) carried out a study which required pigs to lever-press in order to gain access to three different commodities: food, social contact with another pig and a door being opened. As a way of systematically varying the amount of effort required to access the commodities they used a fixed ratio (FR) schedule of reinforcement, where the commodities were presented after a specified number of presses. Figure 7.4 illustrates their findings.

It can be seen that for all animals the amount of food consumed remained approximately constant as the FR value increased. As stated before, the average absolute values of the slopes of the regression lines is a measure of the elasticity of demand and this was 0.02 for food. For contact with another pig, the number of times access was attained declined steadily as the FR values

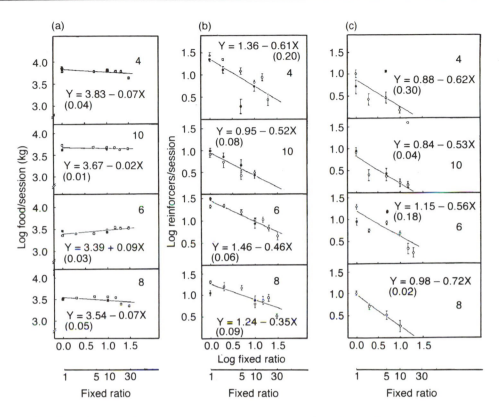

Fig. 7.4. The numbers or amounts of reinforcers obtained by individual pigs (numbers 4, 10, 6 and 8) as a function of the Fixed Ratio (FR) of lever presses required to obtain reinforcement. The reinforcers were (a) food, (b) social contact and (c) door opening. The best-fit straight lines, their equations and the standard errors of the slopes (in parentheses) are also shown. Open circles are data from ascending FR schedules and closed circles are data from descending FR schedules (Matthews and Ladewig, 1994).

increased. The average elasticity of demand was 0.49. The numbers of door openings declined rapidly and systematically with increases in the FR value, with the average elasticity of demand being 0.63. In the words of the authors (p. 717):

> The elasticity coefficients for food were close to zero and similar to those observed with other animals . . . This provides additional support for the notion that items essential for survival have small elasticity coefficients. The coefficient for food was smaller than that for the remaining items and close to the theoretical minimum value (zero) supporting the suggestion that food is the obvious standard against which other items should be rated (Dawkins 1983a).
>
> A rank ordering of the items (from most to least essential) using the elasticity measures gives a sequence of food, contact and door opening. This ordering also makes intuitive sense since food would seem more important than a simple stimulus change such as door opening.

7.4.2. Physiological consequences of behavioural deprivation

A second approach to assess the effect on welfare is to see if deprivation of a particular behaviour has an impact on the physiology of the animal, particularly if behavioural deprivation induces physiological changes that reduce the animal's health or biological functioning (Moberg, 1985a). De Passillé *et al.* (1993) took this approach in examining the motivation of non-nutritive sucking in calves and the effect of sucking deprivation on calves' welfare. They examined whether or not performance of sucking behaviour by calves during milk ingestion influenced the physiological processes involved in digestion.

In order to determine whether non-nutritive sucking by calves after drinking milk affected the secretion of digestive hormones, de Passillé *et al.* (1993) examined the postprandial secretion of insulin and cholecystokinin (CCK) when the calves either could or could not suck an artificial teat. The postprandial increase in both CCK and insulin have been implicated in satiety. The results showed the normal rise in both insulin (Fig. 7.5) and CCK after feeding. However, for both hormones, the postprandial rise was larger when the calves were able to suck the teat after the meal. These results clearly show that the performance of a behaviour associated with feeding can directly influence digestive processes even if the consumption of food is not altered. The authors concluded (p. 1072):

> The results may have broad implications for the welfare and housing of the animals. The widespread metabolic effects of insulin and CCK . . . mean that deprivation of sucking behaviour cannot be assumed to be inconsequential for animal well-being and growth even if this does not affect nutrient intake. Nonnutritive sucking by human infants has been found to lead to increased

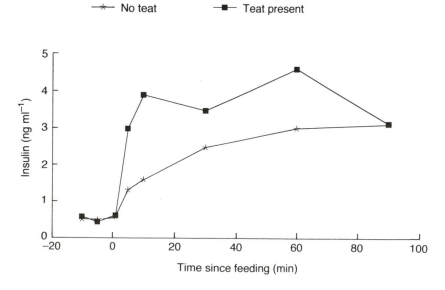

Fig. 7.5. Mean insulin concentrations in hepatic portal vein of young calves after drinking milk. The calves either could or could not suck a non-functional rubber teat after drinking their milk. The figure is based on data in de Passillé *et al.* (1993).

growth . . . An altered pattern of hormone secretion could explain the improved digestion of milk when calves can suck milk from a nipple rather than from a bucket . . . An association between object sucking and secretion of insulin and CCK (and, hence, with increased satiety) may explain the highly persistent nature of this behavior.

7.4.3. Stereotypies

Stereotypies are generally defined as unvarying, repetitive behaviour patterns that have no obvious goal or function (Fox, 1965; Ödberg, 1978). These behaviours have had a high profile in recent years because they are often described as 'abnormal' and thought by many to indicate welfare problems for the animal displaying them (Lawrence and Rushen, 1993). Indeed, stereotypies are most often observed where animals are confined and there are constraints on their ability to perform certain behavioural patterns (Mason, 1991b). This has led to the proposal that stereotypies result from the frustration of specific motivational systems (Rushen et al., 1993a). If this is indeed the case then it indicates that an animal is still motivated to perform the behaviour, that is, there is evidence for behavioural deprivation.

As an example, Keiper (1969) investigated the stereotypies of 'route-tracing' and 'spot-picking' in caged canaries. The birds were housed in cages/aviaries of different sizes, with or without a swinging perch, and either provided with seed which was freely available from dishes or required to 'work' to extract the seed from different devices.

Changes to the cage size and method of feeding had differential effects on the two types of stereotypies. Route-tracing appeared to be a response to restrictions on movement imposed by space allowance because it was consistently less in the largest sized cage (Fig. 7.6). The presence of a perch appeared to disrupt route-tracing physically and thus resulted in a decrease in the occurrence of that stereotypy, but had little effect on spot-picking. In contrast, spot-picking was significantly reduced when birds were required to work for food, but there was no effect on route-tracing in this condition (Fig. 7.7). These results provide support for the hypothesis that stereotypies reflect specific motivation and, therefore, may provide evidence for specific behavioural restriction or deprivation.

So in the study by Keiper (1969), increasing the opportunity for foraging reduced stereotypies in canaries. This approach has also been tried with wild species held in captivity e.g. walruses (Kastelein and Wiepkema, 1989), primates (Lam et al., 1991) and bears (Carlstead et al., 1991).

7.5. Conclusions

- The question of behavioural restriction is one of the most difficult of the scientific issues in animal welfare.
- Farm animals in semi-natural environments have retained much of the behavioural repertoire of their wild ancestors (Jensen, 1986) but many of these 'natural behaviours' cannot occur in intensive systems.

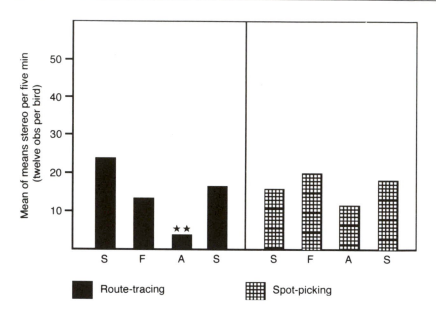

Fig. 7.6. The frequencies of stereotyping for canaries in the standard cage (S), the flight cage (F) and the aviary cage (A). The stars indicate a significant reduction ($P < 0.01$) in route-tracing in the aviary cage (Keiper, 1969).

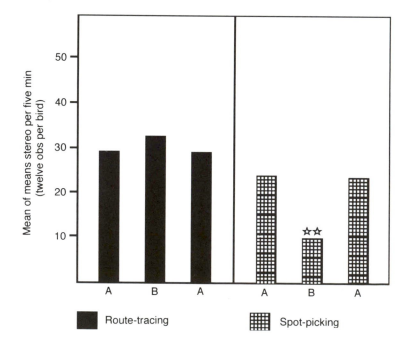

Fig. 7.7. The frequencies of stereotyping for canaries in the control condition (A) and when required to work for their food (B). The stars indicate significant differences ($P < 0.01$) between experimental and control conditions (Keiper, 1969).

- Behavioural restriction is more likely to impair welfare if: (i) the motivating factors result from internal changes in the animal rather than from the animals' environment; (ii) motivation remains high even if the animal cannot perform the behaviour; and (iii) if it is the performance of the behaviour which is necessary to reduce the motivation, rather than the achievement of the consequences of the behaviour.
- Behaviours which originate from internal changes in the animal include nest-building in poultry, which reflects the hormonal changes preceding egg laying. Dust-bathing in poultry, too, shows evidence of internal motivation, though the physiological basis of the motivation has yet to be determined.
- Behaviours the performance of which appears to be important to the animal have been called behavioural needs, but in most cases research has not yet determined which ones fall into this category.
- In a number of cases, achievement of the normal functional consequences, in the absence of the behaviour itself, is not sufficient to reduce the motivation. Providing preformed nests to poultry and pigs does not reduce nest-building, while giving calves sufficient milk does not reduce motivation to suck (Rushen and de Passillé, 1995).
- Evidence is less clear as to whether performance of behaviour is necessary to reduce the motivation, but failure to allow performance of sucking behaviour in calves can influence physiology, and prevention of other behaviour can lead to abnormal behaviour such as stereotypies.
- There is great diversity in motivational systems and it seems unlikely that general principles will be found. It is necessary to investigate the motivational systems underlying each separate behaviour to reach firm conclusions about the influence of behavioural restriction on animal welfare.

PART III
Assessment

Given that welfare is not a simple, unitary variable, it is not possible to *measure* it in the same way that mass or length or time can be measured. David Fraser (1995, p. 113) points out:

> that while science provides many ways to identify, solve and prevent animal welfare problems, science cannot 'measure' the overall welfare of animals because there is no single measure, nor any purely objective way of combining different measures, that eliminates value-related disagreements.

However, welfare can be *assessed* by considering its various aspects and problems relating to them, outlined previously. Part III covers the main approaches to such assessment.

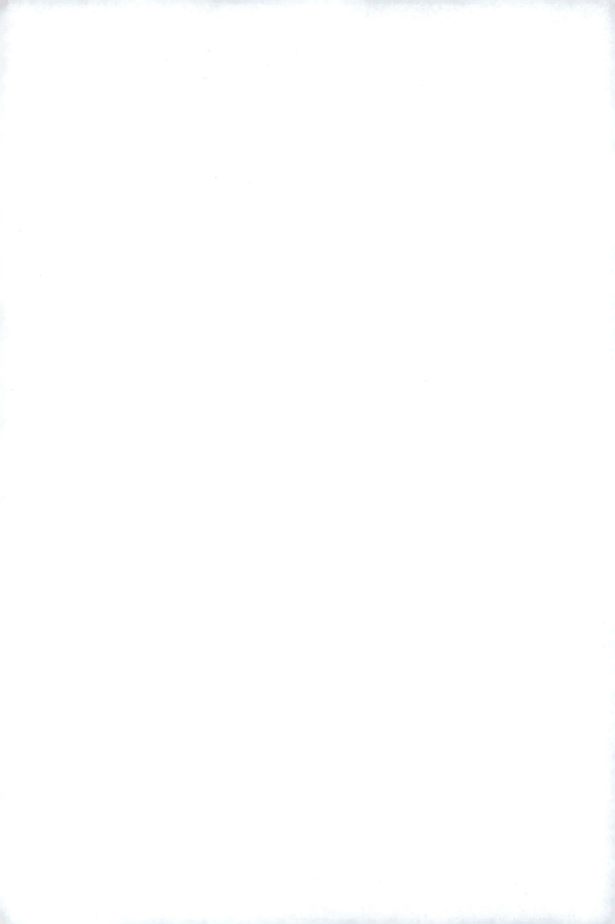

CHAPTER 8
Health and disease

Barry O. Hughes (Roslin Institute, UK) and Peter E. Curtis
(University of Liverpool, UK)

Abstract

Understanding relationships between health and welfare depends on drawing
inferences about subjective feelings such as pain, discomfort and distress.
Zoonotic diseases where symptoms, lesions, behavioural responses and outcomes are similar in humans and animals help to clarify the relationship between ill health and well-being. Quantifying suffering requires careful observation
and consideration of a broad range of indicators, including changes in physiology, behaviour and production. It is especially difficult when animals are in
large groups, or disturbed, or removed from their normal surroundings. In intensive situations suboptimal environmental conditions or increased metabolic
demands either have direct effects on health or can interact with infective
agents or nutritional factors. Stress can play an influential role, often through
its immunosuppressive effects. The resulting widespread, subclinical disorders
have a major adverse effect on welfare. Under extensive conditions climatic
changes, habitat degradation and overstocking can result in ill health through
malnutrition and excessive parasite burdens. The harmful consequences may
extend to free-living animals. The disorders which have the greatest impact in
depressing welfare are either those where an acute disease process causes
extreme suffering, such as contagious bovine pleuropneumonia, or long-term
progressive conditions involving severe chronic pain, such as lameness in dairy
cows, foot-rot in sheep or sheep scab. In many cases effective control, prevention or eradication is possible but hindered by inadequate training, by socio-
economic pressures or by market forces.

8.1. Introduction

The relationship between health and welfare is self-evident. Some people
regard them as almost synonymous: 'Animal welfare has been variously
defined but for practical purposes I find it useful to replace the term with the
words health and well-being' (Ewbank, 1987, p. 4). In suggesting that welfare
includes health, though health on its own does not necessarily imply welfare,
Ewbank was following the lead set by the Brambell Committee (1965, p. 11):

> A principal cause of suffering in animals, as it is in men (sic), is disease. Many
> veterinary witnesses have drawn our attention to this and to the necessity of
> taking it into account fully in assessing the welfare of animals. We have been

Animal Welfare (eds Michael C. Appleby and Barry O. Hughes)

impressed by this evidence and accept the major importance of the disease risk in evaluating the welfare of an animal under any system of husbandry.

Health, though, is more than the absence of disease. It is a positive state of 'soundness of body; that condition in which the functions are duly discharged' (Oxford English Dictionary, 1973, p. 938), where an organism is in a 'sound bodily and mental condition' (Chambers Dictionary, 1983, p. 577). Although veterinary students are taught a list of signs of health, some physical (activity, bright eyes, shiny coat, pricked ears, good appetite) and some mental (alertness, responsiveness, showing interest in its surroundings) it is not always an easy state to recognize. It lies at one end of a continuum, from health through subclinical disease and overt pathological change to death.

Disease influences welfare not only by its effect on the animal's body but also on its mind. Suffering is perceived centrally as pain and distress, and some have argued that all that matters is how the animal feels:

> Our thesis is that animal welfare is dependent solely on the mental, psychological and cognitive needs of the animals concerned. In general, if these mental needs are met, they will cover the physical needs . . . As long as the animal 'feels' all right then its welfare will be all right. Now, of course, usually when an animal *is* ill, it will also *feel* ill, so that taking care of its mental health (i.e. how it feels) will automatically take care of its physical health.

(Duncan and Petherick, 1991, pp. 5017–5018)

This last sentence neatly illustrates the gulf between ethological and veterinary thinking. Many veterinarians would have put it the other way round – that taking care of an animal's physical health will automatically take care of its mental health. A.F. Fraser (1989, p. 332) has pointed out that some veterinary authorities define animal welfare as: 'maintaining appropriate standards of accommodation, feeding and general care, the prevention and treatment of disease'. Fraser himself takes a more holistic view and draws a distinction between physical well-being (clinical health) and psychological well-being (normal behavioural expression). Others go further and, like Duncan and Petherick, recognize that the presence of disease does not necessarily imply poor welfare for the animal:

> Animals cannot consciously assess the implications of their disease states but their owners will do it on their behalf. Many bitches with advanced mammary tumours – and . . . as yet free from . . . secondary growths – can lead full, active and seemingly comfortable lives. Their owners, however, can be . . . distressed, understand the significance of the lesions and act accordingly, i.e. take advice, instigate treatment, request euthanasia.

(Ewbank, 1987, p. 5)

However, Duncan and Petherick's proposition, that we stop focusing on physical events and concentrate on mental ones, is impractical – at present virtually nothing is known about animals' subjective mental processes. Until much more is known about animals' cognitive states, inferences about health and welfare will continue to be drawn using appropriate pathological, physiological and behavioural signs. Nevertheless, we accept that welfare, for animals as well as humans, is as much a state of mind as a state of body, though in practice we have to use the latter to infer the former.

In this chapter we consider how welfare is assessed in terms of health and some of the ways in which it can be adversely affected through ill health: disease, parasitism, malnutrition, injury and genetically-induced disorders. The welfare implications of particular conditions will depend on the extent to which they result in suffering (pain, distress, severe discomfort). We concentrate on farm animals, about which more is known.

8.2. Effect of Disease States on Welfare

Much can be inferred about the impact of a particular disease on welfare by examining its nature, development, course and effect on behaviour. Although the relationship between illness and suffering is one with which clinicians grapple daily, remarkably little has been written on the topic.

Recognition of suffering is central to this question but, even in the case of pain, is far from straightforward:

> Clinical assessment of pain depends mainly upon visual inspection, however, pain may be present which cannot be detected in this way. Acutely painful processes in the limbs or spine are relatively easy to diagnose because they disrupt locomotion. Severity of pain can be assessed by measuring the intensity and frequency of such signs as locomotor activity and posture . . . Three categories of pain may be recognised but uncertainty may remain even after careful observation.
>
> Loeffler (1986, p. 49)

Clinicians emphasize the importance of assessing the behaviour of sick animals but are sometimes uncertain how to interpret what they see. Jackson (1987, pp. 42–44) writes:

> The assessment must mostly be immediate and thus useful measurements of physiological and biochemical stress such as blood cortisol levels cannot be used in the course of practice . . . Quiet observation of the undisturbed animal [is] particularly important in determining whether the animal appears to be in pain. There is some evidence that adult farm animals may experience less pain when suffering from certain conditions than do horses and small animals. The horse suffering from torsion of the bowel appears to experience severe pain, whilst the cow, ewe or sow with a similar problem appears to be less distressed. [Because of] the difficulty of assessing subjective feelings in animal patients . . . it may often be kindest to prescribe analgesia on the assumption that pain is being experienced.

Behaviour often correlates poorly with the apparent severity of the condition.

> Baby piglets may show loud vocal responses to mildly painful stimuli, but does this really indicate pain or is it . . . a defence mechanism against being crushed by the sow? Some animals appear unconcerned by major trauma. The cow with a fractured femur may lie quietly eating or cudding, showing no signs of distress until she attempts to rise. [In contrast] lower limb lameness, joint disease and inflammatory conditions adjacent to the diaphragm are amongst numerous conditions in which pain appears to be a regular feature.

Context can influence animals' reactions and behaviour and thus the conclusions which are drawn. For example, when a companion animal is examined by a veterinarian, it is important to decide whether or not its owner should be present, but the best strategy for each case has to be decided individually. Sometimes the owner's presence calms the animal, so that its responses are more 'normal', whereas in other cases the opposite is true (S. Corr; A.M. Nolan; unpublished).

Rarely is the welfare impact of specific disease conditions systematically considered but Curtis (1990) attempted to do this for poultry diseases. Some (for example, egg drop syndrome, infectious avian encephalomyelitis in adults or sudden death syndrome in broilers) were classified as having little adverse effect on welfare, some (fowl pox, mycoplasmosis, salmonellosis) had intermediate or variable effects while some could cause considerable suffering (Gumboro disease, pasturellosis, *E. coli* infections). This clinical assessment was based on the duration of the condition, the nature of the lesions and the degree of apparent pain or distress evinced by the birds.

8.3. Environment, Disease and Welfare

In agriculture, the advent of intensive production, with its use of controlled environments, antibiotics and effective vaccines, was an unparalleled opportunity to improve welfare by bringing infectious diseases under control. In practice, however, one set of disease risks was exchanged for another.

> The environment of modern housing systems has a major influence on animal welfare and health. Although many classical diseases are controlled today, there remain a variety of environmental disorders which can cause considerable losses in performance and lives. Most of these problems occur in pig, poultry and calf production and include disorders of the digestive and respiratory tracts, cardiovascular system as well as the skin and skeleton. In milking cows, mastitis and lameness are typical disorders influenced by the environment . . . One survey showed that 20% of all suckling pigs and 48% of all weaners died of viral gastroenteritis or coli enterotoxaemia, 21% of store pigs suffered from pneumonia and 34% of fattening pig losses were due to cardiovascular failure . . . Not all diseased pigs show clinical signs that can be detected in the confined conditions of some livestock systems. Often subclinical disease is only apparent at slaughter.

(Hartung, 1994, p. 25).

To illustrate his point Hartung cited an epidemiological survey by Elbers, which showed (Table 8.1) that at slaughter only 29% of finishing pigs were disease-free. The others showed a variety of pathological lesions post-mortem and all had reduced weight gains compared with the disease-free group. These pigs were suffering from ill health of sufficient severity to impair growth. The implications are serious: they suggest that the welfare of the majority of intensively-reared pigs is at risk.

The aetiology of low-grade disease conditions such as these is complex; there is rarely a single cause and their control is correspondingly difficult.

Table 8.1. Proportion of pigs at slaughter showing subclinical lesions and growth rates (relative to 100 for disease-free). Data are from 155 herds with a population of 101,306 (A.R.W. Elbers, cited by Hartung, 1994).

Condition	Percentage	Growth rate
Disease-free	28.6	100
Pneumonia	31.8	94
Pleuritis	18.6	94
Other respiratory conditions	9.3	95
Leg inflammation	3.9	94
Tail inflammation	2.0	94
Liver lesions	1.8	96
Skin lesions	1.7	93
Arthritis	1.4	90

Environmentally evoked diseases are caused by a combination of factors. In a discussion of the aetiology of clinically manifested pig herd diseases . . . Ekesbo lists the following factors which contribute to subclinical disease and interact in the production of clinical disease states: Large herd or group size; Slatted floor in pen; Rough concrete floor surfaces; Unsuitable pen devices, Sow kept confined; No straw; Infection.

(Broom 1987, p. 23)

Ekesbo (1981, p. 254) himself considered that the increased incidence of many diseases in intensive systems was attributable to 'distress factors'. He concluded that the health of pigs was at risk:

when their normal behaviour patterns of feeding, dunging and bedding in separate areas was prevented, when their environment became more barren, with a risk of understimulation, and when they were exposed to overstimulation, for example, through constant noise.

Whereas free-living animals occupy a variable world and can usually select an appropriate microclimate, in controlled environments humidity, air movement and temperature are relatively fixed and animals must tolerate whatever the producer provides. Webster (1994) has classified farm animals as Group I (pigs and poultry) with limited ability to regulate body temperature, and Group II (cattle, sheep, horses) which can regulate it effectively.

The zone of thermal comfort can be described as the thermal state which the animal will select for itself . . . This is undoubtedly narrower than the thermoneutral zone . . . For Group II species most environments within the thermoneutral zone may be considered acceptable on welfare grounds. [However] the recommended temperatures in intensive pig and poultry houses constitute the upper limit of the zone of thermal comfort. It is an interesting paradox that the species most susceptible to heat stress (pigs and poultry) . . . are confined in houses designed to maintain temperature well above ambient by a combination of high stocking density, high insulation and restricted ventilation. As temperature rises above 20°C it becomes at first difficult and then impossible to prevent intolerable heat stress simply by increasing ventilation. Some houses for (especially) broilers are potentially lethal in conditions that may reasonably be expected during a normal English summer.

(Webster 1994, p. 52).

The environmental stresses caused by inimical microclimates, which as well as unsuitable temperatures include dust, ammonia and other noxious gases, are probable factors in the high levels of subclinical disease in intensively housed animals.

8.4. Stress and Disease

The adverse effects on health and welfare of poor environments can be exerted directly or indirectly. Direct effects include inadequate ventilation resulting in airborne infections, slippery floors causing falls and traumatic injuries, and overstocking on a restricted area of pasture resulting in excessive parasitic worm burdens. Indirect effects are subtler, longer term, cumulative, interactive, and are exerted through intervening variables as 'stress'.

Some authorities have explored the reciprocal relationships between stress, welfare and disease. Broom (1987, pp. 22, 23) argues:

> that if the welfare of an animal is poor, the chances that it will be susceptible to disease are often increased . . . The incidence of disease might often be reduced by improving welfare and an inadequate response to disease challenge might imply that welfare is poor.

He draws attention to individual variation and points out that 'when a number of animals live in apparently similar conditions only one or two show signs of disease, or most show disease but only one or two die'. He cites evidence to support the proposition that disease causation is multifactorial.

These multifactorial influences may act through stress mechanisms which inhibit the immune system.

> Animals encountering difficult conditions often show some degree of immunosuppression . . . In all species susceptibility to disease can be increased by biological disturbances . . . Conventionally-housed mice, carrying the Bitner strain of oncogenic virus, developed more tumours than mice housed in cages in which noise, draughts and pheromones from other cages were minimised . . . Rats transferred to individual cages after being kept in groups were compared with rats kept individually since weaning. After dosing with a carcinogen or with adenocarcinoma cells, rats transferred from groups to isolated conditions had greater tumour weights. Such studies would be ethically unacceptable to most people but show that the environment affects the ability of an individual to resist tumour formation.

(Broom and Johnson, 1993, pp. 121,122)

Corticosteroid hormones play a key role. Animals with increased circulating corticosteroids have impaired immune responses: pigs' ability to produce antibodies

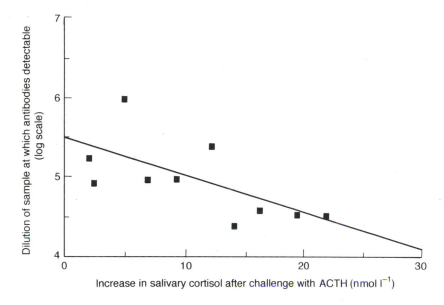

Fig. 8.1. Immune function may be depressed when adrenal cortical activity is high. The antibody level (against tetanus) in sows' colostrum tends to decline with increased cortisol output following ACTH challenge. (From Broom and Johnson, 1993.)

against tetanus declines as salivary cortisol increases (Fig. 8.1). The consequences are clearly seen in Gross and Siegel's classic studies of social stress in chickens:

> When birds which were strangers were put together they displayed, fought and had increased adrenal cortex activity. After such social mixing had occurred, challenge with *Mycoplasma gallisepticum*, Newcastle disease, Marek's disease or haemorrhagic enteritis resulted in greater pathogen levels in the body, greater morbidity and greater mortality than in chickens which were not mixed with strangers . . . Social mixing reduced antibody activity against both viral . . . and particulate antigens. This immunosuppression was probably mediated via increased corticosterone levels and reduced interleukin II production by T cells.
>
> (Broom and Johnson, 1993, p. 127)

The action of stress in promoting disease is, however, not unidirectional. A number of pathological conditions can themselves be potentiators of stress, as Michell (1987, p. 14) has explained:

> Biochemical changes are not only a result of stress but a neglected cause of it in clinical conditions. Disturbances of plasma sodium, calcium, magnesium glucose and pH as well as acetonaemia and the more complicated alterations caused by uraemia or hepatic failure can all cause symptoms which are likely to be stressful. Hypomagnesaemia, often unsuspected, has come under intense scrutiny as a factor aggravating the adverse effects of stress in man and animals. The relationship between stress and disease is thus a sinister commensalism.

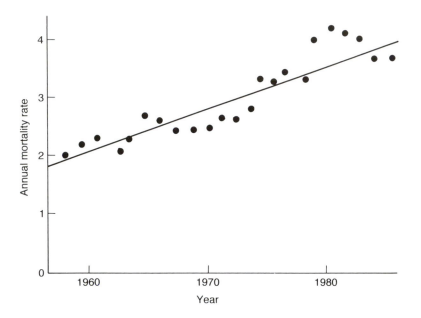

Fig. 8.2. The mortality rate in Danish dairy cows has tended to increase between 1959 and 1983 (From Broom and Johnson, 1993). The values on the *y*-axis represent the number of cows dying on farms each year, expressed in terms of an arbitrary index of mortality.

One disturbing effect of chronic stress is its effect on life expectancy. Broom and Johnson (1993, p. 113), cite a survey of dairy cattle by J.F. Agger:

> Many farmers have reported that the average age to which their dairy cows lived during the 1980s and 1990s was less than that of cows in earlier years. They link this with the higher production rate of modern cows. If a cow exhibits high feed conversion and a high metabolic rate, as a consequence of a high protein diet and selection for such efficiency over many generations, longevity may be reduced. Evidence for such a change in modern cows is indicated by the number of cows in Denmark being sent to rendering plants, which normally occurs after they have died on the farm. Such data [suggest] that the life expectancy of dairy cows was halved between 1960 and 1982 (Fig. 8.2).

Although Broom and Johnson are correct in drawing attention to the increased mortality rate, with its implication that modern cows suffer poorer health, the data do not show that life expectancy has halved. Most cows do not die on farms – their life expectancy is determined not by mortality on the farm but by the age at which the farmer decides they are insufficiently productive and sends them to slaughter. This age, an index of 'burn-out', may also have declined.

8.5. Specific Pathological Conditions as Case-Studies of Suffering

Distinctions can be drawn in welfare terms between disease conditions, depending on how much distress they cause. Some, such as contagious bovine pleuropneumonia, cause extreme suffering. Some, such as lameness or sheep scab, cause long-term suffering through chronic pain or intense irritation. Some, such as the adenovirus disease EDS (egg drop syndrome) 76 of poultry, impair health and production and have a major economic impact, but hardly affect welfare (Curtis, 1990). Zoonoses, especially those which produce analogous lesions, symptoms and outcomes in animals and humans, offer a valuable model for judging the impact of pathological change on welfare (Murray *et al.*, 1995).

8.5.1. Contagious bovine pleuropneumonia (CBPP)

CBPP, an acute septicaemia of cattle caused by *Mycoplasma mycoides*, was a worldwide scourge in the nineteenth century and is still a problem in developing countries.

> There is sudden onset of high fever, fall in milk yield, anorexia and rumination ceases. There is severe depression and animals stand apart or lag behind a travelling group. Coughing, at first only on exercise, and chest pain are evident, affected animals being disinclined to move . . . Respirations are shallow, rapid and accompanied by expiratory grunting. Pain is evidenced on percussion of the chest.
>
> (Radostits *et al.* 1994, p. 911)

Comparable experience of serious respiratory disease by humans suggests by analogy that cattle, which eventually die of anoxia, experience severe distress. Morbidity is up to 90% and mortality can exceed 50%. Survivors suffer marked lung damage and may continue to show symptoms. CBPP causes immense suffering, whether the animals live or die. Vaccination is possible, but eradication by compulsory slaughter is more secure.

8.5.2. Lameness in cattle

This is probably the most important welfare problem in intensively kept dairy cattle. There are two major types, bacterial and metabolic (Peterse, 1986). The former, generally caused by *Bacterioides* spp, is secondary to excessive or abnormal claw loading. The latter is seen as laminitis, where the predisposing factors include nutrition, stress, parturition and flooring, though the initiating event is the absorption of toxic fermentation products from the gut. The adverse effects are readily apparent:

> The welfare implications of lameness in dairy cattle are considerable and in addition to causing great pain and discomfort to the animals it is detrimental to productivity . . . Lame cows entered the parlour later than normal cows and were more restless on their feet. At pasture lame cows lay down for longer and grazed for shorter periods. Lame cows had lower bite rates than normal cows.

> The behavioural differences . . . indicated that lameness had serious effects on
> welfare and productivity.
>
> (Hassall *et al.*, 1993, p. 578)

This condition illustrates the complexity of the aetiological, ethical and practical issues underlying health, welfare and intensive agriculture. It is widely prevalent, chronic, apparently extremely painful causing widespread suffering, and yet almost totally preventable. Causation is multifactorial (Peterse, 1986; Brochart, 1986; Clarkson *et al.*, 1993) and includes the flooring surface (type, design, frictional coefficient), the diet (composition, especially protein and energy content), the feeding system, social factors (group size, density, nature of hierarchy), husbandry (inspection, foot trimming, disinfection régimen, dung disposal) and the arrangement and maintenance of the housing system (cubicles, bedding, self-feeding area, passages, standing areas, presence of standing liquid). If all these risk factors were set at values known to be associated with sound, healthy feet, then the incidence of lameness could be near zero.

In the UK lameness in cows was recognized in 1988 as a welfare rather than a disease problem when the Ministry of Agriculture, Fisheries and Food commissioned a major investigation with 'welfare an important consideration in funding this research', which should include 'the production of control packages' (Clarkson *et al.*, 1993, p. 2).

The problem arises because the economic pressures required to minimize costs result in the adoption of diets, systems, stocking densities and low labour input which result in high risk factor values. The relationship is self-limiting; if the system overall is too intensive then the incidence and severity of lameness will be so high that it begins to depress milk output and thus raises unit milk cost. Potter and Broom (1986, p. 131) focused on the economic benefits of controlling lameness:

> The cost of treatment of these disorders, as well as production losses, could
> more than compensate for any minor saving which might result from crowded or
> otherwise inadequate housing conditions. If the real costs of these losses were
> known, it might be possible to argue in favour of good housing conditions in
> economic terms. The necessity for changes in management practices would then
> be clear to farmers and welfare would be improved without the need to resort to
> arguments based on physiological, behavioural and moral grounds.

Potter and Broom's ethical stance is commendable but optimistic. If market forces oblige dairy farmers to optimize returns then it will be economically advantageous to set the risk factors at the point where the adverse effects of lameness in limiting productivity are just not quite severe enough to begin cancelling out the economic benefits of all the other cost-reducing measures. Surveys of lameness incidence suggest that farmers tolerate high levels: 25% and 20% in two French surveys (Brochart, 1986) or 55 new cases per 100 cows per annum (Clarkson *et al.*, 1993). The best way to limit suffering would be to frame regulations which obliged producers to maintain the incidence of 'lameness', however defined, below some set-point. This requirement to control lameness would then itself become a factor to consider when farmers were taking decisions regarding all the other risk factors.

8.5.3. Infectious foot-rot in sheep

This is another condition which seriously depresses welfare:

> Footrot of sheep is common in most countries where there are large numbers of sheep, except . . . in arid and semi-arid areas. The incidence is highest on good improved pastures during warm, moist periods. In these circumstances as many as 75% of a flock may be affected at one time and lameness be so severe that many sheep are forced to walk on their knees . . . Loss of bodily condition is extreme and this, combined with a moderate mortality rate and the expense of labor and materials to treat the disease adequately, makes footrot one of the most costly of sheep diseases.
>
> (Blood and Radostits, 1989, p. 746).

Not only is this disease so painful that sheep are unwilling or unable to stand, the treatment (paring the hoof to the quick to expose and treat the lesion) causes serious discomfort.

Although it is in the interests of both producers and sheep to control foot-rot, it is widespread throughout temperate parts of the world wherever sheep are densely stocked, because the major organism (*Bacterioides nodosus*) is so ubiquitous and infectious. It can be controlled by passing the flock regularly through a foot bath but, until an effective vaccine is developed, is likely to remain a major problem.

8.5.4. Parasitism

The most salient feature in the link between parasitism and welfare is the importance of the host–parasite relationship. Most parasitic conditions cover a spectrum from inapparent infection at one extreme to severe morbidity/death at the other and the health of the host is dependent on a dynamic equilibrium. For most parasitic diseases, the initial entry and continued presence of the parasite triggers an immune response. Provided the host is healthy, nutrition is adequate, level of challenge is containable and immune response is functional and not impaired by immunosuppressive agents such as stress or certain virus infections, then a balance is achieved and the effects on welfare are minimal.

Parasitic gastro-enteritis (PGE)

> Infestations with the small nematodes . . . are probably the most important single cause of losses, in both calves and sheep. They cause poor growth and death in countries where ruminants are run at pasture the whole year and the disease they cause is characterised by persistent diarrhoea and wasting.
>
> (Blood and Radostits, 1989, p. 1051).

The worms damage the epithelium of the abomasum and small intestine, depress enzyme production and nutrient absorption, and result in loss of plasma proteins, anaemia and ionic imbalances. PGE, a disease of intensive production, occurs where many animals are on limited areas of pasture, so reinfection rates are high. It is a serious welfare problem and control depends on effective pasture management and treatment. The worm eggs are long-lived so paddock rotation is ineffective. The best strategy is to reduce stocking rate, graze sheep and cattle together because the parasites are host-specific, and dose regularly with anthelminthics.

Sheep scab

This disease, caused by a psoroptic mite, is another chronic condition causing considerable suffering. Its incidence depends on the quality of management and it is avoidable or even eradicable. It is an unpleasant disease which produces intense distress:

> In a typical outbreak of sheep scab many animals show itchiness and shedding of the fleece. Some become markedly emaciated and weak and death may occur . . . The mites puncture the epidermis to feed on lymph and cause inflammation, resulting in itchiness.
>
> (Blood and Radostits, 1989, p. 1096)

In the UK, after eradication in 1952 by compulsory sheep-dipping and restrictions on movements from infested farms and areas, it was reintroduced in 1973 and has shown a remarkable resurgence in the 1990s. This is attributable to several factors: removal of movement-restrictions and legally-enforced requirement to dip, coupled with withdrawal of persistent organo-chlorine insecticides and a move away from the dangerous, highly-toxic organophosphorus compounds to safer but less effective ones. The depressing conclusion is not only that complacency can lead to the reintroduction of eradicated diseases but that, even when it is in producers' own interests to maintain effective disease control, self-regulation does not work and external surveillance is necessary. Sheep scab is now a major welfare problem in the UK.

8.5.5. Egg drop syndrome 76

This adenovirus disease affects laying hens, localizing in the shell gland of the oviduct. It manifests by a sudden fall in egg production, loss of shell strength and pigmentation, with many shell-less eggs. The birds are normally healthy but occasionally appear slightly depressed for 48 hours or so (McFerran and Stuart, 1990). The direct effects on welfare are minimal but because egg production is unlikely to recover sufficiently the flock is usually slaughtered and the house repopulated with point-of-lay pullets.

8.6. Culling, Slaughter and Euthanasia

When considering health, disease and welfare it is important also to consider death. The ethics of death are complex but because life is valued death is generally regretted. The term used to describe death itself varies depending on the context.

8.6.1. Slaughter

The routine killing of normal animals is *slaughter*. It leads to ethical concern in the case of compulsory eradication schemes, where healthy animals are killed and their carcasses destroyed because they have been in contact with an animal suffering from a notifiable disease. Here death is regretted not because it causes suffering (the method of killing should be as humane as routine slaughter), nor because the individuals are perceived as being of special value, but because the lives of normal, healthy animals are arbitrarily ended.

8.6.2. Culling

Farm animals are *culled* when it is unprofitable to keep them longer. In some species, like poultry, treatment of individuals is minimal, because it is uneconomic; the cost of handling and treatment exceeds any contribution it might make to profit. Medication is often not an option because of statutory withdrawal periods for meat, milk or eggs. In the larger animals carcass value may be appreciable and this encourages early culling in all cases where condemnation is unlikely.

8.6.3. Euthanasia

Companion and zoo animals undergo *euthanasia*. Here the individual has a value in its own right. It will be kept alive as long as there is any likelihood of recovery. Because of the human–animal bond the owner's interests may involve an element of conflict (the benefit of the animal's continued presence balanced against concern for its suffering), decision taking may be difficult and advice from an impartial authority may be helpful. In the case of zoo animals, particularly endangered species, the value of individuals as sources of genetic diversity may be considerable. Care must be taken that the animal's interests are not subordinated to these other priorities.

8.6.4. Sacrifice

Fewer conflicts arise with laboratory animals, where uniformity of response is an important consideration in experimental design and the use of healthy, normal animals is essential. The term *sacrificed* is often used when an animal is humanely killed during the experiment, implying that the animal's interests are secondary to those of science. Welfare problems can arise when experiments require the controlled induction of ill health. In the UK and some other countries end-points, with euthanasia imposed as soon as they are reached, are agreed under the supervision of an external regulatory authority.

8.7. Nutritional, Metabolic and Genetic Disorders

Not all ill health is caused by infectious disease. Undernutrition or malnutrition can result in stunted growth, debilitation or failure to withstand normal stresses. 'Deficiency of energy is the most common nutrient deficiency which limits the performance of farm animals' (Radostits *et al.*, 1994, p. 1370). Energy deficit can result because of inadequate supply (overgrazing, drought, snow covering, cost) or poor quality or limited digestibility. In spite of constantly growing knowledge of nutritional requirements, deficiency diseases are still

common, because of the complex interrelationships between availability, interactions and absorption:

> The difficulties encountered in making an unequivocal diagnosis of nutritional
> deficiency [are considerable] in the area of trace elements and vitamins. The
> amounts of such substances as Se present in feedstuffs and body tissues are
> exceedingly small and their estimation is difficult and expensive.
>
> (Radostits *et al.*, 1994, p. 1368)

Farming practices, pasture management and selective uptake by plants are
major influences on grazing animals. 'Domination of the pasture by particular
plant species may be important [to the extent] that animals grazing the pasture
may suffer trace element deficiencies' (Radostits *et al.*, 1994, p. 1368). Disorders here, as elsewhere, are often the product of complex interactions. 'Decreased resistance to infection is a clinical consequence of naturally-occurring
Cu deficiency in sheep, which is amenable to treatment with Cu and genetic
selection' (Radostits *et al.*, 1994, p. 1384).

Under intensive conditions metabolic disorders are of most concern. 'Amongst
domestic animals the metabolic diseases achieve their greatest importance in
dairy cows and pregnant ewes . . . The high-producing dairy cow always verges
on abnormality' (Radostits *et al.*, 1994, p. 1311). This is a consequence of
the rapid turnover of fluids, energy and ions; any sudden variation in intake
or output may cause abrupt, damaging changes in the internal environment.
The high prevalence and mortality rate of conditions like hypocalcaemia or
hypomagnesaemia mean they are of major importance in North-West Europe
and in New Zealand.

Genetic selection for production efficiency can have adverse effects on
health. In poultry this selection has affected skeleto-muscular and cardiovascular function. Laying hens selected for high egg number and low maintenance
requirements (which implies a small body mass) can become prone to osteo-
porosis towards the end of the laying cycle, because so much structural bone
has been mobilized for egg shell formation. Such birds have fragile bones and
when caught and transported fractures are common. Some broiler strains selected for rapid growth rate show an increased incidence of tibial dyschon-
droplasia (a defect of chondrocyte differentiation) which, if severe, results in
serious leg abnormalities and lameness. In some heavy-bodied turkey strains
breeding birds suffer from a degenerative hip condition involving cartilage
breakdown, which results in joint damage and lameness. Recent increases in
the incidence of ascites in growing broilers are attributable to hypoxia leading
to cardiovascular insufficiency and eventually heart failure. In all these cases
there are serious implications for welfare, which depend on the duration and
severity of the condition, and the extent to which it results in pain, discomfort,
weakness or distress.

8.8. Wildlife

The argument that free-living animals fall outside human responsibility, so
their health and welfare should not be of human concern, is specious. Most

free-living species are now influenced in some way by human activities and in many cases this influence is malign, often through its effect on their food supply:

> We must begin to discard the 20th century trend to define disease as the result of a collision between a pathogenic agent and a susceptible individual. Until recently zoological medicine was primarily concerned with parasitological and infectious diseases, with specific and identifiable causes. The consequences were an emphasis on cure, not prevention, on individuals rather than populations, and on clinical rather than preventive medicine. The best example of how a narrow interpretation of health and disease in wildlife medicine can be disastrous is in the understanding and diagnosis of the most prevalent disease in free-living populations – malnutrition and starvation.
>
> (Franzmann, 1986, p. 8).

Two examples will suffice: (i) Overfishing in the North Sea has had catastrophic effects, not only on the various species of fish which prey on each other, but also on increased mortality among seabirds such as puffins and guillemots, and is now beginning to affect seal populations; (ii) Amphibian numbers are declining because of impaired reproduction: eggs developing in shallow water are being damaged by increased ultraviolet radiation due to ozone thinning.

8.9. Discussion

The evidence reviewed in this chapter supports the common view that good health is a major determinant of well-being in all animals. It is also clear that sufficient knowledge is available to prevent most of the diseases and disorders that put the welfare of domestic animals at risk. In spite of this, the health of many farm animals, in particular, is suboptimal. This is true of both extensive and intensive methods of production and the underlying reasons are economic, either real or imagined. Economic pressures are often used to justify conditions resulting in poor welfare – some of these could be alleviated at no extra cost.

In developing countries most of the major infectious diseases are under control most of the time; the problem is availability of sufficient forage and feedstuffs, in short supply because of habitat destruction, overgrazing, pasture degradation, climatic variability and the need for cereal grains as human food. Often, more animals are kept than the available resources can support and there are other undesirable outcomes, such as the exclusion and destruction of wild species – inevitably animal health and welfare suffer.

In developed countries the situation is different but in some respects the outcomes are not dissimilar. In both intensive and extensive systems, stocking rates are high and herd or flock sizes large. This is partly a response to market forces (economies of scale) and partly to agricultural policies; in the European Union, for example, sheep production is supported by per capita payments, so hill grazing tends to be overstocked and flock numbers are excessive for adequate supervision. Dairy herds have expanded as milk quota has become a marketable commodity, a higher proportion of grassland is earmarked for the production of winter forage to minimize feeding costs, the available grazing pasture has accordingly shrunk so the danger of poaching has increased and the number of cows per worker has risen with greater automation. As the complexity of the system increases, the time spent on routine tasks expands and the time available to devote to animal care shrinks. Thus even ostensibly extensive systems have become intensified. Under these conditions the health of an individual animal may become a dispensable element. The extreme case is the battery-caged hen, where flock sizes of more than 12,000 birds per person are not uncommon and, if the daily inspection required by law lasted no longer than 1 second per bird, it would still take over 3 hours just to glance at them.

This inability to supervise animals adequately, to pick up early warning signs of disease, behavioural change or stress, to pay meticulous attention to preventive procedures and to carry out immediately all appropriate remedial measures, must be an important factor in the occurrence of so much disease or disorder in intensive systems. The constant time pressure, apart from its adverse effects on animal health and welfare, must also increase the stress imposed on stockpersons and farmers. It may be related to the high rate of suicide in rural workers recently reported in the UK and emphasizes that concern regarding welfare should not be limited to animals but should also be extended to those who look after them.

We shall not end on a note of unrelieved gloom. Recognition of the importance of greater knowledge and awareness is steadily increasing. A telling example comes from the studies of lameness in cattle. In a UK survey of dairy farms there was a strong correlation between the extent of a farmer's knowledge, training and awareness, and a low incidence of the condition in the herd (Mill and Ward, 1994). Much of the information to improve welfare is now available – the next stage is engendering the will to put it into effect.

8.10. Conclusions

- Environmental factors are highly influential in determining the health status of animals; interactions between stress, immune function and disease are increasingly recognized.
- Welfare in intensive systems is of particular concern, because of the minimal attention devoted to individual animals, with growing evidence of many low-grade, subclinical disorders.
- Diseases differ greatly in the suffering they induce, but pathological change is a poor predictor of pain or distress. Disorders of the joints or digestive system seem especially painful; this may reflect our ability to detect behavioural or postural changes, rather than telling us what animals are feeling.
- Causes of ill health other than infective agents play a key part, especially under extensive conditions, where malnutrition can be common.

- Even wildlife species are adversely affected by human activities. The heavy hand of human interference, directed and inadvertent, is now influencing the health and welfare of animals everywhere.
- Veterinarians conducting clinical examinations should attempt to assess how much and in what way disorders influence welfare. This information should be published to increase understanding of the welfare impact of disease processes.

CHAPTER 9
Behaviour

Joy A. Mench (University of California, USA) and
Georgia J. Mason (University of Oxford, UK)

Abstract

The use of behaviour as an indicator of welfare in captive and domesticated animals has generated much discussion and controversy. Nevertheless, behaviour is one of the most easily observed measures of welfare, and can provide excellent cues about the preferences, needs, and internal states of animals. We describe some normal behaviours that indicate at least short-term reductions in welfare, since they have been associated with states like frustration, conflict, pain, disturbance, distress, fear or illness. Because the expression of normal behaviours varies with the situation, the species and the strain of animal, knowledge of species-typical behaviour and of behaviour of individuals and their social groups is a prerequisite for using such behaviours to assess welfare. We also discuss the welfare implications of abnormal behaviours. These are often viewed as indicators of reduced welfare because they are associated with impoverished environments and frustrated motivation, and are correlated with other signs of poor welfare. The relationship between abnormal behaviours and welfare, however, is not simple. The propensity to develop stereotypies depends on interacting factors that may have little to do with welfare, including neurophysiological predispositions. In addition, once established, abnormal behaviours may persist even in enriched environments, and their performance can have beneficial rather than negative consequences for the animal. So what can behaviour tell us about welfare? A great deal – providing that development, causes and consequences for the animal of performing (or not performing) different behaviours are well understood.

9.1. Introduction

The importance of behaviour as a means of assessing welfare in animals was made explicit by the Brambell Committee (1965, p. 10) in its landmark report on intensive farming practices:

> The scientific evidence bearing on the sensations and sufferings of animals is derived from anatomy and physiology on the one hand and from ethology, the science of animal behaviour, on the other . . . we have been impressed by the evidence to be derived from the study of the behaviour of the animal. We consider that this is a field of scientific research in relation to animal husbandry which has not attracted the attention which it deserves and that opportunities should be sought to encourage its development.

Good stockmen and animal managers have always used animals' behaviour as a guide to their health and welfare. The Brambell report, however, stimulated a more formal approach to the study of behaviour of confined animals, which in turn stimulated controversy about what behaviour actually tells us about welfare. Despite this controversy, behaviour is still one of the most easily observed indicators of welfare. Behaviour, after all, is what animals do to change and control their environment, and thus provides information about their needs (Chapter 7), preferences (Chapter 11) and internal states.

In this chapter, we focus on the relationships between behaviour and welfare. We discuss both normal and abnormal behaviours, and provide examples of behaviours indicative of aversive states like frustration, pain and stress. We also mention some pitfalls and limitations of this approach to assessing welfare.

9.2. Normal Behaviour and Welfare

9.2.1. Understanding normal behaviour

The study of normal behaviour can tell us what animals do when frightened, ill, or in pain, as well as when they have abundant resources and are free from predation. Comparisons of free-living and captive animals can show us which behaviour is absent in captivity, and provide cues as to which behaviour might be important for an animal to perform. Finally, ethological studies are vital to understand the functions and welfare significance of otherwise puzzling behaviour, for example the tonic immobility reaction that some animals show in response to frightening stimuli (Chapter 6).

To know what the behaviour of an animal 'means' in terms of its welfare, it is necessary to have a detailed knowledge of the behaviour characteristic of the animal's species. One approach is to attempt to develop an 'ethogram', or catalogue of behaviours (Banks, 1982). Since most captive environments provide animals with only limited opportunities to perform behaviours, observation of animals in more extensive environments is required. As Dawkins (1989, p. 77) points out:

> To ask sensible questions about the extent to which hens in battery cages
> suffer through being deprived of the opportunity to perform certain behaviour
> patterns, we need a baseline against which to compare behaviour in
> intensive systems.

For non-domesticated animals like most zoo animals, the behaviour of wild conspecifics can be studied to determine the range, frequency, temporal patterning and function of the behaviour of individuals, as well some of the social and environmental factors that lead to variation in expression.

The situation is more complicated in domestic animals, where selection has caused changes in behaviour (Price, 1984). Because it can be difficult to determine the precise nature of these changes, feral animals or domestic animals placed in complex 'naturalistic' environments are usually studied in preference to wild progenitors. Stolba and Wood-Gush (1989) carried out one of the most elaborate studies of this type. They observed the behaviour of groups of domestic pigs allowed to range in two large forested enclosures over several years. They then constructed an ethogram of 103 different behavioural elements. They concluded (pp. 423–424) that:

> domestication and rearing conditions had not affected [the pigs'] potential to show a rich repertoire of behaviour. Indeed, the behaviour reported here was seen within 1 to 6 months of release into the Pig Park and resembled that of the European wild boar in wild or semi-wild conditions.

It is sometimes suggested that welfare is promoted if animals are able to perform the activities that most closely resemble the behavioural repertoire of their free-ranging conspecifics. In an appendix to the Brambell Report (1965. p. 79), for example, Thorpe stated:

> While accepting the need for much restriction [of agricultural animals], we must draw the line at conditions which completely suppress all or nearly all the natural, instinctive urges and behaviour patterns characteristic of actions appropriate to the high degree of social organization as found in the ancestral wild species and which have been little, if at all, bred out in the process of domestication.

However, as Hughes (1978, pp. 22–23) and others have pointed out, differences in behaviour between free-ranging and captive environments do not necessarily imply suffering:

> The crucial question now is this – do these changes in quantity, the nature and organization of behaviour indicate merely that [an animal] is an adaptable creature, and has appropriately adapted her behaviour to suit a different environment, or do they show she really does have ethological needs which she is unable to satisfy and therefore becomes frustrated? . . . The mere fact that an animal has an appendage or a behaviour pattern in its repertoire does not mean that it is obliged to make use of it.

Wild animals also show variation in the types of behaviours performed under different circumstances. Tribes of chimpanzees in different areas of Africa, for example, differ in patterns of tool usage and social group formation, differences linked to the requirements of the various habitats in which they reside (Gibbons, 1992). Behaviour of individuals within a particular location can also vary depending on shifting environmental factors like resource availability. Although lions usually hunt in groups, they may also hunt alone or in pairs depending on the size, distribution, and availability of prey (Packer, 1986).

Fraser (1992, p. 100) emphasizes the problems that arise in trying to interpret normal behaviours as indicators of welfare:

> Let me illustrate this with three types of natural behaviour of pigs. First . . . the repertoire of 'separation calls' that piglets give when they are separated from the mother. This is species-typical behavior ('innate,' if you wish), but there is no question in my mind that the calls denote a state of distress from which the animal wishes to escape. Second on the list is panting and wallowing. These, too, are 'innate' behavior that the pig uses to avoid over-heating, but the behavior occurs only under hot conditions. Third is nest building by sows during the day before they farrow. Domestic pigs in a field may make elaborate nests of

branches and grass soon before farrowing. Confined sows become very active during the pre-farrowing period; they may spend many hours performing the movements of nest-building such as nesting and rooting on the concrete floor, and they may even develop abrasions on their faces through these actions. Clearly there is strong nest-building motivation specific to the pre-farrowing sow and not contingent on stimuli from the environment. The point is . . . that a pig's natural behavior includes some things that they want to do (such as building a nest before farrowing), some things they want to do only if the conditions require it (such as panting and wallowing), and some things that they do not want to do at all (such as separation calls). A simple comparison of animal behavior in confined and traditional environments may identify some interesting differences that merit further study, but this approach does not by itself allow us to say which of the differences are positive, negative, or neutral in terms of animal welfare.

Distinguishing among these types of normal behaviour poses some difficult (although not insurmountable) problems. Determining which behaviours animals 'want to do only when conditions require it' rests primarily on determining the functions of particular behaviours. In some cases, this is relatively simple. The wallowing referred to by Fraser above, for example, was seen in the pigs in the Pig Park only when ambient temperatures exceeded 18°C (Stolba and Wood-Gush, 1989), demonstrating that it is a thermoregulatory behaviour and therefore probably unnecessary for pigs in colder or climate-controlled conditions. In other cases, however, assessing the function (or functions) of a particular behaviour can be more complex:

> It has been said that battery cages prevent wing-flapping . . . but perhaps the bird in a cage is not motivated to wing-flap. Wing-flapping is often described as the bird stretching its wings, but . . . it could also be a sexual signal or a social signal or an intention movement to fly. Until we know what wing-flapping is, what causes it, what function it serves, and how it develops and how it has evolved, we cannot say that caging prevents wing-flapping.
>
> (Duncan, 1981b, p. 493)

Determining which behaviours animals want (or need) to do regardless of conditions, then, is more problematical. Duncan (1978b, p. 292) argues that two steps are necessary: 'Look for unusual or inappropriate behavioural changes' and 'Show independently that these are indicative of reduced welfare.' Methods that have been used to demonstrate reduced welfare include assessing motivation and analysing physiological correlates of behavioural changes. These are discussed elsewhere in this book.

Although at present our understanding of the causes, functions and importance for welfare of the normal behaviour of most species is limited, in the section that follows we will provide several examples of ways in which normal behaviour can be used to evaluate welfare.

9.2.2. Behaviour indicative of disturbance, pain, or distress

Wild, feral and captive animals show a number of behaviours characteristic of disturbance, fear or acute distress. Behaviours of this type (which fit Fraser's description of behaviours that animals 'do not want' to perform) include 'escape and avoidance (e.g. rapid locomotion away from a source of stimulation), immobility or protective responses, and distress signals (e.g. calls, odors, facial expressions)' (Archer, 1976, p. 234). Although the response will depend on the situation, behaviours of this sort are indicators of at least a short-term reduction in welfare.

The frequency and intensity of expression of at least some of these behaviours provide information about the distress experienced by the animal. Weary and Fraser (1995a, p. 1047) recorded the vocalizations given by piglets after separation from the sow:

> 'Non-thriving' and 'unfed' piglets called more and used more high-frequency calls, longer calls, and calls that rose more in frequency than their 'thriving' and 'fed' litter-mates . . . If a piglet's calls provide reliable information about its need for the sow's resources, then this calling can be used as a measure of its welfare.

Vocalizations also increase in frequency in other animals when they are hungry, cold or in pain (Weary and Fraser, 1995b).

Because of their clinical and experimental importance, behaviours associated with pain have received much attention. Morton and Griffiths (1985) list signs of pain in laboratory animals, and also demonstrate an important consideration – that responses to pain, distress and disturbance are species-specific. For example, guinea pigs squeal urgently and repetitively when in pain but rarely show aggression, while rats may squeal only when handled or when pressure is placed on the affected area but may also become aggressive. Bateson (1991, p. 832) points out that:

> Species differ greatly in the way they respond to potentially damaging stimulation or to parts of the body that are injured or diseased . . . For instance, many primates often show remarkably little reaction to surgical procedures or traumatic damage . . . The classes of stimuli that are potentially injurious and those that are potentially useful are likely to depend greatly on ecological conditions . . . The same goes for the circumstances in which the animal should take note and respond appropriately in order to reduce the chances of further injury and those in which such incoming information should be suppressed.

An understanding of species-characteristic responses to illness, pain and distress, and the environmental and social factors that modify those behaviours, is important for assessing welfare in captive animals.

9.2.3. Changes in behaviour

Morton and Griffiths (1985, p. 432) make another important point about using behaviour to evaluate welfare: 'Changes in the overall appearance of a group of animals, the way in which they interact and the deportment of an individual may indicate the first signs of abnormality.' Hart (1988, p. 133) discusses the changes in behaviour shown by sick animals and describes their importance to the healing process:

> Behavior associated with being sick can be viewed as representing an all-out effort to overcome the infectious disease, putting virtually all of the animal's resources into fending off the invading pathogens. The behavioral patterns that we commonly see in people or animals that are acutely ill, including complete or

partial anorexia, sleepiness, depression, lack of interest in drinking water and reduction of grooming activity, can be viewed as potentiating the fever or acute phase response by conserving energy . . . the same behavioral patterns might serve to protect a prey animal from predation while it is acutely ill.

The importance of observing behavioural changes in individuals is also demonstrated by studies of beak-trimming in poultry:

> The amount of time spent by the birds in performing certain behaviour
> patterns was substantially altered by beak trimming. Three behavioural
> categories immediately decreased after beak trimming, namely feeding, drinking
> and preening, and it is telling that all these directly involve the beak . . .
> pecking, which also involves the beak, decreased in the beak-trimmed
> group . . . the most obvious characteristic of beak trimming was inactivity,
> reflected in substantial increases in standing throughout the experiment
> and in sitting dozing for one or two weeks.
>
>   (Duncan *et al.*, 1989, pp. 484–486)

Since beak-trimming also results in the formation of neuromas in the stump suggestive of chronic pain (Gentle, 1986), these changes in behaviour appear to be sensitive indicators of the post-procedural pain experienced by the hen.

As Morton and Griffiths (1985) suggest, changes in social behaviours may also provide cues about welfare. Aggression is a normal part of the behavioural repertoire of social species, and aggression which causes injury poses a welfare problem. Increases even in non-injurious aggression, however, may also be associated with reduced welfare. Duncan and Wood-Gush (1971) deprived chickens of food for 24 hours and then provided them with food under a perspex cover. They found an increase in aggression, and suggested that (p. 503):

> Frustration is correlated with aggressive responses in the domestic fowl.
> However, the presence of a bird lower in the social hierarchy seems to be a
> necessary stimulus before aggressive responses are elicited.

Frustration also leads to increased aggression in pigs. Carlstead (1986) fed group-housed pigs at variable intervals. Half were given a reliable signal (a bell) that indicated that the food was about to be delivered, while the other half received unreliable signals. In the latter (p. 35) 'higher aggression [was found] directly after a false signal . . . supporting the hypothesis that unreliable feeding signals produce frustration-induced aggression in grower pigs'. Pain as well as frustration results in increased aggression in a number of species (Morton and Griffiths, 1985).

9.2.4. Suppression of normal behaviour

Ongoing behaviour is often temporarily suppressed and replaced by more appropriate behaviours when animals are disturbed. Under conditions of higher intensity or longer lasting stress, however, certain behaviours may be suppressed even after a disturbance has ended. Behaviours associated with reproduction are one example in some species:

> The expression of both male and female reproductive behavior appears to
> be modified by stress, especially social stress. Although the physiological

mechanisms involved have not been conclusively demonstrated, at least in the
female the response of the adrenal axis to stress seems to be to prevent the
gonadal steroids from eliciting sexual behavior.

(Moberg, 1985c, p. 264)

This was demonstrated in a study by Ehnert and Moberg (1991), in which ewes
were injected with estradiol to stimulate oestrus, subjected to either social
isolation or transportation stress, and then tested for oestrous behaviour.
Transportation (p. 2988) 'blocked the expression of estrus in five of eight ewes
and delayed the expression of estrus in one other'. Isolation had a similar but
lesser effect, delaying or blocking oestrus in four of nine ewes. Suppression of
certain behaviour may therefore provide evidence that the animal has
experienced significant stress.

Behaviours associated with exploration and play (Chapter 3) may also be
affected by stress. In one study of exploration (Arnsten *et al.*, 1985, p. 803):

Naive rats were exposed to one of three stressors (restraint, tailpinch pressure,
high intensity white noise) or to control procedures, and were observed in a
novel environment . . . The average time an animal spent per contact with
stimuli in the environment was decreased significantly with stress.

Similarly, rats shocked and then placed in a novel environment two days later
show 'a decreased diversity of exploration [but no decrease in] general activity
in comparison with animals not exposed to stress' (Rosselini and Widman,
1989, p. 339).

In both studies, the primary effect of stress was to change the character
and range of exploratory activity. Play behaviour, on the other hand, decreases
or disappears entirely under conditions of stress associated with food shortage
or drought (Lee, 1984). Play and diverse exploration may be 'luxuries',
dispensed with during stress.

9.2.5. Normal behaviour out of context

Sometimes in a conflict or frustrating situation activities appear which are
apparently irrelevant and out of context with the activity immediately
preceding them or following them.

(Wood-Gush *et al.*, 1975, p. 184)

An example of such an activity, referred to as displacement behaviour, is
preening shown by hungry domestic fowl in response to being presented with
food covered by perspex. Duncan and Wood-Gush (1972, p. 68) reported that
these preening movements:

were of shorter duration than those in the normal situation, and it was thought
that this accounted for the 'frantic' appearance of the displacement preening.
The pattern of preening also differed in the thwarting situation with plumage
areas which were easy to reach receiving more attention than in the control
situation.

But some displacement activities are seemingly 'indistinguishable in form or
orientation from the same behaviour patterns in normal contexts . . . and their
identification [has to be] based almost exclusively on a contextual analysis'

(Maestripieri, *et al.* 1992, p. 968). Displacement behaviour can therefore be difficult to characterize, and this has caused some controversy regarding its usefulness. In a recent review of displacement activities in primates, however, Maestripieri *et al.* (1992, p. 967) concluded that:

> displacement activities tend to occur in situations of psycho-social stress and their frequency of occurrence is affected by anxiogenic and anxiolytic drugs. In the light of this evidence, it is suggested that displacement activities can be used as indicators of emotional states.

In interpreting displacement behaviours (as well as frustration-induced behaviours like aggression) in terms of welfare, it is important to realize that:

> conflict is a widespread occurrence in animals, and, more importantly, that conflict behaviour patterns may be adaptive, enabling an animal to cope with the conflict and often eventually to resolve it . . . while conflict and frustration do not always indicate suffering, they sometimes certainly seem to . . . [particularly during] prolonged or intense occurrences.
>
> (Dawkins, 1980, p. 75–6)

9.3. Abnormal Behaviour and Welfare

9.3.1. Understanding abnormal behaviour

The behaviour we see in captivity is sometimes so unusual or bizarre, its consequences for the animal so baffling, that comparison with free-living animals does not help us. Such behaviour includes: stereotypies (repetitive behaviour patterns with no obvious function); excessive licking and even eating of hair, wool or feathers; and persistent biting at the tails of other animals – a problem particular to pigs. These sorts of behaviour patterns are usually termed abnormal, and their implications for welfare are controversial.

One controversy relates to the definition of abnormal behaviour. The literal meaning of abnormal is 'away from the norm': statistically rare or different from a chosen population. This is the sense in which several authors have used it (Meyer-Holzapfel, 1968). The animal living free, or in naturalistic conditions of captivity, is usually taken as the 'norm'. However, as Dawkins (1980, p. 77) pointed out:

> The moment a behaviour is labelled 'abnormal' . . . it can become almost impossible not to assume the animal doing it must be suffering, because 'abnormal' is such an emotionally loaded word.

This is because the term is sometimes used specifically to mean pathological, either causing harm to the animal or the product of damage or illness (Schmidt, 1982).

Clearly not all the behaviour that is abnormal in the first sense is also pathological. Behaviours abnormal in the sense of being unique to captive animals include lever-pressing by trained rats, ball-chasing by pet dogs and running in wheels by caged hamsters. And there are even cases in the wild of animals performing unusual behaviour patterns. Macdonald (1992) describes a rash of car vandalism in Switzerland and Germany caused by stone martens that had – for some unknown reason – developed a taste for chewing rubber. Ignition cables, coolant hoses and insulation foam were all liable to be 'martenized'. When not performing these 'statistically unusual' abnormal behaviours, all the animals described here are likely to seem normal, healthy and unaffected by any mysterious pathology.

Nevertheless, abnormal behaviour often gives cause for concern. Even if the animal performing it is not diseased, the behaviour could still be the product of a welfare problem like frustrated motivation. Some authors have even devised scales against which to gauge whether particular levels of abnormal behaviour indicate unacceptably poor welfare (Fig. 9.1).

We now consider the evidence that links abnormal behaviour with poor welfare. We will focus on stereotypies as a large, diverse and much-studied group of abnormal behaviour patterns. The links between stereotypies and welfare have been analysed in three main ways: by identifying the types of environment in which they are most common, by identifying the motivational bases of the behaviour, and by looking for links with other welfare indicators such as physiological signs of stress. We then consider some problematic cases and their implications for attempts to 'read off' an animal's welfare from the levels of abnormal behaviour it displays.

9.3.2. Abnormal behaviour and poor welfare

Environmental effects

Different environments have been compared to see the extent to which they elicit abnormal behaviour. Ödberg (1987) studied jumping stereotypies developed by voles in cages. Half of the cages were bare, while half were filled with leaves and branches. He found that in the barren cages voles were more

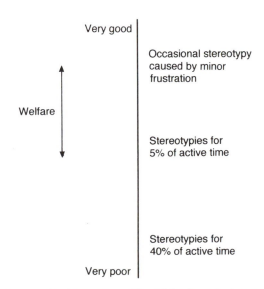

Fig. 9.1. A scale linking the frequency with which stereotypies are performed to welfare (Broom and Johnson, 1993).

than twice as likely to develop this behaviour. In this type of study, groups of animals are deliberately housed in different ways. A related technique uses animals already living on farms or in zoos. The ways in which their environments differ – space, amount of food and so on – are recorded, and the relationships between these and the abnormal behaviours are analysed. This epidemiological approach has been used on the abnormal behaviour of stabled horses (McGreevy *et al.*, 1995). Weaving, wind-sucking and crib-biting were most common in stable-yards where horses were fed a high proportion of concentrates relative to natural forage like hay. Horses allowed visual contact with one another between their stables also developed less abnormal behaviour, particularly wood-chewing.

There are two drawbacks with this 'environmental factors' approach. One is that independent measures of the merits of the environments are necessary. It would clearly be circular to argue that abnormal behaviour reflects poor welfare because it is more common in one environment and that this environment is worse because it is linked with higher levels of abnormal behaviour. The second is that it does not identify the motivational basis of the behaviour. This can mean that which aspect of the eliciting environment is causal remains a puzzle.

Motivational bases

One of the earliest attempts to identify the motivational basis of an abnormal behaviour was that of Meyer-Holzapfel (1968, pp. 482–483), who studied zoo animals. Her close observations revealed that one stereotypy in a lone dingo developed from attempts to return to its pack in the neighbouring enclosure (Fig. 9.2):

> At the beginning, the dingo ran back and forth along the separating trellis, keeping quite close to it; when it turned around at each end of its path, the

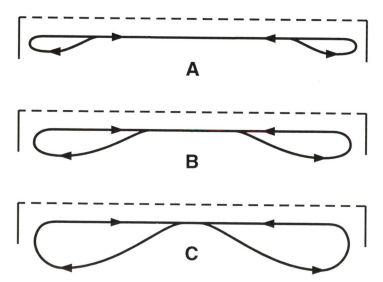

Fig. 9.2. The development of stereotypy in a dingo separated from its pack (Meyer-Holzapfel, 1968).

turns were quite small. In the following days, these paths were paced farther and farther from the trellis. Thus the path gradually took the form of a figure eight.

More recently, Wurbel *et al.* (1996) conducted a developmental study of two strains of laboratory mice. One strain performed a wire-gnawing stereotypy, the other, a jumping stereotypy. Both were found to develop from similar behaviour patterns relating to exploration. In the former, it developed from climbing up at the cage lid, and sniffing between the bars, while in the latter it developed from rearing up at the sides of the cage, and sniffing up towards the cage lid. However, studying development presents some methodological problems, especially in really proving that one behaviour pattern develops from another. For instance, Dantzer (1986, p. 1778) summarized two studies of the development of abnormal behaviour in tethered sows as follows:

> The stereotypies that develop after tethering appear to be derived from re-directed aggressive acts elicited by the environment in which animals are placed (Cronin *et al.*, 1984). For example, pre-feeding stereotypies are built upon elements of re-directed activities consecutive to thwarted attempts to reach the food trolley. (Rushen, 1985b)

However, Rushen's study was careful to distinguish between pre- and post-feeding stereotypies and concluded that most of the behaviours actually stemmed from foraging. Post-feeding snout-rubbing and rooting seemed to represent oft-repeated food-seeking sequences.

These interpretive problems highlight the value of a second means of identifying the motivational bases of abnormal behaviour: through experiment. Terlouw *et al.* (1991) used experiments to show that foraging is indeed the most likely basis for the abnormal behaviour of tethered sows. Half of their subjects were tethered and half were loose-housed in groups. For each type of housing, half were fed 2.2 kg d^{-1} and the other half were fed 4 kg d^{-1}. Behaviours such as sham-chewing before feeding, bar-biting, and chain-chewing were higher in the pigs kept on low levels of food (Fig. 9.3) as was drinking. Housing type, in contrast, had little effect. Tethered sows spent more time standing inactive, and more time in the relatively uncommon post-feeding sham-chewing, but there were no other effects.

Wiedenmayer (1997) similarly carried out a test of a motivational hypothesis. Gerbils in laboratory cages commonly scrabble or dig at the corners. He argued that in the wild these animals dig their own burrows, ceasing to dig once they have achieved a tunnel. So would providing a tunnel – preferably one that leads to a nest – cause corner-scrabbling to cease in captive gerbils? He found that indeed it would, thus showing that the motivation to dig a completed tunnel was behind their stereotypy.

Correlates of abnormal behaviour

The third method of assessing the welfare significance of abnormal behaviour is to see if it correlates with signs of stress or poor welfare. For example, von Borell and Hurnik (1991) found that individual pigs performing the greatest amount of this sort of behaviour had the greatest corticosteroid responses to ACTH. Correlations like these do not distinguish cause and effect – they merely

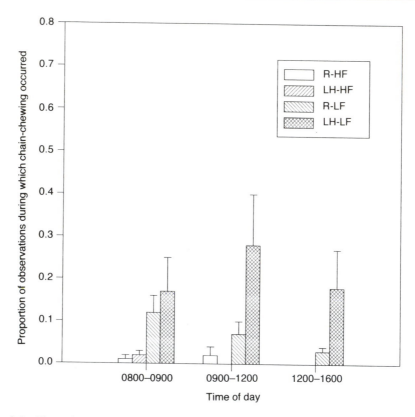

Fig. 9.3. The relationships between housing type, feeding level and chain-chewing in gilts (after Terlouw *et al.*, 1991). R = restrained (tethered), LH = loose-housed, HF = high fed (4.0 kg d^{-1}), LF = low fed (2.2 kg d^{-1}).

tell us when two phenomena co-vary. However, in some cases it is obvious that abnormal behaviour is having consequences which are bad for welfare, such as physical injury. Morris (1964, p. 112) describes one heart-rending case:

> In the case of a hand-reared tigress that repeatedly attempted to move forwards towards her human 'friends', a rather damaging form of pacing developed. The animal pressed forward so hard as it paced back and forth that its nose was rubbed across the bars, like a boy trailing a stick along garden railings. This rapidly produced a large sore patch which became raw until the whole surface of the snout became a sensitive, naked area.

Implications

Abnormal behaviour has been equated with poor welfare because it is often prevalent in environments we judge to be poor, often develops from frustrated motivation, and sometimes correlates with other signs of poor welfare. This might suggest that abnormal behaviour, especially stereotypies, is indeed a reliable indicator of poor welfare, i.e. that individuals with low levels of stereotypy are better off than those with high, and that environments that elicit high levels of stereotypy are worse than those that result in little or none of this behaviour. Unfortunately such suggestions – and simple scales like that in Figure 9.1 – are belied by some problematic counter-examples, as discussed below.

9.3.3. Problems in using abnormal behaviour to judge welfare

Cooper *et al.* (1996) looked further into the jumping stereotypies of caged voles. They transferred voles from barren cages to ones enriched with vegetation and found that 14-month-old voles were more likely than 2-month-old voles to continue performing stereotypies in the new cage. This is clearly a problem for using levels of stereotypy to assess vole welfare. Was welfare of old animals no better in enriched than in barren cages? Or had the behaviour ceased to be a reliable indicator of welfare? Other problematic cases are those in which abnormal behaviour is linked with seemingly poor environments, but other measures show that individuals with the highest levels are not necessarily most stressed. For instance, when heifers are tethered, they show increased levels of corticosteroids and stereotypies such as tongue-rolling. But corticosteroids are no higher in animals with high levels of stereotypy (Redbo, 1993).

Factors affecting levels of abnormal behaviour

Individuals may differ in their abnormal behaviour for many reasons. For instance, fundamental properties of dopaminergic pathways in the brain can affect how much climbing activity mice show when stressed or frightened (Cabib, 1993). Individual differences in physical fitness, levels of hormones such as testosterone and fundamental properties of pathways in the brain can also affect how animals persist in the face of frustration or failure, how likely they are to develop habit-like routines, and thus very possibly their tendencies to develop stereotypies.

For example, aspects of motor-control that might affect stereotypies were surveyed by Mason and Turner (1993, p. 77), who summarized:

> Individuals with a limited ability to generate a range of behaviour patterns spontaneously, or who readily restrict their attention . . . might be more inclined than others to developing stereotypies . . . That animals may differ in their propensities to develop or control behaviour in particular ways has welfare implications, for it suggests that an individual's stereotypy levels are not just a product of how aversive it finds its current environment, but are also influenced by the readiness with which certain behavioural control mechanics come into play.

Factors outside the animal affect its levels of abnormal behaviour, too. The exact stressors the animal is exposed to can affect what sorts of behaviour it displays, how exaggerated and sustained this behaviour is, and how likely it is to develop into something that looks abnormal. For instance, rodents exposed to chronic mild electric shock, or to cold, tend to become immobile rather than to develop stereotypies (Archer, 1979). Social facilitation may also affect the incidence of abnormal behaviour: animals may be more likely to develop stereotypies if their neighbours already perform them (Cooper and Nicol, 1994).

Thus an animal's expression of abnormal behaviour is the product of many interacting factors, some of which have nothing to do with welfare.

Developmental changes

Stereotypies provide a clear case of developmental changes affecting the usefulness of behaviour as an indicator of welfare. Kennes *et al.* (1988) found that stereotypies in voles were not inhibited by the opioid antagonist, naloxone, once over a certain age, and that they were performed outside of the original situation, sometimes in the absence of any apparent conflict. Overall, it seems that as a stereotypy develops it may be performed in a wider range of circumstances. It may therefore be as much a 'scar' of past experience as an indication of current frustration or environmental inadequacy (Mason, 1991a).

Benefits of abnormal behaviour

The final factor to complicate the link between abnormal behaviour and welfare is that in some cases it can actually have beneficial consequences. Cronin *et al.* (1985, p. 530) found that naloxone reduced stereotypy performance in tethered sows and concluded that:

> The performance and maintenance of stereotypies depend on the release of endorphins. These substances may calm the sows . . . Thus, performing the seemingly purposeless stereotypies may function as an effective coping strategy for survival. That these behaviours are present during many hours a day may be related to the dependency-creating properties of endorphins and therefore these stereotypies may be considered as an addictive-like phenomenon.

Although this interpretation has since been criticized, the idea that apparently functionless behaviour may have consequences has remained prevalent in the literature, partly because of the findings of other, more recent, studies. For example, restricted-fed hens that 'spot-peck' have lower corticosteroid levels than those which do not (Kostal *et al.*, 1992). de Passillé *et al.* (1993) studied calves kept away from their mothers and fed on milk from a bucket. These animals sucked at objects, particularly after drinking, and this seemed to have important effects on digestion, encouraging the release of hormones like insulin.

9.4. Conclusions

- Behaviour is one of the most easily observed indicators of welfare: it provides information about animals' needs, preferences and internal states. The study of normal behaviour can tell us what animals do when frightened, frustrated, distressed, ill, in pain, as well as when they have abundant resources and are free from predation.
- Normal behaviour can be divided into three categories: behaviour that animals want to do, behaviour they want to do but only when external circumstances require it, and behaviour they don't want to do.
- No one set of behavioural responses can indicate reduced welfare, though changes in the frequencies of individual and social behaviours or suppression

of behaviours can provide cues about welfare problems. Behaviour that occurs out of context may also indicate disturbance.

- Responses to aversive experiences vary with situation, with species and with strain of animal. Their interpretation requires knowledge of the species-characteristic behavioural repertoire, the functions of behaviour patterns, the contexts in which they occur and the behaviour which is characteristic of groups and individual animals.
- Abnormal behaviour presents difficulties: it is relevant to the study of welfare but is not a straightforward indicator of an animal's emotional state. Sometimes it appears to be closely related to adverse situations where animals are frustrated or restricted, while in other cases it is not seen, or persists even when the environment is improved, or even appears to act to improve welfare.
- Like symptoms in veterinary medicine, abnormal behaviour should be treated as a sign requiring further investigation: it can turn out to be an indication of a harmful process, or neutral, or sometimes even beneficial.

CHAPTER 10
Physiology

E.M. Claudia Terlouw (INRA, Clermont-Ferrand, France),
Willem G.P. Schouten (Wageningen Agricultural University,
The Netherlands) and Jan Ladewig (Royal Veterinary
and Agricultural University, Denmark)

Abstract

Although originally the term 'stress' was used to refer to the physiological responses involved in adaptation to the environment, nowadays the term describes the animal's state when it is challenged beyond its behavioural and physiological capacity to adapt to its environment. The most frequently monitored physiological responses to acute stress are increased secretion of glucocorticosteroids from the hypothalamo–pituitary–adrenal axis into the blood and increased activity of the sympathetic branch of the autonomic nervous system, resulting in increased plasma levels of adrenaline and noradrenaline and increased cardiac output. Due to efficient feedback mechanisms, chronic stress is generally not measurable by changes in hypothalamo–pituitary–adrenal and sympatho-adrenal activity. Chronic stress may, however, affect the regulation of these systems, which becomes apparent when the animal is subjected to acute stress. The sympatho-adrenal response occurs much faster than the hypothalamo–pituitary–adrenal response, and different stressors provoke different hormonal profiles. Acute and/or chronic stress may further induce changes in opioid peptides, insulin, prolactin, growth hormone and vasopressin. Stress may be accompanied by an increase in body temperature, by immunosuppression, by increases in plasma ion levels and reduction in weight gain. Animals tend to differ consistently in stress reactivity.

10.1. Introduction

10.1.1. Physiological responses to challenge

Effective response to environmental challenges is essential to survival. When threatened, an animal increases its alertness and either shows active responses, such as fight or flight, or immobilizes to remain unnoticed. At the same time, physiological changes occur. Changes can occur in plasma concentrations of various hormones, such as glucocorticosteroids, endogenous opioid peptides, catecholamines, sex hormones, growth hormones, thyroid hormones, vasopressin and insulin. These hormonal changes affect cellular metabolic processes, releasing glucose and free fatty acids from the liver and other tissues, and altering their uptake by the brain and muscles. Initially, the non-specific response to any demand from the external and internal environment on the

Animal Welfare (eds Michael C. Appleby and Barry O. Hughes)

animal's system was called 'stress' (Selye, 1932). Nowadays 'stress' has a negative connotation, often describing the animal's state when it is challenged beyond its behavioural and physiological capacity to adapt to its environment (Fraser *et al.*, 1975). Despite this shift in meaning, measurements of stress are principally based on physiological indices of activation, including the gluco-corticoids and catecholamines. Cardiac output (heart rate, blood pressure), a major determinant of the blood circulation and thus of the availability of energy substrates, is influenced by environmental challenge and is also used as a measure of stress.

The secretion of glucocorticosteroids (cortisol and corticosterone) is controlled by the corticotropic releasing hormone (CRH) which is released from the hypothalamus into the portal veins of the pituitary. CRH stimulates the secretion of adrenocorticotropic hormone (ACTH) from the frontal lobe of the pituitary (adenohypophysis) into the general circulation. After reaching the adrenals, ACTH stimulates ACTH receptors of the adrenal cortex, causing the release of glucocorticosteroids into the bloodstream. The system is often referred to as the hypothalamo–pituitary–adrenal (HPA) axis. The presence of glucocorticosteroids in the blood is necessary for a wide range of physiological functions. Johnson *et al.* (1992, pp. 117–118) write:

> Glucocorticoids exert many different effects, including effects on cardiovascular function, metabolism, muscle function, behaviour and the immune system. These effects can be grouped into two categories defined as permissive and regulatory . . . 'Permissive' effects of glucocorticoids function to 'permit' other hormones to accomplish their function at a normal level, and are observed primarily in the resting state and may span the resting and stress states. The permissive role of glucocorticoids is crucial for maintenance of homeostasis at the basal state. 'Regulatory' effects of glucocorticoids are exerted only by stress-induced levels of these hormones.

Johnson and co-workers refer to Munck *et al.* (1984), who 'hypothesized that the regulatory effects of stress-related elevations of glucocorticoids may be necessary to prevent over-reaction of the central nervous, immune and other systems, which, if unchecked, may lead to injury'. They go on to emphasize the carefully controlled regulation of the system (p. 118):

> Several closed feedback mechanisms regulate the secretion of glucocorticoids. There is a major feedback loop in the hypothalamic–pituitary axis. Thus, circulating glucocorticoids act on the pituitary directly to inhibit ACTH secretion, as well as on the hypothalamus to suppress secretion of CRH. Additional feedback loops include the inhibitory effect of ACTH, β-endorphin and CRH on the hypothalamic CRH neurons. These mechanisms enable the organism to maintain a stable blood level of glucocorticoids at all times, while simultaneously providing an emergency override, via the central nervous system, to respond to stressors.

The term 'stable' means 'within the normal limits'; like many other hormones, CRH, ACTH and glucocorticosteroids are secreted in an episodic fashion. Secretory episodes are unevenly distributed over the 24-hour period (circadian variation). Furthermore, ACTH and glucocorticosteroids are secreted in a pulsatile fashion: the 24-hour sinusoidal waveform contains many small peaks (ultradian variation, lasting less than one day) (Ixart *et al.*, 1987).

Release of catecholamines (adrenaline and noradrenaline) depends on the autonomic nervous system, which is the involuntary nervous system that controls vegetative functions such as the digestive system, the cardiovascular system, respiration and thermoregulation. It consists of the (ortho)sympathetic and the parasympathetic nervous systems which have opposing effects. Activation of the sympathetic inhibits digestive functions and stimulates cardiac output, whereas the parasympathetic does the opposite. Plasma noradrenaline is principally released by the nerve endings of the sympathetic nervous system and, to a lesser extent, the adrenal medulla, which is a specialized end organ of the sympathetic system. In contrast, adrenaline is almost exclusively secreted by the adrenal medulla.

Stress influences the balance between the sympathetic and parasympathetic systems; depending on the situation, the type of stressor and the individual, the relative activity of either the sympathetic or parasympathetic will be increased. This new balance determines the change in heart rate; stress may either increase (tachycardia) or decrease (bradycardia) heart rate. When stress is prolonged, the sympathetic input usually outweighs the parasympathetic input; consequently, an initial bradycardia often returns to basal levels or becomes a tachycardia. In any case, a stress-induced prolonged increase in heart rate is maintained mainly by increased plasma adrenaline secreted by the adrenals. The exact mechanisms that underlie the control of cardiac output and the release of adrenaline from the adrenal medulla are still to be elucidated.

10.1.2. History

At the beginning of the century, Cannon (1914) demonstrated that the sympatho-adrenal ('sympathetic adrenal medulla') system is necessary to meet external challenges. He showed that physical and emotional disturbances trigger the same physiological responses. The important role of the glucocorticosteroids in the stress response was first recognized by Selye (1932), who found that many different noxious stimuli provoke a rise in plasma corticosterone levels in rats. Partly in contrast to Cannon's earlier statement, Selye postulated that glucocorticosteroids are the prime mediators of the physiological response that helps the animal adapt to stress. Because of the apparent generality of the physiological response, he formulated his classic theory of the General Adaptation Syndrome (GAS). Later, Selye's theory was criticized by Mason (1974) because it was predominantly concerned with physical stressors, and ignored the psychological dimension of stress. Mason pointed out that most of Selye's experiments incorporated psychological stressors that explained the similarity of the physiological responses he observed. There is now much evidence showing the importance of subjective assessment by the animal of a given stressor. For example, Weiss (1970, 1971) found that rats that could control and/or predict the occurrence of an electric shock showed less pronounced stress responses than counterparts with no control or warning signal. Current research generally acknowledges that the animal's appraisal of the stress is a major determinant of the stress response. Furthermore, both the sympatho-adrenal and hypothalamo–pituitary–adrenal response are important measures of the stress response.

10.2. Effects of Acute Stress

10.2.1. Hypothalamo–pituitary–adrenal axis

Domestic animals are often subjected to stressful procedures. For example, it is common to dehorn young cattle, which involves capture, restraint in a crush and removing the hornbuds, usually by burning. The animals resist strongly throughout the procedure. To investigate stress caused by dehorning, Wohlt *et al.* (1994) measured plasma cortisol responses to this procedure in 4–5-week-old Holstein calves. The main objective was to compare the amount of stress caused by two different electrical instruments; a conventional dehorner requiring application for 1 to 2 min, and a recently developed dehorner that within milliseconds heats to 816°C and needs to be applied for only 10 s. The authors removed the first and second hornbud on two different days, with one day in between. Using a balanced design, they examined the effect of the successive dehornings, as well as differences between removal of the left and right hornbud. Dehorning caused an increase in plasma cortisol for one hour, reaching a maximum 15 min after dehorning. The increase was greater on the second occasion (a fivefold increase) than on the first (fourfold). There was a significant difference between the left and the right hornbud, with a smaller cortisol increase when the right hornbud was removed than when the left one was removed. There was no difference in cortisol response with respect to use of the different dehorning instruments.

The increase in plasma cortisol in response to dehorning suggests that the procedure was aversive to the calves. Other observations may help to assess the degree of aversiveness. An interesting observation is the higher response during the second dehorning, compared to the first. Research on laboratory animals has shown that reaction to repeated stressors depends on a number of factors, such as intensity, duration, number of repetitions, and frequency of the application (Natelson *et al.*, 1988). With less intensive stressors, the response decreases upon repeated exposure, whereas with more intensive or painful stressors, the stress reaction increases upon repeated exposure (Konarsky *et al.*, 1990; Pitman *et al.*, 1990). The increased response to the second dehorning observed by Wohlt *et al.* may indicate that the dehorning procedure was a severe stressor, probably because of the pain that accompanies the burning of the hornbud. Such severe pain may also explain the lack of difference in cortisol response between the use of the two different dehorning instruments. The difference in response between dehorning of the left and right hornbud suggests a lateralization in pain receptivity, a phenomenon also observed in humans (Bryden, 1982).

Wohlt *et al.*'s (1994) experiment included a control treatment where the calves were separated from their conspecifics, handled, and physically restrained in a crush, but not dehorned. The control treatment was accompanied by a two-fold increase in cortisol that also lasted one hour. These results show that part of the effects of the dehorning procedure was simply due to the handling and isolation of the calves. It is obvious from the extent of the different cortisol responses, however, that the dehorning procedure was more stressful than the handling and the restraint.

Measurements of cortisol are valuable in stress research, not only for the ease of the technique, but also because cortisol shows a graduated response, depending on the severity of the stressor (Kvetnansky *et al.*, 1984), as is demonstrated by the study of dehorning. Comparing the cortisol increase of a group of animals subjected to a series of stressors can be a useful means to assess their aversiveness. Parrott *et al.* (1988, p. 382) compared the response of castrated rams to several acute stressors. In their experiment:

> The control procedure involved momentarily holding one of the free sheep in the communal pen for the purpose of blood collection. Restraint was applied by suspending an animal in a canvas sling in a corner of the pen. Isolation was achieved by carrying a sheep to a pen in a nearby small hut.

Blood was collected by jugular venipuncture. Two samples were obtained during the pre-treatment period (–60 and 0 min). The treatments were imposed at 0 min, and subsequent sampling took place at 5, 15, 30, 60 and 120 min. The results showed that plasma cortisol levels at –60 and 0 min were similar and did not differ between treatments. Levels tended to rise subsequently for all treatments. In the control animals plasma cortisol was increased at 5, 15 and 30 min (Fig. 10.1). In the animals subjected to restraint and isolation, the overall increment in cortisol was higher than during the control conditions, with the most pronounced effects during the isolation treatment. The results need to be interpreted with care. The interval between the first and second sample was 60 min, whereas between the second and third sample it was 5 min. The higher cortisol levels in the third than in the second sample in the control conditions could therefore be explained by stress induced by the second sampling. This elevation was transient, lasting only 30 min. These results are of interest, because they show that different stressors elicit cortisol responses of different amplitudes and because they show that plasma cortisol can show a rapid and transient increase. Secretion of glucocorticosteroids by the adrenal cortex may be a relatively slow process and, depending on the species and duration of the stressor, maximal values are often reached only 20 to 90 min after application of the stressor (von Borell and Ladewig, 1992; Rushen *et al.*, 1993b; Janssens *et al.*, 1995). Other studies, however, have found more rapid changes. Von Borell and Ladewig (1992) found in pigs that cortisol levels doubled 10 min after intravenous administration of ACTH. Similar rapid changes occur in rats and cattle after exposure to a stressor (Nakao *et al.*, 1994; Rots *et al.*, 1995).

Stress factors must be studied individually, in order to assess the contribution of each to the overall stress response. Parrott *et al.* (1988) separated different sources of stress: suspension in the canvas sling took place in a corner of the home pen, thus avoiding additional stressors induced by isolation or exposure to a novel environment. In contrast, isolation was achieved by carrying the animal to another arena, thereby possibly introducing additional

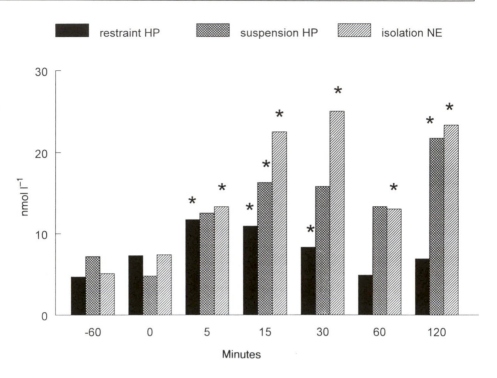

Fig. 10.1. Plasma cortisol responses to human restraint in the home pen (HP), to suspension in the home pen and to isolation in a novel environment (NE). The data show that hormonal responses depend on the type of stressor. Comparisons were made between average pre-treatment levels and individual post-treatment levels, using a two-tailed paired t-test (*= $P < 0.05$). Modified after Parrott *et al.*, 1988.

stress due to handling, transport and an unfamiliar environment. Such effects may have contributed to the stronger cortisol increase during the latter treatment compared to the suspension.

Measurements of plasma cortisol may help to improve husbandry procedures by avoiding unnecessary stress. Work by Nakao *et al.* (1994) has shown that the animal's physiological and motivational state may influence its perception of the aversiveness of certain procedures. Vaginoscopy was followed by an increase in cortisol only when adult Holstein-Friesian cows were in the luteal phase of the reproductive cycle, not when they were in oestrus. On the other hand, rectal palpation caused a 1.5-fold increase lasting 25 min, independently of the reproductive cycle. Artificial insemination (AI) caused a similar increase, attributed to the effects of accompanying rectal palpation. Given that stress can reduce fecundity (Dobson and Smith, 1995), it may be advisable to avoid rectal palpation during AI.

10.2.2. Sympatho-adrenal system

Measurements of heart rate and of plasma (nor)adrenaline have also been used to estimate stress caused by practical husbandry procedures. Lay and co-workers (1992) compared the effect of hot-iron and freeze branding of 8-month-old calves on heart rate and plasma catecholamine. Animals were captured and restrained in a crush for 5 min prior to branding. Control conditions consisted of handling, restraining and sham-branding the animals. Analysis of the results showed that heart rate varied over time for all treatments. The authors report (p. 333) that 'All calves' heart rates decreased below the pre-branding mean by 10 min post-branding.' During the first 6 min after introduction into the crush, heart rate varied between 100 and 110 beats min^{-1}. Thereafter, heart rate was lower, varying between 90 and 100 beats min^{-1}. They found no differences in heart rate between treatment and control groups, and, as they state, this can at least partially be due to the high initial heart rates of the animals. However, hot-iron branding provoked an increase in plasma adrenaline within 30 s after branding which lasted for less than 30 s. The transient increase probably reflects the stress due to pain caused by the branding. Closer inspection of the data reveals that this transient rise in adrenaline was accompanied by a non-significant increase in heart rate. Unfortunately, the authors do not report any analysis of correlations between adrenaline levels and heart rate. It is possible that there was also an effect of freeze branding, as the authors state (p. 333): 'At 0.5 min post-branding, heart rate of freeze branded and hot-iron branded calves tended to be higher than that of sham-branded calves.' Both treatment and control situations were accompanied by an increase in plasma noradrenaline levels, but no differences were found between the groups. Whereas adrenaline often reflects psychological stress, noradrenaline is more closely correlated with the physical activity of the animal (Henry and Stephens, 1977; Scheurink et al., 1989). The overall increase in noradrenaline is, therefore, likely to be caused by struggling.

The combined exposure to handling, restraint and social isolation may have caused a rise in heart rate which masks the putative effects of branding. The effect on heart rate of social isolation without influence of other stressors has been elegantly tested by Hopster and Blokhuis (1994) in dairy cows. By removing the social group, except for the experimental animal, from the home pen, they avoided all additional influences of handling and exposure to an unfamiliar environment. Hopster and Blokhuis found that basal heart rate (76–105 beats per min) showed a 30 to 116% increase when the social group was removed. Similar experiments on domestic chicks, with glucocorticosteroids as a measure of stress, gave comparable results (Jones and Harvey, 1987).

10.3. Effects of Chronic Stress

Domestic and zoo animals are often exposed to long-term stress and its effects on a variety of physiological variables have been extensively investigated. Generally, overall plasma glucocorticoid and catecholamine concentrations rise only briefly. For example, the effect of initial tethering on heart rate in pigs lasts only for several hours (personal observations by Schouten and Rushen). Initial tethering of bulls and female pigs caused an overall increase in basal plasma cortisol that lasted only a few days (Becker *et al.*, 1984; Ladewig and Smidt, 1989). Some physiological changes may last longer. Janssens *et al.* (1995) found that after 2 months' tethering, pigs showed similar overall basal cortisol levels to their loose-housed counterparts. However, tethered pigs showed higher levels in the evening than controls, leading to a flattening of the circadian rhythm of cortisol secretion. The difference had disappeared after 3 months of tethering. Some scientists (Becker *et al.*, 1984, 1989) interpret such physiological adaptation in terms of psychological adaptation to the aversive conditions. However, others have shown that the physiological adaptation is only apparent. As discussed below, the functioning of the controlling systems may change due to long-term stress.

10.3.1. Hypothalamo–pituitary–adrenal axis

The responsiveness of the adrenal cortex can be tested by measuring its secretion of glucocorticoids in response to ACTH administration. After repeated intravenous administration of ACTH the glucocorticoid response to the dose increases over time (Johnson *et al.*, 1992), indicating an increased capacity of the adrenal cortex to secrete glucocorticosteroids. Chronic stress may have a similar effect. The cortisol response to ACTH administration was significantly higher in pigs after tethering for three or four months than before (Janssens *et al.*, 1995). Changes in the functioning of the HPA axis also become evident when long-term stressed animals are subjected to an acute unfamiliar stressor. Janssens *et al.* (1995) subjected female pigs to 15 min of restraint by a rope noose applied to the upper jaw to immobilize them (nose-sling). Pigs tethered and fed restrictively for 11 weeks showed a stronger cortisol response to the test than loose-housed controls. Similar results have been obtained for leopards in a zoo: changing from a regular to a randomized feeding schedule led to an increase in glucocorticoid output (Carlstead *et al.*, 1993).

Increased adrenocortical responsiveness after long-term housing stress is not found in all cases. Ladewig and Smidt (1989), when comparing the adrenocortical response of bulls kept free on deep straw and bulls kept tethered for 5 weeks, observed that tethered bulls had a lower adrenocortical response to ACTH. The direction of the changes in adrenocortical responsiveness due to chronic stress may depend on factors such as sex, species or ontogenetic aspects. An alternative explanation is also possible. Ladewig and Smidt reported that tethered bulls, although lying down for the same total duration each day, changed position half as often, probably because being tethered made it more difficult. In large animals, changing position is an energy demanding activity. The higher energy expenditure in loose-housed bulls may have led to a more reactive HPA axis, resulting from frequently changing demands. In this case, the difference in adrenocortical responsiveness is unrelated to the physiological adaptation of the tethered bulls.

It is of interest to know whether changes occur also at the pituitary level. Such changes can be tested pharmacologically by injecting CRH into the ventricles of the brain and by measuring the ACTH response. Due to technical difficulties, little information is available for larger animals at present. However, when subjecting tethered and loose-housed pigs to acute stress, Janssens *et al.* (1995) found that, while the cortisol response did not differ between groups, tethered pigs showed a reduced ACTH response, indicating that changes may have occurred at hypothalamo–pituitary level.

10.3.2. Sympatho-adrenal system

Research on humans and monkeys suggests that chronic stress may facilitate cardiovascular disease (Sapolsky, 1990; Sundin *et al.*, 1995). Other pathological conditions may occur in humans and animals, such as immune suppression, ulceration of the digestive tract and reduced growth (Weiss, 1970, 1971; Morrow-Tesch *et al.*, 1994; Ekkel *et al.*, 1995). The sympatho-adrenal system plays an important role in these stress-induced pathologies. As in the case of the activated HPA axis, chronic stress is not accompanied by changes in easily measurable variables from the sympatho-adrenal system, such as heart rate and plasma catecholamine. However, there is evidence that the control of cardiac function may change due to chronic stress. Schouten *et al.* (1991) and Schouten and Rushen (1993), comparing heart rates of pigs tethered for 1, 2 or 6–8 months with loose-housed controls, found no effect of housing on basal heart rate, but a significant effect on heart rate after food delivery. Tethered pigs showed a greater increase in heart rate in response to feeding than loose-housed pigs, which increased with duration of tethering. These observations suggest a change in the balance of sympathetic and parasympathetic activity, apparent during challenge. Schouten *et al.* (1991) subsequently studied the relative inputs of the sympathetic and parasympathic systems, by blocking the sympathetic with the β-adrenergic receptor blocker, carazolol. Administration of carazolol reduced the basal, pre-feeding heart rate in all treatment groups, but the effect was more pronounced in tethered than in loose-housed pigs. Post-feeding heart rate was also much more reduced in tethered than in loose-housed pigs. Furthermore, the effects of the blocker increased with increasing duration of tethering (Fig. 10.2). Thus, the pre-feeding effects show that even under non-challenging conditions, tethered pigs have a higher sympathetic activation than loose-housed pigs. The post-feeding effects show that the greater increase in heart rate after feeding in tethered pigs is primarily due to an increase in sympathetic activation. The lack of effect of housing condition on basal heart rate indicates that the increased sympathetic activation was counterbalanced by an increased parasympathetic activation. Food delivery is a major source of arousal in tethered pigs (Terlouw *et al.*, 1991, 1993) and the more pronounced effects of carazolol on heart rate after rather than before feeding reflect an over-reactivity of the sympathetic to food delivery. The housing-induced differences in heart rate regulation appear not to be related to poor physical condition due to lack of exercise, because the basal heart rate would also have been affected. Furthermore, when the tethered sows were released and loose-housed, the differences persisted, albeit to a lesser degree.

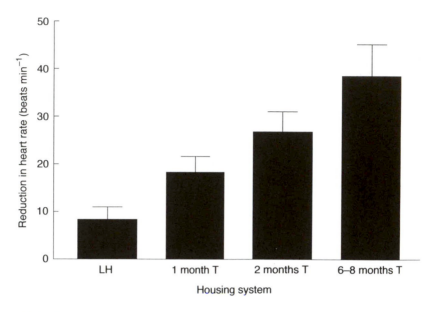

Fig. 10.2. Reduction in post-feeding heart rate calculated by subtracting heart rate following carazolol injection from heart rate following saline injections in sows loose-housed for 1 month (LH) or tethered (T) for 1, 2 or 6–8 months. The data show that the sympathetic activation increases with time since tethering. After Schouten *et al.*, 1991.

The effects of chronic intermittent stress on adrenal medulla functioning have been studied in laboratory animals (Kvetnansky *et al.*, 1984; de Boer *et al.*, 1990). As Johnson *et al.* (1992, p. 120) describe:

> Chronic intermittent stress is associated with changes in the adrenal medulla including increased activity of enzymes involved in catecholamine biosynthesis, increased rates of synthesis and elevated tissue concentrations of catecholamines. Chronic intermittent stressors appear to affect catecholamine release during subsequent exposures as a function of the familiarity, strength and predictability of the stressor. Thus, exposure to a homotypic (familiar) mild and predictable stressor in a chronic intermittent fashion results in a reduced sympathetic, sympathomedullary response over time. In contrast, following chronic intermittent stress, exposure to an acute heterotypic (novel) stressor results in an enhanced sympathetic, sympathomedullary response.

The changes in sympathetic/parasympathetic control on heart rate in long-term tethered pigs demonstrated by Schouten *et al.* (1991) show that long-term stress may influence sympatho-adrenal functioning in this species, too.

10.4. Combined Measurements

10.4.1. Hypothalamo–pituitary–adrenal axis and sympatho-adrenal system

The HPA and sympatho-adrenal axes are not independent; on the contrary, the two systems influence each other, both centrally and peripherally. At the central level, CRH, secreted by the hypothalamus, not only stimulates the release of ACTH from the pituitary, but also the activity of target neurons in the brain, for instance in the *locus coeruleus* (Valentino *et al.*, 1986), which plays a major role in the control of the activity of the sympatho-adrenal system. Furthermore, adrenaline released from the adrenal medulla stimulates secretion of ACTH by the pituitary, thus amplifying the initial response of the HPA axis. Although ACTH is the most important factor in the control of glucocorticoid secretion from the adrenal cortex, there is increasing evidence that sympathetic activation enhances the sensitivity of the adrenal cortex to ACTH (Charlton, 1990; Delbende *et al.*, 1992). Possibly through a stimulation of the blood flow through the adrenal gland (van Oers *et al.*, 1992) the reverse effects also occur: glucocorticosteroids diffuse to the adrenal medulla, where they increase the adrenaline : noradrenaline ratio.

When an animal is stressed, release of glucocorticosteroids is relatively slow, because it is mediated by blood factors, whereas increases in heart rate and release of adrenaline and noradrenaline take place within seconds, because they are under direct nervous control of the autonomic nervous system. This is illustrated by the work of Niezgoda *et al.* (1993), who studied simultaneously the response of the sympatho-adrenal and HPA axes to short-term stress in sheep. Sheep with jugular catheters were subjected to a 30-min restraint stress applied by a human, and blood samples were taken 30 min before, and 2, 5, 15 and 30 min after the start of the restraint. Blood samples were also collected from unrestrained control animals. The controls showed no fluctuations in plasma catecholamine or cortisol. In restrained sheep, adrenaline and noradrenaline increased immediately, whereas plasma cortisol started to rise after 5 min, and were clearly elevated only 15 min after the start of the restraint (Fig. 10.3).

10.4.2. Other indicators of stress

Measurements of hormones other than those described above can be used to determine stress responsiveness. A useful hormone is prolactin, which is secreted into the general blood circulation by the median eminence of the hypothalamus. In rats, prolactin rises in response to various stressors (Kant *et al.*, 1983; Dantzer *et al.*, 1988). Parrott *et al.* (1994) subjected sheep to a number of different stressors and measured prolactin, cortisol and catecholamine responses. The treatments consisted of capture and brief restraint in the home pen (control); 60 min standing in a pen filled every day with water to a depth of 25 cm with another animal visible in an adjacent pen; 60 min standing with a companion sheep in the oscillating pen of a transport simulator; and 60 min solitary confinement in a pen inside a hut away from the barn. They found different response patterns for the different treatments. Plasma cortisol

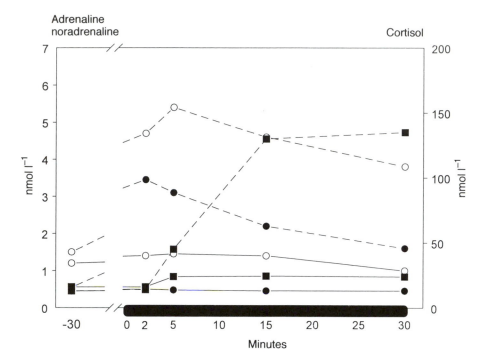

Fig. 10.3. Plasma adrenaline (filled circles), noradrenaline (open circles) and cortisol (squares) during 30 min of restraint (0–30 min dotted lines) or during control conditions (solid lines) in sheep. The data show that the sympatho-adrenal axis responds much faster than the hypothalamo–pituitary–adrenal axis. After Niezgoda *et al.*, 1993.

rose 2- to 3-fold in response to all treatments, apart from the control treatment, reaching a maximal level between 20 and 30 min after start of application of the stressor. In contrast, isolation was the only stressor to influence noradrenaline secretion, with a (non-significant) 1.5-fold increase. Plasma adrenaline increased in response to transport simulation and isolation, peaking 10 min after the onset of the stressor (4.5-fold for transport and 3.5-fold for isolation). Water stress was accompanied by a transient, but significant 2-fold increase in adrenaline, also reaching a maximum after 10 min. Prolactin was influenced by transport simulation, with a 2-fold increase between 10 and 20 min. Prolactin levels decreased slightly during water stress, perhaps due to cold-induced inhibition. The authors conclude (p. 238):

> The results of this short study suggest that physical stress of transport simulation had a greater effect on cortisol, prolactin and adrenaline release than any of the other treatments, whereas the only procedure affecting noradrenaline concentrations was the psychological stress of isolation.

The latter observation is unusual, because plasma noradrenaline concentrations are assumed to reflect changes in physical activity (Henry and

Stephens, 1977; Scheurink *et al.*, 1989). The different qualitative and quantitative characteristics of the stressors are reflected in different hormonal patterns.

In pigs, prolactin increases in response to acute restraint (Klemcke *et al.*, 1987). The effect of repeated application of a painful stressor on prolactin and other hormones has also been assessed in pigs (Rushen *et al.*, 1993b). Pigs were subjected to 15-min restraint with a nose-sling, applied daily over 9 days. Blood samples were taken every 15 min, starting 15 min before the restraint, on the 1st and 9th day of the experiment. When stressors are painful, habituation does not occur. Accordingly, HPA responses did not differ between the 1st and 9th restraint: initial and final restraint led to a maximal 10-fold increase in plasma ACTH at 15 min and a 4-fold increase in plasma cortisol at 30 min. Both hormones reached basal levels 85 min after the beginning of the restraint. Prolactin changes were similar to cortisol changes but less pronounced: a 2-fold increase 30 min after the beginning of the restraint reached basal levels at 85 min. Growth hormone, which changes during chronic stress in several species, including laboratory animals (Kant *et al.*, 1983), did not show clear responses to restraint in the study of Rushen *et al.*, because of great individual variation. Thus, while plasma prolactin measurements may distinguish between qualitative aspects of different stressors, growth hormone may be less suitable, at least in pigs.

Psychological stress may cause other physiological changes. Stress-induced hyperthermia, a rise in body temperature, may be induced by various stressors, such as mild restraint in rats (Terlouw *et al.*, 1996), and the anticipation of a school exam (Marazziti *et al.*, 1992) in humans. In rats stress-induced hyperthermia is not merely a secondary effect of stress-induced physiological changes, rather, it reflects activation of the immune system (Kluger *et al.*, 1987). At present, it is not known whether stress-induced hyperthermia occurs in farm animals. There are some indications, however, suggesting that the rise in body temperature in farm animals observed during handling and transport is, at least partially, a stress response. Observations show that the hyperthermic response is more pronounced in animals that have an increased stress reaction, in terms of cortisol and heart rate, and thus, that this response may be part of the stress reaction (Terlouw *et al.*, 1994). However, this hypothesis needs to be confirmed by more detailed studies.

Other immune functions may show reduced responsiveness as a result of stress. For example, lambs showed reduced lymphocyte responses to antigen challenge after restraint (Coppinger *et al.*, 1991; Minton *et al.*, 1992). While immune suppression was apparent after 6 hours of restraint, the effect became more pronounced after repeated restraint over 3 consecutive days. Similarly, pigs subjected to 5 min of nose-sling stress showed decreased lymphocyte counts (Dubreuil *et al.*, 1993), mixing and transporting of pigs was accompanied by a reduced immunoresponse to an intradermal injection of the antigen phytomagglutinin (Ekkel *et al.*, 1995) and pigs subjected to long-term social stress showed a reduced immunoresponse to pokeweed mitogen (Morrow-Tesch *et al.*, 1994). The effects of stress on immunoreactivity are not always unidirectional; depending on the duration and the intensity of the stress an increase, rather than a decrease of immunoreactivity may be found (Dubreuil *et al.*, 1993).

Despite extensive studies, the exact mechanisms underlying the immuno-suppressive effects of stress are still not known. It is known that glucocorti-costeroids may cause immunosuppression and at least part of the suppressive effects of stress on immunoresponsiveness may be due to increased activity of the HPA axis (Munck *et al.*, 1984). Several studies on farm animals are in accordance with this hypothesis. Thus, Ekkel and co-workers (1995) showed that pigs with a stress-induced reduction in immune functioning had higher saliva cortisol levels. However, Minton and co-workers (1995, p. 812) have shown that: 'Increased plasma cortisol measured during restraint and isolation stress cannot alone account for reduced lymphocyte proliferative responses'. Lambs were subjected to one of three treatments: restraint and isolation stress, in-fusion with cortisol to increase plasma cortisol levels similar to those in lambs subjected to restraint and isolation stress, and control. While lymphocyte re-sponses to phytomagglutinin and other antigens were lower in stressed than control lambs, no differences were found between control and cortisol injected lambs. At least in this species, stress-induced immunosuppression appears to depend on other mechanisms.

Some types of stress may induce responses that are strongly influenced by the physical or physiological consequences of these stressors. Food deprivation may be accompanied by physiological changes related to the altered meta-bolism, including plasma cortisol, free fatty acids, glucose and β-hydroxy-butyrate (Parrott and Misson 1989; Warriss *et al.*, 1989; Knowles *et al.*, 1994). The effects of water deprivation can be assessed by vasopressin (which regulates water metabolism), plasma osmolality and plasma hematocrit values. Muscle fatigue may be assessed by measuring plasma creatine phosphokinase, an enzyme which is involved in muscle metabolism (Komulainen *et al.*, 1995). Stress may affect many blood plasma characteristics. For example, 5 min of nose-sling stress in pigs was accompanied by increases in plasma sodium, pot-assium, calcium, phosphorus, cholesterol and glucose, and a decrease in plasma free fatty acids (Dubreuil *et al.*, 1993). Stress may also influence the partial pressure of O_2 and CO_2 in the blood owing to effects of the sympathetic nervous system on respiratory frequency, depth of inspiration, and on the release of red blood cells from the spleen into the bloodstream (Mormède, 1988; Dubreuil *et al.*, 1990). Some of the observed changes are due to the psychological component and some to the physical component of a stress response. Scheurink *et al.* (1989) found that when rats swam for the first time, plasma adrenaline increased more than after habituation to swimming. Noradrenaline showed the opposite effect: rats accustomed to the procedure showed a greater increase than rats swimming for the first time.

Finally, indirect measurements may be used to assess stress. For example, pigs reared under specific stress-free conditions (avoiding mixing and transport-ing) had increased average daily weight gains (Ekkel *et al.*, 1995).

10.5. Individual Differences

Differences between individuals in their behavioural and physiological responsiveness to aversive situations appear to be consistent; that is, individual responses to different stressful situations are correlated (Lyons and Price, 1986;
Lawrence *et al.*, 1991). Consistent individual differences have been observed
in laboratory animals, goats and pigs (Lyons and Price, 1986; Bohus *et al.*,
1987; Lawrence *et al.*, 1991). Pigs differ consistently in their cortisol response to ACTH challenge, indicating variable sensitivity of the adrenal cortex
(Hennessy *et al.*, 1988; von Borell and Ladewig, 1992; Zhang *et al.*, 1992).
Von Borell and Ladewig (1992) determined behavioural activity in the home
pen, open-field behaviour and the adrenocortical response to ACTH in male
pigs, aged 10 to 30 weeks. Individual variation in behavioural responses was
large: for example, at the age of 18 weeks, the proportion of time that individuals were active in the home pen varied between 30.2 and 60.4%. Similarly
large individual variation was found for ACTH challenge; at the age of 16 weeks,
cortisol responses to ACTH varied between 82.8 and 192.8 ng ml^{-1}. Individuals remained consistent in their behavioural and physiological responses
when subjected repeatedly to the same test, showing that differences were due
to basic individual characteristics that remained stable over time. The physiological and behavioural responses were correlated: pigs with high ACTH
responsiveness showed more locomotion and vocalized more during the
open-field test and were less active in their home pen.

The mechanisms underlying the above correlations are still to be elucidated.
In their classic review, Henry and Stephens (1977) distinguish two categories
of behavioural responses to stress: the fight/flight response, where the animal
responds actively, and the conservation/withdrawal response, where it immobilizes. These two categories are accompanied by different physiological profiles.
The fight/flight response is characterized by relatively high sympatho-adrenal
reactivity and relatively low HPA reactivity. In contrast, the conservation/
withdrawal response is characterized by relatively high HPA-reactivity and
relatively low sympatho-adrenal reactivity.

The work by Henry and Stephens was predominantly on laboratory
animals and humans. Their hypothesis may be generalized to other species;
Dantzer and co-workers (1980) found a negative correlation between plasma
cortisol and behavioural activation during extinction sessions of panel pressing
for food in young pigs. Von Borell and Ladewig's (1992) findings in pigs are,
however, contradictory to Henry and Stephens' model, because they found a
positive, rather than a negative, correlation between increased HPA reactivity
and behavioural activation during stress. Research is in progress to elucidate
further the relationship between behavioural and physiological individual differences in pigs (Mendl *et al.*, 1992; Hessing *et al.*, 1994a).

Individual differences in behaviour are related to characteristics of the central nervous system. For example, Terlouw *et al.* (1992) injected female pigs
with amphetamine, which stimulates the central dopaminergic systems, resulting in behavioural activation. By measuring the behavioural response to
amphetamine, they obtained a measure of the sensitivity of the dopaminergic

systems. The pigs were then tethered and fed restrictively for 50 days. Under these conditions, pigs often develop stereotypic activities, consisting of excessive drinking and persistent chewing on the tether chain, but showing large individual differences (Terlouw *et al.*, 1991). Those pigs that were less responsive to amphetamine tended to develop more stereotypic activities when tethered and fed restrictively, indicating that the development of stereotypic activities may be related to the sensitivity of central dopaminergic systems. Behavioural differences in mice are similarly correlated with central dopaminergic sensitivity (Benus, 1988). Other work on laboratory animals and pigs has shown that individual differences in behavioural responsiveness are related to differences in the sympathetic/parasympathetic balance, with behaviourally active animals showing a predominantly tachycardiac response when exposed to acute stress (Bohus *et al.*, 1987; Hessing *et al.*, 1994a). These observations suggest that individual differences in behavioural and physiological responsiveness to stress originate at least partially from differences at the central level.

10.6. Combining Behaviour and Physiology

For accurate interpretation, behavioural and physiological measurements need to be considered together. An animal showing no overt behaviour may simply be resting, or it may be behaviourally inhibited due to high arousal. Similarly, changes in physiological variables, such as an increase in heart rate, may be due to stress, or may be provoked by supposedly pleasant events, such as food delivery and sexual activity (Bloom *et al.*, 1975). An integrated approach is needed to study potential sources of stress and their impact on animal welfare. The relatively recent approach of combining individual behavioural and physiological characteristics in the analysis is a helpful advance. It enables us to study individual strategies in stress responses and adaptation to stress, and contributes to our understanding of the underlying mechanisms.

10.7. Conclusions

- Acute stress affects a large range of physiological variables. Stress responses usually measured are: (i) plasma glucocorticosteroids, which reflect the activity of the hypothalamo–pituitary–adrenal axis; and (ii) plasma adrenaline and noradrenaline, and heart rate, which reflect the activity of the sympatho-adrenomedullary system.
- Chronic stress is generally not measurable by changes in the hypothalamo–pituitary–adrenal axis or in the sympatho-adrenomedullary system, due to efficient feedback mechanisms. Chronic stress may affect the regulation of these variables.
- The physiological stress response depends on the type, the intensity and the duration of the stressor, as well as on the characteristics of the animal.

CHAPTER 11
Preference and motivation testing

David Fraser (University of British Columbia, Canada)
and Lindsay R. Matthews (Ruakura Agricultural Centre,
New Zealand)

Abstract

Since the early 1970s, scientists have used preference tests (tests that require animals to choose between two or more different options or environments) as a means of answering questions about animal welfare. Preference tests have been used to establish animals' preferences for common housing options such as ambient temperature, illumination and preferred types of bedding and flooring; to improve the effectiveness of devices such as loading ramps and nest boxes; and to clarify how strongly animals avoid various aspects of confinement and methods of restraint.

To use preference research to answer questions about animal welfare, three issues need to be addressed. First, we must ensure that experiments do adequately reflect the animals' preferences. The preferences of an animal are likely to vary with the animal's age and experience, the time of day, environmental conditions, and the animal's on-going behaviour; therefore, preference experiments must be comprehensive enough to identify the relevant sources of variation. Experiments must also avoid confounding preference with familiarity, and avoid spurious results arising from the use of particular testing procedures and response measures. Second, to draw inferences about animal welfare from preference research requires that we establish how strongly an animal prefers a chosen option, avoids an unpreferred one, or is motivated to perform a certain behaviour (nest-building, exploration) that is prevented in some environments. Various methods to assess preference and motivation strength have been proposed. Third, the environments preferred by an animal will often, but not always, promote its welfare in the sense of health and psychological well-being. However, preferences may not correspond to welfare if the choices fall outside the animals' sensory, cognitive and affective capacities, or if animals are required to choose between short- and long-term benefits.

Future priorities for preference testing include more emphasis on identifying the factors underlying animals' preferences, greater integration of preference research with other indicators of animal well-being, more reliance on the natural history of the species as a source of hypotheses about environmental preferences, and greater use of preference research in the design of animal environments.

This is contribution 96–31 of Agriculture and Agri-Food Canada's Centre for Food and Animal Research

11.1. Introduction

According to legend, Saint Francis of Assisi once approached a fierce wolf that had been terrorizing the Italian town of Gubbio, and offered the animal a choice: rather than continue in its wild ways, the wolf could choose to live within the town walls as a sedate and well-fed citizen. The wolf accepted the latter option and lived happily in the town for some time, but eventually the wolf's wild nature proved hard to reconcile with the choice it had made, and it fled from the town in misery and disgrace (Bruckberger, 1971).

Preference tests are commonly used as a tool in the study of animal welfare. Fundamental to this research is the assumption that animals make choices that are in their own best interests, and that a knowledge of the preferences shown by animals will help us understand and improve their welfare. However, the story of Saint Francis and the wolf suggests that this assumption is not always so straightforward. This chapter reviews the use of preference testing in animal welfare research, and attempts to answer the question raised by the story of Saint Francis and the wolf: under what conditions do the choices made by an animal serve as a reliable guide to its welfare?

11.2. Early Use of Preference Testing

The naturalistic study of animal behaviour is an important precursor to preference testing. The fact that birds perch on branches or wires, and that mice burrow in fields or walls, provides information about the environments that these animals prefer. If collected in a systematic and quantitative way – for example by identifying the sizes of branches that birds do and do not use for perching – such observations can be a starting point for designing animal environments and a source of hypotheses for more controlled preference experiments.

Similarly, traditional laboratory studies of behaviour have provided significant insights into animals' preferences, although such work was often done as basic research on animal motivation. For example, S.A. Barnett and colleagues monitored the movements of rats and mice in a residential maze where food, water, nesting material, and other resources were available in different compartments. The apparatus was used to study how exploration, feeding and other behaviour is influenced by deprivation, genetic differences and different stages of the reproductive cycle (Barnett and McEwan, 1973; Barnett and Smart, 1975; Cowan, 1977). Such methods (Fig. 11.1) are now being applied more specifically to questions about animal welfare (Nicol, 1986; Blom *et al.*, 1992).

Surprisingly, the formal proposal to study animals' environmental preferences as a component of animal welfare research arose from a British parliamentary committee. The ethologist W.H. Thorpe was one of the members of the 'Brambell Committee' formed in the United Kingdom to investigate the welfare of intensively housed farm animals. In his appendix to the committee's report, Thorpe (1965) proposed what became an agenda for using scientific

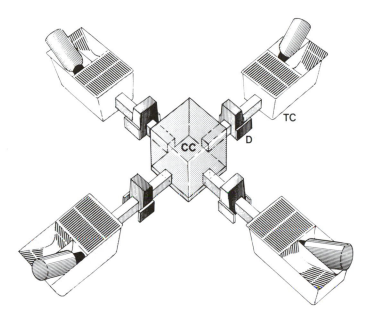

Fig. 11.1. A four-choice housing system for preference tests with mice, as described by Blom *et al.* (1992). The apparatus includes four test cages (TC) radiating from a central cage (CC). Four detector units (D), using red light emitting diodes, record the movement of animals along the passageways leading to the test cages. Behaviour in the cages was also monitored by video recording.

research to resolve animal welfare issues. He mentioned physiological studies of stress, indicators of pain and discomfort, studies of motivation that might be thwarted in confined animals, and research into the cognitive powers of animals. He also mentioned the intriguing possibility of 'asking' animals about their environmental preferences. The example that Thorpe cited was a chance observation:

> In the early part of 1964 a group of African buffalo were captured in a region of Kenya where their natural existence was no longer tolerable or possible, and were taken for release in the Nairobi National Park . . . During the process of transport and preparation for release, they were of course kept in pens or yards much like those in which domestic cattle are kept. When the time came for their release in the new environment, they showed many signs of distaste for it. They would return toward human habitations toward nightfall and try to enter the paddocks where they had been. One even tried to walk through the french windows of the office of the Director of the Kenya National Parks. The natural assumption is that the unfamiliar National Park, reeking of lion, leopard and other dangerous and uncomfortable neighbours, must have seemed a very unfriendly place; far inferior to the luxurious though restricted quarters they had become used to inhabiting!

(Thorpe, 1965, pp. 73–74)

Thorpe concluded that because these animals had experienced a range of living conditions, we could legitimately 'ask' them which they preferred.

Appropriately enough, the first actual experiment using preference testing to resolve a farm animal welfare issue arose from one of the more specific recommendations of the Brambell Committee. The committee had concluded that the flooring materials used for hens in cages were often unsatisfactory. The committee was particularly critical of 'chicken wire' flooring (fine-gauge wire netting of a hexagonal pattern) which, it suggested, 'the bird's foot is not well adapted to grip' (Brambell, 1965, p. 21). Instead, the committee recommended that the cage floor should consist of a heavy-gauge rectangular metal mesh.

To obtain the hens' own view of this recommendation, Hughes and Black (1973) tested the preferences of hens for different types of flooring. They housed hens in cages consisting of two sections, each floored in a different material (Fig. 11.2). They offered various materials in pair-wise choices, and simply observed how much time the birds spent on the different flooring products. The results indicated that the hens had no strong preferences or aversions for the different materials, but their overall preference was for, rather than against, the fine-gauge 'chicken wire' which the Brambell Committee had deemed unsuitable.

Other early preference testing tried to answer broader questions. Dawkins (1977) used preference testing to ask whether hens prefer battery cages to large pens or outdoor runs. In one experiment she gave hens free access to cages and to larger pens for 12 hours, and observed the time that the hens spent in each environment. Perhaps surprisingly, the hens spent considerable time in the cages. She then did a series of trials in a T-maze where turning in one direction caused hens to spend the next 5 minutes in a battery cage, while turning in the other direction led to 5 minutes in an outdoor run. With this procedure, the hens tended to select the outdoor run.

Since these early examples, environmental preference testing and related measures have been used for an impressive variety of purposes in animal welfare research. Simple uses include establishing preferences for ambient temperature (Morrison *et al.*, 1987), for illumination levels (Baldwin and Start, 1985; van den Broek *et al.*, 1995), and for common materials such as types of bedding (Hunter and Houpt, 1989; Blom *et al.*, 1993) and flooring (Marx and Mertz, 1989). The methods have also been used to identify which design features of animal housing and handling equipment are significant to the animals themselves. Such knowledge has allowed more effective design of loading ramps (Phillips *et al.*, 1989), nest boxes (Hurnik *et al.*, 1973), roosts (Muiruri *et al.*, 1990) and other equipment. The methods have also been used to assess how strongly animals seek to avoid noise and vibration (Stephens *et al.*, 1985) and various forms of restraint (Rushen, 1986a).

Despite these successes, preference testing has remained a controversial tool in animal welfare research. In fact, the ink had barely dried on the earliest reports of preference testing when debate broke out over what we can actually conclude from the technique. Initially Duncan (1978a), and subsequently others (e.g. van Rooijen, 1982; Hutson, 1984), provided many criticisms of preference testing, and these stimulated major changes in how preference tests

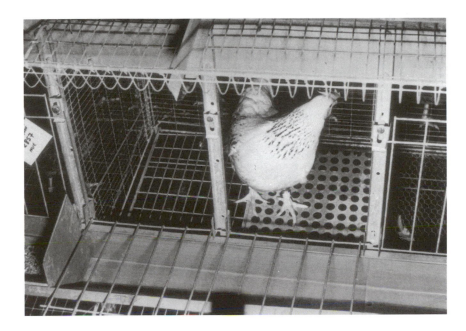

Fig. 11.2. A floor preference experiment with hens conducted by Hughes and Black (1973). The hen is housed in a double cage where she can move freely between two cages floored in different materials. The amount of time spent in each cage was recorded by direct observation using a time sampling method.

are conducted and interpreted (reviewed by Dawkins, 1980, 1983b; Duncan, 1992a; Fraser *et al.*, 1993; Fraser, 1996). Three main issues are involved, two of them mainly methodological and one mainly conceptual, as we describe in sections 11.3 to 11.5 below.

11.3. Ensuring that Experiments Adequately Reflect Animals' Preferences

The first and most basic concern is that preference experiments must accurately capture and identify the animals' true preferences, and this requires attention to several points about how we design and conduct preference research.

11.3.1. Asking suitably complex questions

One criticism of the early preference research is that simple experiments of the type described above underestimate the complexity of animals' environmental preferences. On the surface it might seem reasonable to ask whether pigs prefer pens with straw bedding or pens with bare concrete floors. However, in an initial experiment designed to answer this question (Fraser, 1985), pigs gave very inconsistent results, and further research showed that the pig's degree of preference for straw depends on a variety of factors. Specifically, pigs appear strongly attracted to straw for foraging, but are relatively indifferent to the presence of straw when using a feed or water dispenser; they either prefer or avoid a straw-bedded surface for resting, depending on whether the environment is cool or warm; and preference for straw increases sharply just before parturition when sows normally make nests (see Steiger *et al.*, 1979; Fraser, 1985; Marx and Mertz, 1989; Fraser *et al.*, 1991; Arey, 1992). To deal with this complexity, we need not a simple experiment to determine whether pigs prefer straw, but a more comprehensive study of how the preference is influenced by features of the environment and by the animal's condition and behaviour. Even when the ultimate objective is to decide what kind of housing is best on average for a certain type of animal, research methods that ignore relevant variables are likely to give contradictory results.

Asking more complex questions about animal preferences puts certain demands on experimenters. First, experiments must cover sufficient variation to monitor animals' preferences under a range of fluctuations in both the environment and the animal's condition. Brief tests in a T-maze, as used in the 1970s, have given way to methods such as continuous video or electronic monitoring over periods of days or weeks. For example, van den Broek *et al.* (1995) electronically monitored the movements of gerbils during 48-hour periods in an apparatus that provided different levels of illumination in different compartments; they found that the animals had a clear preference for low light intensities for sleeping but not at other times. Second, experiments should be designed so that individual differences and other variability in the animals' responses can be interpreted. Nicol (1986) noted that when given a range of cage sizes, hens invariably spend some time in the less favoured cages. She proposed that these differences might occur because preferences genuinely vary between individuals or over time, or simply because the birds tend to move about, monitoring the environment periodically, or for other reasons. These different possibilities can be tested with appropriate experimental designs.

11.3.2. Avoiding spurious results

In a given experiment, the particular apparatus or response measure used may have unexpected effects on the preferences that animals show. Fig. 11.3 illustrates a case where different procedures – both designed to test whether sows would prefer a narrow or wide enclosure for farrowing – resulted in contradictory results. Experiments described by Baxter (1991) used four solid, parallel partitions to create three open-ended stalls of different widths in the centre of a large room. Sows housed in this room for farrowing tended to use the narrowest stall more often than the wide ones, and Baxter (1991, p. 12) concluded 'that sows have a significant preference for small farrowing sites.' Phillips *et al.* (1992) used an apparatus consisting of three farrowing stalls radiating from a central hub area. Under these conditions, sows showed a very strong preference for the widest stall ahead of narrower alternatives. Why did the two experiments give contradictory results? The stalls used by Baxter (1991) were enclosed by solid walls on two sides and were open at the ends; therefore, the narrow stalls provided more visual enclosure than the wider ones

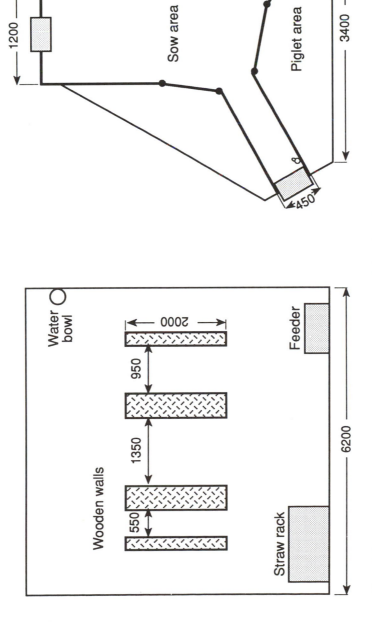

Fig. 11.3. A plan of experimental apparatus designed to test the size of enclosure that sows prefer for farrowing. At left, a large room with four solid, wooden partitions forming three open-ended stalls 550, 950 or 1350 mm wide (from Baxter, 1991). Sows placed in the room could choose to farrow in any stall at will, or in other parts of the room. At right, three farrowing stalls, 450, 750 or 1200 mm wide, radiating from a central area where the sow could exit from one stall and enter another (from Phillips et al., 1992).

and may have been preferred for this reason (see Phillips *et al.*, 1991). Alternatively, the fact that sows could walk straight through the stalls used by Baxter (1991), but had to back out of those used by Phillips *et al.* (1992), might have affected their choice of stall width.

A further concern arises when an animal is required to perform some 'instrumental' or 'operant' response (i.e. a task such as pressing a lever or pecking a key) in order to obtain a reward (see Lagadic, 1989). Certain instrumental responses are appropriate for certain types of reward but not for others (Hinde and Stevenson-Hinde, 1973). For example, it is natural for hens to find food by pecking and to enter a new area by walking. However, in an experiment by Lagadic and Faure (1987), hens were required to peck a key in order to activate a motorized barrier and thus enlarge their cage. In such an experiment, can we trust the result as a true reflection of the hen's motivation to have additional space? Or would alternative responses (e.g. walking rather than pecking) have given different results? The traditional instrumental responses used by experimental psychologists studying motivation for food and water (key-pecking, lever-pressing) often bear little natural relation to the kind of rewards used in research on animal welfare; hence, such methods need to be carefully investigated and validated.

These various examples illustrate the need for 'constructive replication', whereby the main features of an experiment are repeated using somewhat different methods, to ensure that the conclusions are not unduly influenced by a particular experimental apparatus or the manner in which a preference is expressed.

11.3.3. Determining the effects of experience on preferences

Experimental designs also need to take account of the animals' previous experiences (Hughes, 1976b; Petherick *et al.*, 1990). In the simplest cases, animals may show a temporary avoidance of, or attraction to, unfamiliar options, but these temporary reactions must not be used to infer longer-term preferences. For example, Dawkins (1980) noted that hens housed in cages tended, in initial preference trials, to select a cage over an outdoor run, but a few minutes of exposure to the run was enough to overcome this initial reaction.

In other cases, preferences may undergo longer-term change as the animals gain experience of the different options. For example, Phillips *et al.* (1996) housed sows for three weeks in a preference apparatus where the animals could choose to be on different types of flooring. Initially the sows strongly preferred concrete flooring, with which they were familiar, to metal and plastic products. However, this preference waned after several weeks as the animals gained experience of the different alternatives. In this case, the animals may have needed prolonged exposure to the options to become confident in walking and going through their normal postural changes on the different surfaces.

11.4. Assessing the Strength of Animals' Preferences

A preference shown by an animal in a choice experiment may be a weak preference, like a preference for grapes over cherries, or a strong preference, like a preference to live in a house rather than a dungeon. Denying animals access to their preferred options presumably affects welfare more if the preference is strong rather than weak. Thus, in addition to establishing what an animal prefers, we also need some indication of preference strength. As expressed by Dawkins (1983b, p. 23):

> Just because an animal prefers one thing to another or chooses one set of conditions over another, this cannot be taken to mean that it necessarily suffers if it has to make do with its least preferred state . . . What we need is a way of calibrating the various signs of welfare and suffering in a quantitative way.

A related concern arises from the experimental designs used in most preference testing. As noted by Fraser *et al.* (1993, pp. 108–109):

> In most other types of research, the variation attributable to the treatment is compared with extraneous variation, due to individual animals or groups, to location effects, time effects, and so on. In preference tests the different options are usually presented to the same animals at the same time and in almost the same place.

Consequently, preference tests generally minimize extraneous variation, and may detect statistically significant differences even where the magnitude of the preference is small.

In the simplest approach to establishing preference strength, experimenters have tried to determine whether a preferred environment is sufficiently rewarding that an animal will learn to perform some operant or other instrumental response to obtain access to it. For example, having established that hens prefer floors with litter instead of bare wire, Dawkins and Beardsley (1986) tested whether hens would learn to peck a key or break a photobeam to gain access to a cage with litter. If the animal can be trained in such a way, then the motivation to be in that environment must be more than trivial.

Such experiments, however, do not provide a quantitative scale for comparing the strength of different preferences. Consequently, Dawkins (1983a) proposed that we might assess the strength of one preference by 'titrating' it against a second, well understood preference for a reward such as food. In one experiment, Dawkins trained hens to enter two cages from a common choice point. One cage contained litter (to permit dust-bathing) but no food, while the other contained food but no litter. Dawkins then required the hens to choose between the two cages after zero, 3 or 12 hours of food deprivation. The results suggested that the hens' motivation for dust-bathing, under the given conditions, was about as strong as their motivation to eat when food had been withheld for 3 hours.

In a further refinement, Dawkins (1983a, 1990) proposed that motivation testing could be blended with a concept used by economists to assess the importance of a commodity to human consumers:

> Commodities for which a given percentage increase in price results in a decrease in the quantity demanded are said to have *elastic demand* and are sometimes

> called luxuries; those for which a given percentage increase in price results in little change in the quantity demanded are said to have _inelastic demand_ and may be called necessities . . . Elasticity of demand is a key concept for the study of animal welfare . . . because it shows how important different environments or commodities are to the animals themselves.
>
> (Dawkins, 1990, p. 6)

To apply this concept to animals, a commodity such as food can be provided in response to some work ('price') that the animal has to perform, and the 'price' can then be varied experimentally. Commodities that are very important to the animal should show relatively inelastic demand; that is, the animal should work harder and harder to maintain a given level of reward if the reward is very important. By establishing the elasticity of demand, we should be better able to judge the importance that animals attach to food, companionship, bedding, exercise and other features. Technical and other difficulties in using the method have been noted by Dawkins (1990), Dantzer (1990), Mench and Stricklin (1990) and others.

In research to date, various methods have been used to vary the 'price' that animals must pay for commodities. Matthews and Ladewig (1994) used an _operant response_ to vary price. In their experiment pigs were required to press a nose-plate to receive either food or social contact with another pig. As the number of presses needed to obtain food was increased from 1 to 30, the pigs compensated by pressing more and more, and thus obtained a fairly constant amount of food. When social contact was the reward, the pigs failed to compensate for the increasing price and received fewer rewards. An alternative approach is an _obstruction test_ which requires animals to overcome some obstacle in order to gain access to a reward. Petherick and Rutter (1990) described a computer-controlled push-door that they used to measure the amount of 'work' that hens would expend to obtain food, and Duncan and Hughes (1988) used a similar method to measure hens' motivation to enter a nest box for laying. The dangers of obtaining spurious results because of artefacts are discussed by Petherick and Rutter (1990). In _limited time tests_, the experimenter increases the price of commodities by reducing the amount of time available to obtain them. For example, Dawkins (1983a) placed hens for several hours per day in an apparatus consisting of one cage furnished with food and water, and a second, adjoining cage containing only litter. She gave the birds 2, 4 or 8 hours in the apparatus, and they had no access to food or litter at other times. When the birds had 8 hours in the apparatus, they spent considerable time with the litter, but when time was limited to 2 hours, the birds reduced the time they spent with litter in order to feed.

Finally, measures of motivation strength can also be applied to situations that animals avoid. For example, Rushen (1986a) used _aversion testing_ to assess the welfare implications of electro-immobilization of sheep. Electro-immobilization involves use of a pulsed, low-voltage current passed through the body to immobilize an animal. Some veterinarians had claimed that the technique reduces the distress that animals experience during restraint for procedures such as shearing. Rushen trained sheep to move along a runway to a pen where they were restrained in various ways with and without electro-immobilization. He showed that over repeated trials, sheep that received the electrical treatment at the end of the runway became more difficult to move along the runway than those that were restrained without electro-immobilization. The usefulness and validity of various behavioural measures of aversion are discussed by Rushen (1986b) and Rutter and Duncan (1991, 1992).

11.5. Clarifying the Link between Preferences and Welfare

Even when we have accurately identified an animal's preferences and assessed their strength, we need to clarify the conceptual issue of how an animal's preferences relate to its welfare. For this, we need to be reasonably clear on what we mean by welfare.

For present purposes, we will consider two key components of animal welfare (see Chapter 2). The first is based on the *subjective experiences* of the animal and involves reasonable freedom from prolonged or intense pain, discomfort, frustration and other unpleasant states, together with positive experiences such as comfort and contentment. The second component is based on the *biological functioning* of the animal and involves freedom from disease, injury, and malnutrition, and other threats to normal health and survival.

Presumably an animal's preferences are closely linked to its subjective experiences at the time of making the choice. For example, we assume that animals will in general seek out environments in which they find comfort, contentment and other positive experiences, and will avoid environments in which they suffer. As noted by Dawkins (1980, p. 91): 'Animals may not be able to talk, but they can vote with their feet and express some of what they are feeling by where they choose to go.'

However, the link between preferred environments and positive subjective experiences may break down if the short-term and longer-term consequences of the choice are in conflict. As Duncan (1978a, p. 198) noted:

> Animals . . . cannot be expected to weigh up the long-term consequences of their decisions as would human beings, and make rational choices accordingly. In fact there is an increasing volume of evidence . . . to show that animals prefer an immediate reward compared to an equal or even larger reward sometime in the future.

Duncan's example involved hens which are given 'trap-nests' in which to lay eggs. After entering a trap-nest, the bird cannot escape until it is released by a handler and thus may remain trapped without food, water and social contact for several hours after oviposition. The fact that hens continue to use the nests does not necessarily mean that they do not mind being held in the trap-nests, nor that their preference for laying in a nest box outweighs their aversion to being restrained. Rather, the hens' behaviour on entering the nest may simply reflect their motivation at the time, and not the future consequences of the action.

The link between preferences and the biological functioning of the animal is perhaps more complex. For an animal of a wild genotype developing and living in an environment similar to that in which the species evolved, we expect natural selection and ontogenic development to produce a set of environmental preferences that promote the health and survival of the individual and its offspring. Exceptions may arise, however, if an artificial environment creates challenges for which the animal's evolution and ontogenic development have failed to prepare it, or if the animal has been genetically altered in relevant ways through selective breeding.

The simplest problems arise if animals are exposed to potential dangers or benefits that are beyond their sensory and affective capacity. Many fish species successfully avoid being harmed by certain aquatic pollutants, such as copper, simply by swimming away from contaminated water (Giattina and Garton, 1983). However, fish generally fail to avoid certain other contaminants, such as phenol, selenium, even at levels that cause serious damage or death (Giattina and Garton, 1983; Hartwell *et al.*, 1989). Presumably the fish never evolved or developed the capacity to detect these contaminants, and in these cases their preferences fail to protect their health.

A similar limitation may occur if a choice requires a level or type of cognitive ability that the animal does not possess. Rats rapidly learn to avoid a poisoned food on the basis of its flavour, but not if colour or pellet size is its distinguishing feature (McFarland, 1985). In this case the rats presumably can detect all the distinguishing stimuli, but do not readily associate symptoms of poisoning with the visual properties of the food.

As these examples show, an animal's preferences will not always promote its welfare in the long term. Perhaps the best safeguard is to base preference research on the types of choices that the species arguably evolved the capacity to make, and that the individual animals are accustomed to making in their normal lives.

11.6. Future Directions for Preference Research

For the future, we propose that preference and motivation research needs to develop in four directions. First, instead of simple, empirical comparisons of different environments or materials, preference research needs to identify the primary factors influencing the preferences that animals show. Two approaches have been used for this purpose (Fraser *et al.*, 1993). In a *multivariable approach*, preferences or preference rankings are established among a large number of options which differ in numerous features, and statistical analysis is used to indicate which features are most closely related to the animals' preferences. For example, Farmer and Christison (1982) established the preferences of young pigs for a variety of flooring products, and also measured many attributes of the products, including the amount of traction they offered, the degree of heat loss through the material, and the abrasiveness of the surface. Statistical analysis then showed that weaned pigs tended to choose high-traction floors, whereas very young piglets chose floors that would not conduct heat away from the body (Christison and Farmer, 1983). Alternatively, in a *serial factor approach*, a series of preference experiments is conducted, each one testing preferences for different levels of a single design feature. For example, Phillips *et al.* (1988) exposed pigs to ramps of different designs. In one experiment, the ramps differed only in slope; in another they differed only in level of illumination; in another they differed in width, and so on. The animals showed clear preferences when the slope and traction of the surface were varied, but they seemed indifferent to variation in other features. By using such methods to identify the primary factors mediating animals' preferences, we have a better chance of extrapolating appropriately beyond the particular range of options tested.

A second challenge will be to integrate preference research with other measures used in animal welfare assessment. In theory, animals kept in environments that they strongly prefer ought to experience less discomfort and frustration, and this should lead to lower levels of stress, and perhaps greater health, longevity and reproduction. However, most preference research to date has been done somewhat in isolation from other types of animal welfare research, and the wider animal welfare impacts of providing animals with preferred environments have been too little studied.

Third, a knowledge of the natural history of a species could be better used to provide guidance for preference research. The environments preferred by sows for farrowing are probably quite similar to the nest sites that sows seek in nature (Phillips *et al.*, 1991). Likewise, features of cage design preferred by laboratory rodents, of perches preferred by birds, or of enrichment devices preferred by captive primates may well resemble the features of such items used by those species or their wild ancestors living in natural environments. Thus, a knowledge of natural history could help investigators identify potentially important variables in advance, and the power of controlled experimentation could then establish the relative importance to the animal of the variables that characterize the environments they use in nature.

A fourth challenge will be to make better use of environmental preference testing in the design of new animal environments. Duncan (1992b) suggested that many 'alternative' systems of animal production, designed to meet animal welfare concerns in the 1970s and 1980s, were actually more inspired by public perceptions of animal welfare rather than the 'real needs' of the animals. Concerning systems for hens, he noted:

> During this era, two approaches dominated. One was the 'back to nature' approach which advocated keeping hens on free-range or semi-extensively in spite of the fact that the associated problems of predation, exposure to inclement weather, parasite infestation and general disease control were still within living memory. The other was the 'let's build them a palace' approach which tried to incorporate every conceivable requirement into the birds' environment.
>
> (Duncan, 1992b, p. 476)

In contrast to these approaches, a solid understanding of animals' environmental preferences and the strength of those preferences should allow us to design environments that cater to the priorities of the animals themselves.

11.7. Coda

So, when the wolf of Gubbio chose to live in the town rather than in the wild, could we have concluded that its choice provided objective information about its welfare, and that the wolf would live a happier life in the town? As a preference test, this situation was seriously flawed in two respects. First, the choice offered to the wolf failed to take account of the complexity of the animal's environmental preferences; the town might meet the wolf's needs at certain times but not others. Second, the choice, with its requirement to balance the immediate advantages of a free dinner against the long-term constraints of urban living, probably fell outside the animal's ability to weigh up present and future outcomes. These deficiencies may not have troubled Saint Francis, as he could allegedly converse with animals in their own languages. For those of us who lack this gift, the careful design of environmental preference tests will remain an important manner of understanding an animal's reactions to the environments in which they are kept.

11.8. Conclusions

- Preference and motivation testing provide useful information on the reactions of animals to methods of handling and housing and to other features of their environment.
- The environmental features preferred by an animal are likely to vary with its age and experience, its reproductive state, its on-going behaviour and other variables. Preference research must be comprehensive enough to identify these sources of variation.
- To draw inferences about an animal's welfare from preference research, the strength of the animal's preferences needs to be known. Various methods to assess preference and motivation strength have been developed.
- Great care is needed over the methods of preference and motivation testing. Particular test procedures or response measures may have unexpected impacts on the preferences that animals show. Research must also avoid confounding preferences and familiarity.
- Animals' preferences, as revealed by preference tests, often identify environmental features that will promote their welfare. However, the link between preferences and welfare may break down if the choices offered in preference tests fall outside the animals' sensory, cognitive and affective capacities or if animals are required to choose between short-term and long-term benefits.

Acknowledgements

We are grateful to Peter Phillips and Brian Thompson for their collaboration in preparing Fraser *et al.* (1993), on which portions of this chapter are based, and to Dan Weary and Allison Taylor for helpful comments on the manuscript.

We thank the publishers of *Canadian Journal of Animal Science*, *Applied Animal Behaviour Science*, and *Farm Building Progress* and the respective authors of the articles for kindly allowing material to be reproduced in the figures. David Fraser was on the staff of the Centre for Food and Animal Research, Agriculture and Agri-Food Canada, during the preparation of this chapter.

PART IV
Solutions

Some solutions to the welfare problems covered previously are obvious, but not implemented because of competing priorities. Solutions need to be practicable. One point that emerges from the chapters in Part IV is that prevention tends to be more practicable than cure. Some problems can be cured – one important example is use of analgesia to control pain, discussed in Chapter 5 – but many other problems are difficult or impossible to cure once established, such as some of the stereotypic behaviour patterns considered in Chapter 9. The chapters in Part IV consider animals' physical and social environments, their interactions with humans and the advantages and disadvantages of genetic selection. It will become clear, of course, that these are not independent.

CHAPTER 12

Physical conditions

Michael C. Appleby and Natalie K. Waran
(University of Edinburgh, UK)

Abstract

Where there are problems for welfare caused by the physical environment it is common to make specific changes, attempting to tackle a specific problem or to promote a specific advantage. These changes may be effective in preventing injuries or disease, but such measures are not always implemented (usually for economic reasons) and where implemented may cause other problems: for example, concern for hygiene often leads to animals being kept in barren conditions. Numerous ways have also been tried to diversify feeding methods, but specific changes to the environment often have widespread effects, some of which may be detrimental. Thus a change to the floor surface may affect diverse aspects of animals' behaviour and welfare. A more general approach is therefore appropriate. One area where this is being applied is in handling and transport, when animals encounter environments which are wholly new to them. Two complementary techniques being used here are description of the conditions and their effects on the animals and investigation of animals' perceptions of those conditions. For environments where animals spend more time, several studies have attempted a 'biological approach' in which they consider biological functioning while avoiding simplistic assumptions of 'natural is best'. We consider as examples the Access System for calves, Family Pens for pigs and Modified Cages for laying hens. To produce commercial designs from such studies, however, it will be necessary to justify every feature of detailed specifications.

12.1. Introduction

The physical environment in which animals live is critical to their welfare. It is relevant to observe, then, that the environment of all animals throughout the world is influenced to a greater or lesser degree by humans: there are no longer any completely wild animals living in a wholly natural environment. The principles of this chapter therefore apply to all animals, including those for which human influence is indirect or slight. However, it is mostly concerned with animals for which we have a major influence on their physical environment. For example, Jongebreur (1983, p. 265) discussed housing design and welfare in livestock production:

> It is quite evident that developments in the field of housing and management do influence the behaviour and welfare of the animals. During the application of

these new developments however there has been a lack of knowledge of the interaction between housing systems and animal behaviour. A more comprehensive meaning of the often mentioned term 'good husbandry practice' specially related to modern systems requires more research in this field. A more detailed description of the physiological and ethological needs of the animals kept for farming purposes in accordance with established experience and scientific knowledge can contribute much to better and more appropriate designs of housing and equipment systems.

Two points emerge from such discussions. First, an understanding of problems is essential if solutions are to be found, particularly if they are to be general, not specific to one situation. This chapter should therefore be read in conjunction with previous chapters which considered problems. Second, many of the problems and many of the solutions relate to behaviour – more so than to other factors relevant to welfare. The extent to which performance of behaviour is itself important for welfare was discussed in the chapter on Behavioural Restriction. Jensen and Toates (1993, p. 177) comment as follows:

> In considering ethological needs, it is essential to understand the consequences to the animals of not being able to perform a certain behaviour . . . Ultimately, what should guide our welfare considerations is the degree of suffering an animal will experience if a certain behaviour is impaired.

So the emphasis on behaviour does not imply that other factors are less important. Rather, it occurs because behaviour is the interface between the animal and most aspects of its environment. Thus injury is not itself a behavioural welfare problem, but it occurs or is prevented partly through behaviour. And for those welfare problems which are not mediated by behaviour, such as some diseases, behaviour is important as a symptom in detecting the problem and in assessing the effectiveness of any cure.

Assessment of effectiveness is vital, partly because there may be different solutions available to the same problem. We can not simply assume that our supposed solution has worked. Furthermore, solving some problems creates others. For example, McGregor and Ayling (1990) tried to provide a more varied environment for laboratory mice than standard cages. Presumably a welfare problem was thought to be caused by 'the rather stark environment of a standard laboratory holding cage' (p. 280). They had to abandon the attempt because (p. 277):

> Male CFLP mice were quicker to show signs of aggression in both large wooden cages and standard plastic holding cages to which objects such as bricks and extra sources of food and water had been added.

For this sort of reason, a single change to the environment often turns out to be inadequate – to necessitate other associated changes and perhaps compromise on certain characteristics which cause problems. We shall consider specific changes first: those which have attempted to tackle a specific problem or to promote a specific advantage. One important example which illustrates many of the principles will then be considered in more detail, namely methods of feeding. After this we shall consider whole environments; first the special case of environments for handling and transport – because during these procedures the environment is new to the animals and all-important – and then general approaches to environmental design. We should also point out that changes to the environment made for reasons unconnected with welfare will have effects, and we shall consider some such changes in passing.

12.2. Specific Changes

A considerable amount is known about environmental design and management in relation to reduction or avoidance of specific physical welfare problems of injury and disease. This is particularly true in agriculture, where such problems reduce profit, and there are valuable books on the subject such as those by Curtis (1983) and Wathes and Charles (1994). For example, Nilsson (1992, p. 100) has emphasized that in prevention of injury, softness of the floor is important (although he has also stressed that different characteristics and effects of floors interact, as will be discussed below):

> The softness of the floor is of greater importance for a larger animal than a smaller one, as the contact pressure to the lying area is relatively greater, with the animal's surface theoretically proportional to its weight raised to the power of 2/3. For this reason, dairy cows are especially interesting to study.
>
> Lying areas for dairy cows must have a certain degree of softness to lessen the incidence of injuries and to provide comfort. Studies of this problem showed that the incidence of injuries decreases with an increase in the softness of the floor in standings used for tied dairy cows (Fig. [12.1]).

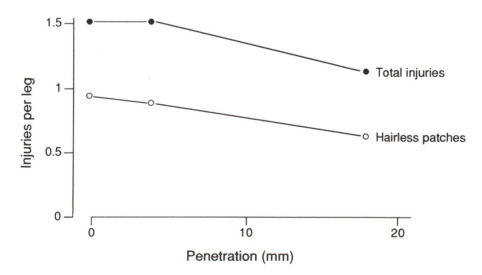

Fig. 12.1. Number of observed injuries (hairless patches, swellings and wounds) according to the softness of the floor material (measured with a 100 mm diameter steel sphere). Investigation of 44 tied dairy cows during three winter housing seasons (from Nilsson, 1992).

Similarly, Curtis (1983, p. 261) points out that number of animals per room and the ventilation system have major effects on the incidence of pneumonia:

> Sometimes a single environmental modification can be associated clearly with some aspect of animal health, so disease management is simpler than usual. Such is the case with the transverse formation of ventilation system now widely adopted in the Dutch pork industry (Proc. 29th Ann. Mtg, Eur. Ass. Animal. Prod., 1978, p.M-P/4.05/1).
>
> In the transverse formation, growing-finishing hogs are kept in rooms holding only 80 to 120 animals. These rooms are arranged on both sides of and perpendicular to a common central corridor. Air moves into the rooms from that corridor and out through exhaust fans at the other end of the respective rooms. During periods of cold weather, the ventilation air can be tempered in the corridor before entering the rooms, thereby greatly buffering external temperature fluctuations. When compared with hogs kept in the traditional sort of house, where air enters the animal space directly from outdoors, only half as many hogs from transverse-formation houses have pneumonic lesions in their lungs at the time of slaughter.

However, there are two major reservations to make about such measures to reduce injury and disease. Firstly, measures known to be effective are often simply not used, for various reasons including economics, as emphasized in the chapter on Health and Disease. Secondly and in contrast, such measures may be adopted irrespective of deleterious effects on other aspects of welfare. Most obviously, concern for hygiene often leads to animals being kept in barren, near-sterile conditions: this is one reason for use of cages for hens, flat-deck crates for piglets and washed concrete floors for zoo animals. In fact it sometimes turns out that the concern for hygiene is exaggerated. Thus it used to be common – and still is in some zoos – for monkey cages to be washed out regularly to avoid infection; this restricted many aspects of behaviour such as time spent on the ground. Chamove *et al.* (1982, p. 316) tried adding floor litter:

> In the present study, using [8] species, aggressive behavior was reduced by a factor of 3 with woodchips and by almost 10 times with grain or mealworms added to the litter. All negative behavior decreased by a factor of over 5 when food was added to the woodchips. Time spent on the ground almost doubled with woodchips, and more than doubled when food items were added to it. These effects occur in monkeys of various ages . . .
>
> In addition, there is no evidence that using woodchips presents a health hazard. As the litter matures, the woodchips become increasingly more inhibitory to bacterial survival. This self-sterilizing action makes it likely that the mere presence of an absorbent litter greatly reduces the probability of disease spread due to fecal contamination.

Where animals are kept in barren conditions, the need has arisen for making changes to ameliorate the associated problems. For example, when piglets are kept in simple pens aggression is a problem, particularly if they are regrouped. McGlone and Curtis (1985, p. 22) provided 'hides' at the side of the pen: recesses big enough for a piglet's head and shoulders. These proved effective in reducing aggression:

> Typically, two pigs would fight for awhile, then one would enter a hide, thus ending the fight. After standing for several seconds in the hide, the pig often

would lie down, with its head remaining in the hide. The ratio of time pigs spent standing or lying while in the hide was not quantified, but it was clear that pigs usually lay while their heads were in a hide. Because pigs do not fight while lying, it was to be expected that, as hide use increased, fighting would decline, and attack duration was indeed reduced when hides were available. This was especially so during the first 30 min after regrouping; although pigs spent less than 3% of this time with head-in-hide, attack duration was reduced by 42%.

With other welfare problems associated with behaviour, methods of prevention are more debatable, as mentioned in the introduction. For example, Baxter (1983) suggested that it might be possible to provide farrowing sows, usually kept in barren pens, with an environment which makes it unnecessary for them to perform nesting behaviour. However, Arey et al. (1991, p. 61) found that this suggestion was not borne out:

> When pre-formed nests were presented to six sows on the day before farrowing, straw removal was reduced, straw carrying and pawing remained the same. Rooting, lying and the duration of nest building increased. Nest building is highly motivated behaviour in sows and the performance of the activities themselves appears to have a significant role in reducing the motivation. Nesting material appears to be a key factor both in the regulation and performance of the behaviour.

So in this case the change needed to the environment has been identified, namely provision of nesting material and sufficient space to use it.

Space restrictions, with associated effects on behaviour, are sometimes applied not because they are necessary in themselves but to achieve some other result. For example, metabolism crates are used for collection of urine and faeces. However, a thoughtful approach may allow the result to be achieved in another way. Carlstead et al. (1992, p. 167) showed that close confinement was unnecessary for urine collection from felids, as follows. A similar approach could probably also be used for many animals; for example, pigs also have habitual urination and defecation sites.

> For experiments 1–3, 16 adult male and 8 adult female domestic cats were housed individually in stainless steel, laboratory cages . . . Each cage contained a 15-cm-wide shelf, water and food bowl and a double layered plastic litter pan. The top pan was punctured with 0.5-mm-diameter holes and contained 0.5 liter of nonabsorbent cat litter which allowed urine, but not feces, to pass through to the lower pan . . . For experiment 4, all felids were housed on exhibit at the National Zoological Park, Washington, DC, with the exception of leopard cats that were maintained initially at the NIH Animal Center. An adult female Geoffrey's cat was housed with a male in an indoor exhibit (3 × 3 × 3 m) that was furnished with . . . two aluminium pans. On 8 different days the female was observed between 9:00 am and 12:00 pm to urinate in one particular pan, and freshly voided urine was obtained on these occasions.

It has already been emphasized that a specific change to the environment may have widespread effects. Similarly, provision for one aspect of animals' behaviour or welfare may affect many other aspects. We shall now consider in more detail one such area which influences among others nutrition, use of time, use of space and social interactions, namely feeding methods.

12.3. Feeding Methods

Feeding is one of the behaviour patterns most controlled by humans when animals are maintained in captive environments. Despite the benefits of such control over the intake of food there are also clear disadvantages when animals have difficulties adapting to environments different from those in which their behaviour evolved. So although in production terms the effectiveness of an environment can be judged in terms of efficiency of food intake, the design of the environment often leads to problems in which individuals within the system are compromised in some way:

> In modern husbandry systems, pregnant sows typically receive all of their food for 24 h in one or two small concentrate meals. This food allowance primarily supplies requirements for maintenance, with only a small additional allowance for growth of maternal tissue and conceptus. The level of feed provided is well below the voluntary intake of the animal and most of the observed aggression in stable groups is related to feeding.
>
> (Martin and Edwards, 1994, p. 64)

When the environment is modified to solve such problems, the aim of the change is generally to encourage animals to feed in a more natural manner. The first step to any change is therefore an investigation of the probable causes of the problems. For example:

> Feed related aggression depends on both the accessibility of the feed and the space around the feeding area. Outdoor sows have more space available than housed animals, and their food is typically distributed over a greater area. It is possible that the problems [of aggression] experienced by low-ranking sows may be less pronounced.
>
> (Martin and Edwards, 1994, p. 64)

In fact, such modification of the environment may not only lead to reduction in undesirable food related behaviour such as high levels of aggression, but may also increase food conversion efficiency.

Modifications can range from a total change in environment as in the example above to small changes in the way food is offered. For example the diet itself can be modified to make it more palatable using flavourings or more bulky to increase gut fill. Thus sugar beet or chopped straw added to concentrate feeds can lead to a decrease in vulva biting in sows (van Putten and van de Burgwal, 1990). An understanding of the way food preferences develop can also aid effective feeding. Some ruminants are naturally neophobic which presents a problem when they are offered novel supplemental foodstuffs during winter months:

> Reluctance to eat new foods can cause economic losses for livestock producers because of reduced animal performance and increased time to market.
>
> (Provenza *et al.,* 1995, p. 84)

Conversely, some animals have a natural tendency to sample feeds separately, and this has been used in development of methods of choice feeding. In a series of experiments with young pigs, Kyriazakis *et al.* (1990, p. 198) concluded that:

> Pigs selected their diet, the composition of which changed systematically as they grew, in a directed manner. The quantity eaten and the composition of the diet selected appeared to reflect the pigs' requirements for maintenance, growth and fattening.

This approach has been extended in some studies where animals are required to work for access to their choice of food. Various feeding devices have been designed with the aim of increasing species-specific feeding behaviour and decreasing behavioural management problems such as stereotypies. One such device, the Edinburgh Food Ball, was designed for sows and is now being adapted for other animals. When pushed by the sow it delivers small food rewards randomly in time and space. The results of the study demonstrate that:

> Food deprived gilts will interact with a foraging device (expressing foraging type behaviour) over long periods of time in the presence of straw bedding. These results suggest that food restriction in sows gives rise to heightened feeding motivation, and that, when given the opportunity, they will express this feeding motivation as foraging behaviour.
>
> (Young *et al.*, 1994, p. 245)

In addition, the authors claim (p. 246) that: 'One criterion of good animal welfare, the expression of a time budget similar to that expressed by free-ranging conspecifics, has been fulfilled.'

However, feeding enrichment devices may not always solve feeding problems, and it is often important to evaluate quantitatively the effects of such devices on a variety of behaviour patterns because it may be that the device leads to an increase in negative, rather than positive, behaviour. For example, it is known that hens prefer to obtain food by performing a simple operant response, even in the presence of free food (Duncan and Hughes, 1972) but the provision of an operant feeding device for deep litter hens did not have the expected result:

> Hens are clearly willing to use operant feeders, whether because of behavioural 'need' or an information-gathering theory of motivation, but in the absence of conventional ad libitum feeders it seems that arousal levels and frustration became too high, resulting in feather pecking and loss of condition. It is concluded that operant feeders are unsuitable for use by themselves.
>
> (Lindberg and Nicol, 1994, p. 225)

There is also the problem of habituation, when an animal becomes accustomed to the device with the result that usage declines over time, and sometimes the results of enrichment studies are unexpected.

It is often difficult to see that there are feeding problems amongst group-housed animals. Individual feeding behaviour may be overlooked in farming environments where group feeding or growth efficiency is measured. The solution to many feeding problems lies in a knowledge not only of species-specific feeding behaviour and requirements, but also in a sound knowledge of the range of behaviour patterns the animal needs to perform.

12.4. Handling and Transport

Handling or transporting animals involves changes to their whole environment, or at least to many of its most important aspects, to the extent that it is
common for welfare to be compromised in all the areas indicated by the Five
Freedoms (Farm Animal Welfare Council, 1992). This is despite the fact that
welfare problems such as fear during handling or injuries during transport are
often also problems for the owners. Of course, methods of handling and transport are often influenced to some extent by experience and knowledge of
animals – for example, consider the knowledge involved in using a dog to herd
sheep. However, only recently has this approach been taken systematically,
and then only for farm animals (Perry, 1990; Grandin, 1993a). Grandin's
book is a particularly important collection of papers on this topic. For example, Hutson's chapter on 'Behavioural principles of sheep handling' (1993,
p. 133) lists what he regards as important characteristics of the animals with
respect to handling:

> These four characteristics of the sheep – vision, flocking behaviour, following
> behaviour and intelligence – form the basis of all behavioural principles of sheep
> handling. I will consider these principles in relation to the three key elements of
> an integrated sheep handling system – the design of the handling environment,
> the handling technique and the reason for being handled – the handling
> treatment. [Concerning design, I] recommended that the most crucial design
> criterion was to give sheep a clear, unobstructed view towards the exit, or
> towards where they are meant to move. This often becomes more evident by
> taking a sheep's eye view of the facility.

Nevertheless, prior knowledge of biology and behaviour in other circumstances will not be enough to plan a system or to predict its effects on the
animals. To give just one example which could probably not have been predicted, Matthews (1993, p. 269) reports that 'deer remain settled in padded
crushes for up to 60 min provided the shoulders of the animal are well restrained'. Thus empirical work is necessary. As with other work on welfare this
has involved the two complementary approaches of describing the conditions
and their effects on the animals and of investigating animals' perceptions of
those conditions. One particularly clear example of the descriptive approach is
work which has been done on the conditions experienced by broilers transported by lorry. Mitchell and Kettlewell (1993, p. 226) examined these conditions and developed the index of Apparent Equivalent Temperature (AET) to
express the interaction of temperature and relative humidity (RH) in causing
heat stress. They then made recommendations for avoidance of heat stress in
practice:

> High thermal loads were observed in the [lorry's] core on warm summer days
> in the open configuration even when the vehicle was in motion, and when
> stationary the risk of heat stress increased. When the curtains were closed
> temperatures and humidities in the thermal core were greatly elevated.
> On 'mild' winter days local temperatures of >30°C were occasionally recorded
> accompanied by RH of >80%. These conditions may precipitate 'paradoxical
> heat stress' during the 'cold season' . . .

In support of these studies laboratory simulations identified combinations of temperature and RH producing equivalent biological responses . . . From the findings, values of AET were determined which would result in minimal (<40°C), moderate (40–65°C) and severe (>65°C) physiological stress . . .

In associated studies a method of on-line monitoring of the conditions within the thermal core of commercial vehicles was developed and, by incorporating the information from laboratory simulations, was used as the basis of a warning system indicating the risk of thermal stress during journeys.

Work on animal perceptions of situations involving handling or transport has included preference or aversion testing and operant techniques. Rushen (1986a, p. 391) examined the aversiveness of electro-immobilization in sheep:

Compared with allowing the sheep to run freely through the race, both physical restraint and electro-immobilization increased the time required to run through on subsequent occasions, suggesting that both treatments were aversive. The longest running times were recorded from the immobilized sheep, and considerably more time had to be spent pushing these animals up the race. These results suggest that electro-immobilization is a more aversive experience for sheep than simple mechanical restraint. The attachment of the electrodes and the necessary extra handling appeared to make no significant contribution to this aversiveness. Furthermore, sheep remember this experience for some 12 weeks.

Stephens and Perry (1990, pp. 50–51) used the operant approach to test response of pigs to vibration and noise in a transport simulator:

All the pigs learned to press the switch panel which turned the transport simulator off. The animals usually began to make responses during the first training session of 30 min and by the fourth session they kept the apparatus switched off for about 75% of the time . . . These experiments clearly demonstrate that young growing pigs find the vibration to be aversive and that the pigs responded behaviourally to terminate the vibration of their pen.

This sort of work is being used to identify methods of handling and transport which have less impact on welfare than those currently in use. To summarize:

The ease of animal handling is determined by a combination of the animal's previous experience, the facilities and personnel involved, and the normal behavioural characteristics of the species. All these factors should be considered in the management of animals which will be handled and transported. Although research has identified some of the important aspects of animal handling, numerous questions remain which will gradually be answered as attention continues to be directed to this subject.

(Gonyou, 1993b, p. 17)

However, it has to be said that implementation is not just limited by unanswered questions. It also depends on practicality, expense and the relative priority given to welfare. Indeed, this whole area of management requires more thought than it has previously been given: for example, such issues as whether pre-slaughter transport is necessary at all or whether animals could be slaughtered on the farm deserve much more attention.

12.5. General Approaches

We have emphasized that specific changes to the environment are rarely specific in their effects. For example, although Nilsson (1992) showed that floors for cows must be soft to prevent injury, they must not be too soft because (p. 100) 'animals experience a very soft underlay as being unstable for standing on. They must have a firm footing for the hooves.' Indeed (pp. 94, 107):

> When developing new floors, consideration must be given to many factors, the most important of which is to maintain and improve animal health. The most important physical properties of the walking and lying surfaces in livestock buildings are: thermal comfort, softness, friction, abrasiveness . . .
>
> It is obvious that the optimal values of all the floor properties are difficult if not impossible to fulfil simultaneously. Instead the aim must be to work out a compromise which as much as possible fulfils the different demands . . . Other important properties of the floors in livestock houses are mechanical strength, cleaning ability, toxicity, pathogenicity, etc.

The theme of this book is that welfare is increasingly an explicit aspect of any such compromise. Probably the most widely used concept in achieving this has been that of 'environmental enrichment': environmental enrichment has been attempted in many contexts, including farms, laboratories and zoos. However, while the concept of environmental enrichment is a general one, too often the actual changes made have been specific rather than part of a general approach, and success has been variable: we have already pointed out one example where 'enrichment' of the environment caused an increase in aggression (McGregor and Ayling, 1990). In other words, the concept has often been applied uncritically, as Newberry (1995, p. 230) points out:

> The term 'enrichment' implies an improvement. However, the term is frequently applied to types of environmental change . . . rather than the outcome . . . In this paper, I define environmental enrichment as an improvement in the biological functioning of captive animals resulting from modifications to their environment.

Newberry goes on to stress the importance of a biological approach (p. 235):

> Enrichment attempts will fail if the environmental modifications have little functional significance to the animals, are not sufficiently focused to meet a specific goal, or are based on an incorrect hypothesis regarding the causation and mechanisms underlying a problem.

So what is involved in a biological approach? Newberry points out (p. 230) that:

> Many authors advocate providing an environment which promotes natural behaviour. However, because there is no single standard for natural behaviour or a natural environment, it is often unclear what is meant by natural behaviour . . . If the objective is environmental enrichment, it is necessary to describe the desired behaviour and explain how the animals will benefit from exhibiting that behaviour.

Furthermore, description of an environment as promoting natural behaviour does not necessarily imply that welfare has been increased. However, at least one well-known example of environmental enrichment in zoos which is often cited as promoting natural behaviour does avoid the pitfall of assuming that no further justification is necessary. Nash (1982, p. 211) describes the relevant behaviour as stimulating and rewarding rather than natural:

> This study examines tool use by a colony of captive chimpanzees at an artificial termite mound. The mound, constructed of concrete, simulates the termite mounds which are used as food sources by wild chimpanzees who extract the termites using grass or twig-type tools . . .
>
> The artificial mound proved to be a viable simulation of the naturally occurring mounds, with most of the chimpanzees exploiting the food in the mound by using tools over the period of study . . . The artificial mound provides the chimpanzees with a stimulating and rewarding activity.

In fact it is often not the case that 'natural is best'. Thus Grandin *et al.* (1987) have shown that providing 'toys' for pigs affects their behaviour not just at the time but also later while being handled, when they are less excitable and easier to drive. Similarly, Webster (1995, p. 176) makes a robust proposal for the development of automatic milking for cows (in combination with other aspects of the environment):

> The development of automatic milking systems using robots for placing the teat cups offers an exciting opportunity to rethink the husbandry of dairy cows in a way that could be consistent both with increased productivity and with improved health and welfare. The cow that can, without having to queue, enter an automatic milking station of her own volition four to six times daily to be fed and/or milked as appropriate will certainly have the potential to produce more milk. She may also be less prone not only to mastitis but also to lameness because of the reduced distension of the udder. However, her demand for nutrients will increase and any welfare problems associated with an imbalance between nutrient supply and demand will become worse. Thus a robot that milked cows four to six times daily may reduce the stresses on the udder but it would only improve overall welfare if feeding and management were also modified to ensure: (1) the diet was of sufficiently high quality to provide the extra nutrients required to meet the increased yield; (2) the diet was balanced to achieve stable fermentation and so avoid the stresses of ruminal acidosis and laminitis; (3) the ration was supplied in such a way that it could be eaten in not more than eight hours per day so as to avoid conflict between the cows' motivation to eat and their motivation to rest.

In considering further what may be involved in a biological approach to environmental design, and the success of such an approach, we shall consider three projects which have resulted in actual proposals for systems for farm animals: for calves, pigs and laying hens. Webster (1995, p. 188) and colleagues worked on an alternative to crates for veal calves:

> We called our approach the Access system. Calves wearing transponders were reared in groups of 14 to 20 in straw yards and given access to a computer-controlled feeding station which dispensed rationed amounts of milk replacer and a small amount of solid feed containing sufficient digestible fibre to stimulate

rumen development. All the calves had to learn was that a teat would appear in one station if they were due for a milk feed but would not appear if they had already had enough; similarly for the solid ration. All calves acquired these basic computer skills within two days. The Access system has, to date, only been used on an experimental scale but it did show that when calves are given just enough of the sort of solid food necessary to normalize rumen development, enteric diseases can be reduced to the low level considered acceptable in normal calf rearing units. Furthermore, since enteritis triples the risk that calves will subsequently contract pneumonia, respiratory infections were normalized as well. Simply put, the calves were now healthy because their development was normal and because they were healthy they could be run in groups.

This is interesting because it considers the interaction between different aspects of welfare: nutrition, health and behaviour. It is worth pointing out here, though, that this would make it difficult to draw up detailed specifications for a commercial form of the system – which has not yet been attempted – because individual features of the system such as space allowance, flooring, feeding and so on will all have interrelated effects. It might well be that without such specifications, producers would 'cut corners' and save costs where they could and the performance of the system would become less reliable.

The difficulty of commercialization is also clear in what is probably the best-known study which has attempted a biological or ethological approach. Stolba and Wood-Gush (1984, pp. 297–298) observed free-ranging pigs and used the observations to design the 'Edinburgh Family Pen System' for pigs:

> Ethological minimum requirements were determined from observations of adult and juvenile large-white pigs in semi-natural enclosures, in increasingly restricted and in conventional conditions. Obligatory features in the environment which consistently enabled the pigs to perform their frequent or regular sequences of behaviour were the design factors for the enriched pens. Each is composed of a nesting, an activity and a rooting area and includes a corridor connecting 4 neighbouring pens. Such a unit houses 4 familiar sows with their fattening offspring, a boar and replacements. Basic features of social structure of the outdoor reference groups were maintained in such pig families. The social contacts in stable family groups enhance the synchrony of heats and lactational oestrus. Thus 2.3 litters/year may be obtained if sows are well fed before mating. As there is no weaning check, the growers reach bacon weight for market around 155 days of age. The system shows what basic ethological research may contribute to reach practical housing conditions which meet the main behavioural requirements of a species.

This study has been outstandingly successful in raising the issue of welfare in farm environments and in encouraging the production of other designs, especially for pigs. However, although development of the system continues this is involving considerable change to the original design. This is because in trying to identify all important aspects of the environment at the same time, the project failed to obtain detailed scientific evidence that any one of those aspects was essential. The system as designed was not directly competitive with existing systems, so there was commercial pressure to compromise on space allowance and provision of various features.

In other words, whatever the approach to designing a system, if it is going to be developed commercially every feature of it has to be justified by exhaustive 'testing to destruction'. Appleby and colleages have attempted to do this in development of the Edinburgh Modified Cage for laying hens by adopting what they call (Appleby, 1993, p. 67) 'a stage-by-stage, systematic approach to cage design.' Thus (pp. 72–74):

> The Edinburgh project started with a pilot trial which compared prototype cage designs with conventional controls. These designs all included perches and nest boxes; some also had dust baths . . . A series of trials then examined facilities separately, to consider their use by the birds and their effects . . . Current trials demonstrate that these possibilities can be combined in practical designs for groups of four or five birds, with few production problems and with benefits for welfare compared to conventional cages.

The trials mentioned have included models with larger group sizes, smaller space allowances and different facilities, all of which had problems relative to the recommended design, so the project is making progress towards detailed specifications (Appleby and Hughes, 1995). Commercial adoption, however, still naturally depends on a combination of economics and legislation.

12.6. Compromise

While welfare is increasingly considered in environmental design for animals, it is never the sole criterion and rarely the primary one. Thus Nilsson (1992, pp. 107–108), despite the importance of his work for welfare, concluded for farm animals that:

> In the end it is the economical consideration that is most important. The net profit resulting from better animal health, higher output and reduced labour – and straw – costs must be compared to the cost of a better floor construction.

We may disagree with that conclusion but we can see that in a commercial context there will be others who do not. In other contexts such as zoos economics may not be primary but there are still other criteria in addition to welfare. Thus the passage quoted above from Nash (1982, p. 211) continues:

> The artificial mound provides the chimpanzees with a stimulating and rewarding activity, interest and enjoyment for the public, and an opportunity for researchers to study tool use under more controlled conditions than are possible in the field.

However, such compromise should not be regarded as wholly negative, because economics and other similar factors can not be divorced from environmental design, and can be used to establish priorities between varied demands for both humans and animals (Appleby, 1997; Chapter 16).

12.7. Conclusions

- An increasing number of projects attempt to apply a biological approach to environmental design. However, there have still been few coordinated projects on the effects of environmental design on welfare, and probably none which are comprehensive.
- Issues which should be taken into account in such projects include the possibility of different solutions to the same problem. For example, there may potentially be both 'natural solutions' (such as keeping a litter together at weaning) and 'imposed solutions' (making up groups of mixed size, not matched size).
- There is no general principle that 'natural is best' but certain aspects of natural environments may be important, such as controllability, predictability (or conversely stimulation such as variability) and complexity.
- One major aspect which has been consistently underemphasized is the effect of experience on animals' responses to physical conditions, which means that welfare has to be considered over the whole lifetime.

CHAPTER 13
Social conditions

Mike Mendl (University of Bristol, UK) and Ruth C. Newberry
(Washington State University, USA)

Abstract

By comparing the structure and dynamics of evolved social groups with those
commonly observed in managed groups of captive animals, we describe how
the latter may lead to the occurrence of animal welfare problems. Solving
these problems is particularly challenging because it is usually more difficult to
predict how animals will respond to each other than it is to predict how they
will respond to changes in the physical environment. One approach is to start
from first principles and design social environments which allow the expression
of the types of behaviour and social organization that seem to be important for
social harmony in natural groups. For example, housing animals in relatively
stable groups, and allowing them the freedom to separate themselves from the
main group, to select which individuals they associate with, and to avoid others,
may help to promote harmonious social life. This approach requires basic
research into the species' social organization under unconstrained free-ranging
situations, and takes time to develop into a practical and viable alternative
to existing systems. An alternative approach is to tackle welfare problems by
altering existing social environments. We suggest that this trouble-shooting
approach is most likely to be successful when the species' social structure and
abilities are taken into account before solutions are devised, and when the
causes of problems, rather than their symptoms, are addressed.

13.1. Introduction

From an animal welfare perspective, the social environment of captive animals
presents us with a dilemma. On the one hand, social companionship is potentially the most effective way of enriching the lives of animals in captivity, a
point clearly made by Humphrey (1976, p. 308):

> [The monkeys] live in social groups of about eight or nine animals in relatively
> large cages. But these cages are almost empty of objects, there is nothing to
> manipulate, nothing to explore; once a day the concrete floor is hosed down,
> food pellets are thrown in and that is about it. So I looked, and seeing this
> barren environment, thought of the stultifying effect it must have on the
> monkey's intellect. And then one day I looked again and saw a half-weaned
> infant pestering its mother, two adolescents engaged in a mock battle, an old
> male grooming a female whilst another female tried to sidle up to him, and

> I suddenly saw the scene with new eyes: forget about the absence of objects,
> these monkeys had each other to manipulate and explore.

Humphrey's intuition that relationships with other individuals are a major source of comfort and entertainment to captive animals is supported by evidence from a variety of species. For example, captive primates show lower levels of abnormal behaviour in the presence of companions than when isolated (Bernstein, 1991), and horses (Feh and de Mazieres, 1993) and talapoin monkeys (Keverne *et al.*, 1989) appear to calm companions by grooming them.

On the other hand, the damage that animals can inflict on each other by intimidation, overt aggression and cannibalism gives rise to serious animal welfare concerns. Unfortunately, it is often difficult to predict the situations in which conspecifics will injure or otherwise damage each other:

> The range of possible reactions to social stimuli is considerably greater than to
> inanimate stimuli, going from enthusiastic and lasting acceptance to extreme
> injurious aggression. In general, it is easier to predict what an animal will do with
> something new than with somebody new.

Visalberghi and Anderson's (1993, p. 5) statement is a challenge to all those concerned with solving socially induced animal welfare problems. Can we gather and use knowledge about social behaviour such that our manipulations of the social environment have more predictable and beneficial outcomes? Before addressing solutions, we first need to consider what the problems are and how they arise. We do this here by discussing the evolution of group living, and contrasting the structure and dynamics of groups living in their natural environment with those of captive groups.

13.2. Evolution of Group Living: the Dynamic Structure of Natural Social Groups

The evolution of social groups can best be considered in terms of the costs and benefits to individual group members. Suggested benefits include dilution of predation risk and enhanced abilities to detect predators, keep warm, defend resources, and locate and catch food. Potential costs of group living include increased competition with group members for resources and an increased risk of contracting parasites or contagious diseases. For each individual, evolutionary theory predicts that the decision to join or leave a group depends upon the relative pay-off (benefits minus costs), in terms of inclusive fitness, of solitary or group living (Pulliam and Caraco, 1984).

Vehrencamp (1983) has modelled the conditions under which different levels of cooperation or despotism should occur in animal groups when individuals are free to join and leave the group. Despotic behaviour results in increased variation or bias in the fitness of individuals within the group (p. 667):

> Selection acts simultaneously on the stronger, dominant members of the group
> to secure more resources for themselves at the expense of subordinates, and on
> subordinates to leave the group when excessively manipulated if they can do

better elsewhere. When it is to the advantage of the dominant to maintain the group, the dominant will ultimately be limited in the degree of bias it can impose by the options available to subordinates outside the group.

Thus, in natural groups, we expect high-ranking individuals to moderate the amount of competitive pressure they exert on low-rankers, because low-rankers can leave when options outside the group become relatively more beneficial. Decisions to join or leave groups are likely to be affected by a variety of factors including predation pressure, resource availability and distribution, and the individual's ability to compete with others in the group.

In line with these predictions, the group structure of free-living animals is fluid and varies both within and between species, ranging from loose aggregations of individuals to long-term, cohesive groups. Members immigrate and emigrate, and there are seasonal and short-term changes in group size and composition and fusion and fission of groups. For example, male feral domestic fowl switch between territoriality during the breeding season and a hierarchical group structure during winter. The females associate in groups with the males during winter and separate to rear their broods in summer (McBride *et al.*, 1969).

13.3. The Constrained Structure of Managed Social Environments

The social environment of laboratory and farm animals and, to a lesser extent, zoo animals is often characterized more by human concerns such as effective use of space and uniformity of group membership than by consideration of the evolved social structures and abilities of the species. The resulting constraints on social behaviour may have detrimental welfare consequences. Clearly, there are dangers in arguing that the welfare of captive animals is good only if they show the same behavioural organization and repertoire as they would show in free-ranging conditions. It becomes even more problematic to relate the behaviour of domestic animals to that of their wild ancestors. However, although domestication has altered the threshold and frequency at which some behaviour patterns are expressed (Price, 1984), domestic animals appear to retain the basic social characteristics of wild conspecifics. For example, the social behaviour of domestic pigs living in a semi-natural environment strongly resembles that of the European wild boar (Stolba and Wood-Gush, 1989). It thus seems likely that domestic animals are predisposed to deal most effectively with the range of group sizes and structures typical of their species, and that the freedom to make decisions about when to join or leave groups and which animals to associate with remains an important feature of their social environment.

Keeping individuals of group-living species in isolation, either temporarily or permanently, clearly limits social behaviour. Isolation often gives rise to a physiological stress response (Reite, 1985; Parrott, 1990), suggesting that the experience is unpleasant. Rearing young animals in isolation from birth also places them at a competitive disadvantage when later grouped with more socially experienced animals (Le Neindre *et al.*, 1992). Furthermore, rearing females in isolation can disrupt their future maternal behaviour (Berman, 1990).

Problems also arise when groups are created by introducing unfamiliar individuals in a confined space and in unnatural combinations. When unfamiliar individuals are suddenly forced together, the level of aggression can be much higher than that observed when unfamiliar individuals encounter each other under more natural conditions (Jensen, 1994). Even if there is no physical contact or injury, individuals may show a marked stress response, and can die, if placed in the enclosure of an established group. These effects may be related to the lack of opportunity for the animals to escape. They may also be related to the group composition. For example, in many species, creating groups of adult males when they would not naturally form such groups results in serious and sustained aggression (Love and Hammond, 1991). Placing young animals together in the absence of their mothers or other older individuals may also give rise to elevated agonistic behaviour (Le Neindre *et al.*, 1992).

Once groups are established, the design of housing systems usually prevents animals from emigrating in response to high levels of aggression. Therefore, high-ranking individuals may be able to exert more pressure on others than they would in free-living groups (Vehrencamp, 1983), with potentially damaging welfare consequences for low-rankers. This problem is exacerbated when resources are limited and groups are housed in unstructured enclosures with no opportunities for avoidance. Rumbaugh *et al.* (1989, p. 360) showed that, for captive chimpanzees at least, there may be a simple solution to this problem:

> In the wild, chimpanzees vary their choice of companions as they move from place to place, yet most captive enclosures are designed so that chimpanzees are always together, either in a large arena, or in cages. Aggressive encounters diminish when chimpanzees have a series of areas they can go to, ideally furnished with doors they can shut behind them if they wish.

Evolved communication mechanisms between conspecifics are often overlooked in managed social environments, with potentially adverse welfare consequences. For example, Algers and Jensen (1991) observed that fan noise disrupted vocal communication between sows and piglets during nursing and reduced milk intake by the piglets. In groups of male mice, Gray and Hurst (1995) found that the presence of male odours within the cage stimulated aggression when the mice were returned to the cage following removal for cage-cleaning and other procedures. They recommended that the mice be returned to completely clean cages following handling to minimize aggression problems.

Although captive social environments can create problems, intra-group competition and destructive social behaviour are not always artefacts of captive housing. Socially induced stress, cannibalism, infanticide and fatal fights also occur in nature. We need to understand the environmental conditions that evoke these behaviour patterns so that we can avoid inadvertently creating situations in captivity where they are likely to occur. In the following sections we consider different approaches to tackling or pre-empting welfare problems in the captive social environment.

13.4. Designing Husbandry Systems Using Knowledge about Species' Social Organization

The rationale of this approach has been to develop an understanding of the species' 'natural' social structure, as observed under conditions similar to those in which it evolved, and then to design a novel husbandry system which incorporates key features of this structure. The underlying assumption is that a 'natural social environment' promotes social harmony and good welfare. This is a debatable point (Dawkins, 1990). Nevertheless, as argued earlier, knowledge of natural social behaviour can be used to enhance the welfare of captive animals.

A seminal example of this approach is the work of Stolba and Wood-Gush (1984, p. 289) on domestic pigs. They suggested that 'a housing system only needs to guarantee relatively few but selected key stimuli and main behaviour elements in order to prevent the impairment of welfare'. Key social stimuli were identified by studying groups of pigs breeding and rearing young in semi-natural environments of varying size and complexity. Social features common to these environments were incorporated into the new housing system. Characteristics of this 'family pen' system included stable core groups of similar size and composition to those observed in the semi-natural conditions, provision of area sub-divisions and enough space to allow individuals to avoid some group members and associate with others, natural weaning, and the policy of avoiding abrupt introduction of new group members. The system eliminated the need to separate and re-mix sows before and after farrowing, and thus avoided the intense aggression that occurs at this time (Edwards and Mauchline, 1993). Keeping sows and piglets in family groups also prevented the social trauma associated with early weaning and the abrupt mixing of unfamiliar, weaned piglets (Jensen, 1994).

A similar approach was used to develop a new group housing system for rabbits (Stauffacher, 1992). Provision of a relatively complex social environment for rabbits appeared to prevent the disturbed reproductive behaviour, infanticide and unstructured behaviour seen in singly caged individuals. Perhaps as a consequence, a breeding success rate of 89% was achieved compared with conception rates of only 30 to 70%, and pup mortality of 30%, in separately caged females.

These findings support the idea that systems designed in this way can reduce welfare problems in the social environment. However, uptake of these systems at the commercial level requires that they are easy to manage, productive and economically viable, or that they are imposed by legislation. The pig system has suffered from some production-related problems that have impeded its introduction into the industry. Ironing out these problems is essential for this approach to be completely successful (Chapter 12).

13.5. Solving Socially Induced Welfare Problems in Existing Husbandry Systems

In contrast to the painstaking procedure of designing social environments from first principles, a more common approach has been to seek solutions to social problems by altering specific features of existing systems. However, constraints of existing systems mean that attempted solutions may be less than ideal. Perhaps more importantly, there may be a tendency to tackle symptoms in a trouble-shooting manner, rather than focusing on the actual causes of the problem. For example, cannibalism in poultry and pigs is often controlled by amputation of the beak tip or tail, respectively, and by keeping the animals in dim lighting. These procedures limit expression of the behaviour without addressing the underlying motivation to perform the behaviour.

In this section we address a serious welfare problem that occurs when animals are re-grouped: the high level of aggression that is associated with mixing unfamiliar animals. This problem has received detailed attention in both pigs and primates.

13.5.1. Treating symptoms

A number of researchers have attempted to reduce mixing-related aggression in pigs by administering psychoactive drugs such as tranquillizers, by timing mixing to coincide with periods of low activity, or by providing food or fresh straw to distract pigs from new group members. The rationale appears to be to engage the pigs in another activity to override the motivation to fight. Thus the symptom is tackled without any deep understanding of the cause.

These studies have produced conflicting results, perhaps partly due to the use of different experimental designs and pigs of different ages. Often, the techniques postpone rather than eliminate mixing-related aggression. Petherick and Blackshaw (1987, p. 609) note that:

> Azaperone reduced agonistic behaviour in mixed, weaned pigs during the period of sedation but, once the effect of the drug had worn off, the treated pigs showed the same level of agonistic behaviour as the untreated group. This might be expected as they still had to establish their dominance hierarchy.

However, Gonyou (1993c, p. 111) suggests that the dose is important:

> Pigs given too high a dosage of azaperone lose both sensory and motor function and fail to familiarize themselves with other pigs during the period the drug is in effect.

The drug amperozide has also been used to reduce aggression between newly mixed growing pigs (Gonyou et al., 1988), although it has adverse side-effects (Barnett, 1993) and failed to decrease aggression-related injuries in newly mixed sows (Barnett et al., 1993).

Similarly equivocal findings relate to the effects of time of day on mixing-related aggression. Barnett et al. (1994a) noted that mixing sows at sunset reduced aggression immediately following grouping, but had no effect on injury scores three days later. They summarized a common problem (p. 344):

> In this experiment aggressive interactions were only recorded immediately
> after grouping and around feeding time on the following day . . . and it is
> possible that aggression was merely delayed.

13.5.2. Understanding causes

It seems that agonistic behaviour is almost inevitable when unfamiliar animals
from highly social species are forced together (Fraser and Rushen, 1987),
probably due to an evolved tendency to deter rapid intrusions into the group.
Victory in the ensuing fights may give individuals priority of access to resources
and hence confer fitness advantages. However, fighting can be a very costly
activity and this has led to the idea that animals should avoid fighting unless
they have a good chance of winning (e.g. Enquist and Leimar, 1983). Therefore, they should be able to assess each other's fighting abilities. Rushen
(1990, p. 135) has explored this idea in studies of pig aggression:

> In initial fights, young pigs seem unable to make such judgements. However,
> they appear to be able to judge the relative fighting ability of an opponent from
> events that occur during a fight . . . The reduction in fighting . . . occurs because
> the pigs accumulate information about relative fighting ability . . . Thus, the
> initial fighting between unacquainted pigs is motivated by uncertainty about
> relative fighting abilities and can be considered a form of social exploration.

Although young pigs of similar size may not be able to assess each other's
competitive abilities without fighting, more experienced animals may have this
ability. Kennedy and Broom (1994) reported that gilts pre-exposed to a group
of sows received less aggression than non-exposed animals following mixing.
Perhaps the pre-exposure period, which simulates the gradual integration of
group members that occurs in natural environments (Stolba and Wood-Gush,
1989), allows some assessment and familiarization which acts to decrease
uncertainty and related fighting behaviour.

The greater the asymmetry in relative ability of unfamiliar pigs, the shorter
a fight is likely to be. Support for this prediction was provided by Rushen
(1987) who showed that if the weight difference between pigs was large
enough the duration and severity of fighting following mixing was reduced,
perhaps by facilitating assessment of relative abilities. Rushen also noted that
the presence of a dominant individual could inhibit aggression between subordinates. Adult boars are dominant in wild and feral groups and their presence helps to minimize aggression when domestic sows are mixed (Barnett
et al., 1993; but see Luescher *et al.*, 1990). Similarly, McGlone (1990, p. 102)
showed that the boar pheromone androstenone could decrease fighting
amongst young pigs:

> I must conclude that androstenone does not operate as a relevant pheromone,
> but rather as a super-male odor. Prepubertal pigs are less likely to attack an
> animal that smells like an adult.

Similar phenomena have been observed in other species (Petit and Thierry,
1994).

Recent research has further extended the idea that asymmetries between
individuals may decrease aggression. In this work, animals have been mixed

according to their behavioural, rather than physical, characteristics. Hessing *et al.* (1994b) reported that, when pigs categorized as aggressive or unaggressive were mixed together, they rapidly developed a stable social order, helping to minimize aggression and maximize growth rates in newly formed groups. The proposal that some populations may achieve social stability only when they contain a mixture of individuals with differing behavioural attributes (Mendl and Deag, 1995) is another idea based on a fundamental understanding of social behaviour which can be used to enhance welfare in animal groups.

13.5.3. *Establishing social relationships amongst captive primates*

> Despite the seeming consensus regarding their social disposition, nonhuman primates in laboratories are usually kept in single cages.
>
> (Reinhardt, 1990, p. 7)

For many primate species, the mixing of unfamiliar animals is not simply an unfortunate consequence of the design of husbandry systems, as is often the case for agricultural animals. Instead, it may be actively encouraged as a way of enriching the lives of individuals that have either been housed in isolation or removed from their pen-mates, both of which are known to lead to responses indicative of stress and depression-like states (Reite, 1985). The risks of wounding and social distress are often given as reasons for avoiding mixing, and indeed some attempts to combine groups or individuals have resulted in serious fighting, injury and even death. However, systematic studies by Reinhardt and colleagues (1989, p. 275) on methods of pair-formation in rhesus monkeys yielded the following observations:

> 1. Young rhesus monkeys, 12 to 18 months old and of both sexes, tend to inhibit aggression in singly caged adults of both sexes . . .
> 2. Individually caged adult rhesus monkeys can be paired with each other without major risk of trauma if they are given the opportunity to establish clear dominance–subordination relationships prior to their first direct encounter.

The former means that socially isolated adults can be provided with a young companion with little risk of aggression occurring. The latter suggests that adult rhesus monkeys, like adult pigs, are able to assess each other's abilities without direct physical contact. Once one individual has signalled subordinance a successful introduction of the animals is possible. Bernstein (1991) warned that if pre-exposure did not result in clear dominance it could actually exacerbate fighting following mixing because 'animals may threaten one another with impunity. This kind of "habituation" leads to an increasing animosity as the animals build a history of aggressive exchange'. In his studies of mixing animals into larger groups, he concluded (p. 331) that 'adding individuals one at a time is generally the least desirable procedure'. Instead, he recommended that several individuals should be introduced together into a group, or even that a large number of completely unfamiliar individuals could be put together at once (p. 332):

> Although the chaos and disorganization may shock the human observers and the impression will be of a riot with enormous amounts of fighting, no single animal will be the target of an organized attack.

The observed low levels of overt aggression during the studies of Reinhardt (1991, p. 7) suggested that 'Dominance relations amongst rhesus monkeys are determined principally by visual means, probably as a result of prior learning.' Therefore, it is important to provide adequate opportunities for the animals to learn to use and interpret social signals before attempting to group unfamiliar animals. Social isolation during early life is clearly detrimental to subsequent social abilities in several primate species (W.A. Mason, 1991, p. 327). Even macaques raised alone with their mother 'appear to have later difficulties accommodating to life in a social group'. Ideally, they 'should be provided with ample peer experience . . . preferably in compatible groups of four or more animals'.

Compatibility between potential pen-mates has not only been assessed by analysing dominance relationships. For captive gorillas in zoos, Gold and Maple (1994) suggested that detailed assessments of 'personality' might be useful as a management tool. They subjectively rated selected behavioural characteristics of nearly 300 gorillas. Four factors describing aspects of individual behavioural style, 'extroverted', 'dominant', 'fearful' and 'understanding', were identified in subsequent analysis. On the basis of these a database was created which could be used to match animals that are moved between zoos:

> For example, suppose the [Gorilla Species Survival Plan] was considering the formation of an additional bachelor group and was deliberating over potential candidates . . . It is known that males with a history of aggressiveness have trouble living in an all male situation. Sociable males, on the other hand, tend to adapt easily to a bachelor group situation . . . The [Gorilla Behavior Index could be used] to look at the ranges of profile scores of males . . . This analysis could lead to the selection of a male . . . with a comparatively high extroverted score . . . and a comparatively low dominant score.
>
> (Gold and Maple, 1994, pp. 515–516)

An understanding of individual behavioural characteristics and their stability may help to pre-empt problems caused by mixing unfamiliar animals. In addition, it may shed light on the intriguing observation that some pairings of animals seem to be immediately successful while others lack this chemistry and result in damaging social strife (von Holst, 1986; Wiepkema and Schouten, 1990).

Of course, once groups are established, it is important to ensure that the welfare of group members is not impaired by social factors. For example, during the two years following successful mixing, about 10–15% of rhesus monkey pairs became incompatible (Reinhardt et al., 1989). In such situations, removal of aggressive individuals may be required. However, there are alternative solutions which we discuss in the next section.

13.6. Solving Problems in Established Social Groups

13.6.1. Providing opportunities for avoidance

In established groups, one important way of ensuring that individuals do not constrain the behaviour of fellow group members or adversely affect their welfare in other ways, is to provide animals with opportunities to avoid each other. For example, avoidance of aggressive or cannibalistic individuals may be easier in larger than smaller enclosures. However, merely increasing the available space may not be effective if that space is open and unstructured, allowing individuals to pursue others unchecked. At high stocking densities, the frequency of agonistic behaviour may actually increase rather than decrease when space is increased (Al-Rawi and Craig, 1975).

The impact of increased group size within an enclosure on opportunities for avoidance is unclear. In chickens kept in pens of a fixed size, the frequency of agonistic pecks and threats decreased with increasing group size and stocking density (Estevez et al., 1997). By contrast, Al-Rawi and Craig (1975) reported increased agonistic behaviour with increased group size and enclosure size in adult laying hens. Also in laying hens, damage due to feather-pecking and cannibalism tends to be more severe as flock size and enclosure size increase (Engström and Schaller, 1993).

Apart from methodological differences between studies, understanding relationships between space and agonistic behaviour is complicated by the intertwined effects of enclosure space, group size, stocking density and access to resources. Thus, to alter stocking density, it is necessary to alter enclosure size or group size, which in turn alters access to resources. To control for all of these factors requires large experiments that may not be practically feasible for anything other than relatively small enclosures and group sizes. Yet the social structure of animals is likely to differ between small groups, where dominance hierarchies based on individual recognition are possible, and large groups, where other rules governing social behaviour may predominate.

Escape and avoidance can clearly be aided by adding protective cover to enclosures, such as barriers and perches. An effect of visual cover in reducing aggression has been reported in a number of species (Chamove and Grimmer, 1993; Whittington and Chamove, 1995). In pigtail macaques, Erwin et al. (1976, p. 321) report that:

> Decreased frequency of agonistic behaviour in the presence of the concrete cylinders, as contrasted with basic frequencies in the usual captive environment among stable groups, suggested that the barriers helped reduce aggression by providing cover for aggressed animals. Subjects began using the barriers immediately upon their introduction to sit on or in, and aggressed animals frequently avoided their aggressors by hiding in the cylinders.

They noted that the presence of cover was effective only for stable groups. 'The availability of cover was not sufficient to overcome the effects of typical macaque hostility towards strangers' (p. 322). By contrast, opaque barriers and pop-holes in which the head can be hidden appear to be effective in reducing aggression among pigs following mixing (McGlone and Curtis, 1985).

Newberry and Shackleton (1997) observed that chickens in large, stable groups preferred partial rather than solid visual barriers. They suggested that these barriers may allow animals to hide but, at the same time, to monitor events on the other side of the barrier. This result indicates that attention must be given to the specific design features of protective structures. Thus, in aviary housing systems for laying hens, where serious problems with cannibalism and feather-pecking can occur (Engström and Schaller, 1993), the long, continuous rows of closely spaced perches may not provide adequate opportunities for individuals to avoid each other. Tree-like structures would probably be more effective in this case.

13.6.2. Manipulating resource distribution

There are other ways to prevent individuals from adversely affecting the welfare of fellow group members. Ideally, a managed social environment will provide all group members with ways of obtaining resources without the need for competition. To achieve this, we need to be aware of the conditions which stimulate competition. Aggressive competition for a resource (such as food or females) will tend to occur when the resource is defensible, as when food arrives in small quantities (Bryant and Grant, 1995) or is dispersed in a limited number of defendable patches (Pulliam and Caraco, 1984). Even if food is provided *ad libitum*, despotic individuals may be able to monopolize access to feeders, as in the case of computerized feeding stations for sows where low-ranking individuals may be intimidated by the presence of an aggressive sow lying at the entrance. In captive green iguanas, the ability to monopolize heat sources probably accounted for the faster growth of high-ranking individuals compared to their cage-mates (Alberts, 1994).

By contrast to aggressive competition, scramble competition will occur for a resource which is not easily defendable, as when a supply of food arrives at a single location accessible to many animals (Milinski and Parker, 1991). In this case, faster eaters, and stronger animals which are able to withstand pushing at the food patch, will be able to eat more food than their weaker group-mates. Solutions to this problem include distributing resources to prevent monopolization by particular individuals and desynchronizing activity to reduce competition. For example, from ideal free distribution theory, we can predict that when food is thinly dispersed over a large area and arrives simultaneously at all locations, animals will spread out evenly with a minimum of competition (Milinski and Parker, 1991). The uniformity of spread may be enhanced if animals can use an easily identifiable cue, such as trough length, as a reliable predictor of food availability. Alternatively, it may be possible to train individuals to feed at different times by signalling when they are allowed to feed. More generally, allowing lower-ranking individuals alternative ways of gathering resources can help to ensure that differences in competitive ability do not lead to differences in welfare (Mendl and Deag, 1995).

13.7. Other Solutions to Social Problems

Genetic selection may provide a long-term solution for reducing undesirable social behaviour (Chapter 15). This approach could take advantage of heritable variation in behavioural characteristics such as aggressiveness, again emphasizing the potential importance of understanding individual differences in social behaviour. For example, it may be possible to reduce cannibalism and feather-pecking in laying hens through artificial selection against beak-inflicted injuries (Craig and Muir, 1993). If these damaging behaviour patterns were eliminated, there would no longer be any need for partial beak amputation.

Consideration should also be given to the selection pressures created by the social environment in which breeding animals are kept. The current commercial practice of housing breeding poultry in single-bird cages relaxes selection on social behaviour traits and may contribute to social problems when offspring are group-housed. If breeding birds were housed in groups and selection was based on high and uniform reproductive output by all members of the group, there would be selection against competitiveness which leads to within-group variation. In fish, Ruzzante (1994) points out that artificial selection for growth rate could inadvertently provide a selective advantage for aggressiveness if selection is practised on groups with a limited or monopolizable food supply (but see also Nielsen *et al.*, 1995, who found no evidence for this effect in pigs). This problem can be avoided by conducting selection programmes under conditions where food is unlimited and easily accessible by all group members.

Specific social abilities such as social learning may also be used in a positive way to enhance animal welfare and production. For example, farm animals are often fed a series of diets at different stages of development, but set-backs in growth may occur at the time of a diet change due to reluctance to try new foods. If certain group members are trained to eat the new food, the rest of the group may acquire a preference for this food quickly due to observational learning or social facilitation (Galef, 1993; Nicol and Pope, 1994). Social learning abilities could also be exploited to enhance the use of new equipment (e.g. electronic feeders).

13.8. Conclusions

- Most attempts to solve social problems in captivity have focused on modifying existing management systems.
- There have been fewer attempts to devise social environments based on a deep understanding of social behaviour.

> One reason may be that social experiments carry greater risks than introducing an inanimate object or device into a cage. Social encounters in particular can be dangerous and require extensive, careful monitoring
>
> (Visalberghi and Anderson, 1993, p. 4)

- Although the social environment sometimes seems a complicated source of trouble, it is also the most important source of stimulation, interest and comfort in the lives of many captive animals.
- For group-living species it is important to devise ways of providing an appropriate social environment rather than resorting to social isolation to avoid problems.

Acknowledgements

This chapter was written while Mike Mendl was at the Scottish Agricultural College (Edinburgh) and Ruth C. Newberry was at the Pacific Agriculture Research Centre of Agriculture and Agri-Food Canada. The authors thank the Scottish Office Agriculture Environment and Fisheries Department and Agriculture and Agri-Food Canada for support, and Dr Linda Keeling for reviewing an earlier draft of the manuscript.

CHAPTER 14
Human contact

Paul H. Hemsworth (Victorian Institute of
Animal Science, Australia) and Harold W. Gonyou
(Prairie Swine Centre, Canada)

Abstract

Human–animal interactions have profound effects on the behaviour and
physiology of farm animals. Regular interactions can result in the animals
developing fear responses to humans, which can have large motivational and
emotional effects on the animals. As a result of stress responses, high levels of
fear of humans can depress both the welfare and performance of farm animals. Our knowledge of human–animal interactions is still limited, but several
avenues for improving animal welfare exist.

Tactile interactions by humans may be either positive or negative in nature
and it is important not only to make all interactions as positive as possible, but
to ensure that the number of negative interactions is kept low relative to the
number of positive interactions. Where a procedure involves negative interactions by humans, it may be possible to eliminate the procedure altogether,
accomplish it mechanically and thus remove the human association, or compensate for the negative interactions by additional positive interactions. If negative
interactions are necessary, their effect may be reduced by prior manipulation
of the animals to improve their response to this human contact. This may be
accomplished by genetic selection for more docile animals or prior positive
handling, perhaps either at sensitive periods of the animals' lives or on a regular
basis. Rewarding experiences at the time may also alleviate the aversiveness of
the situation.

In situations in which animals are fearful of humans and thus the attitude
and behaviour of the stockperson towards the animals are likely to be negative,
the stockperson's commitment to the surveillance of, and the attendance to,
welfare issues can be questioned. Selection and training procedures which
target the attitude and behaviour of stockpeople offer considerable opportunity
to improve animal welfare.

14.1. Introduction

In most forms of animal management, including that of laboratory and zoo
animals as well as on farms, there are regular periods of contact between humans and animals which, at times, may be intense (Fig. 14.1). Human intervention is necessary at least to monitor conditions and the health of the animals
and often to impose routine husbandry procedures. Even in an intensive

Animal Welfare (eds Michael C. Appleby and Barry O. Hughes)

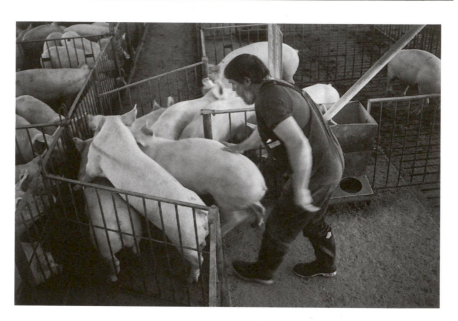

Fig. 14.1. Human–animal interactions are common in modern animal production systems and may have marked behavioural and physiological effects on the animals with consequences for productivity and welfare.

production system such as egg production, in which environmental conditions, provision of food and water and egg collection are automated, there is regular contact associated with inspection of the automated systems and of the health and welfare of the birds. The level of fear of humans displayed by animals in these systems is variable, but high levels are often found. As discussed in Chapter 6, fear may have adverse effects on the productivity and welfare of farm animals. One of the first reports of the significance of the relationship that develops between humans and animals was by Seabrook (1972a) when he concluded that 'The most significant differences between high and low achievement dairy herds was not in the routine used, but in the relationship that existed between the herdsman and his cows.' Although human contact is recognized as influential in affecting fear and thus the welfare of animals, only limited research has been conducted to identify those stimuli involved and how to quantify and reduce their effects.

Although some contact between humans and animals is necessary when caring for animals, it may be possible to manage this contact in such a way that the threat to animal welfare is reduced. This may include a reduction in human–animal contact, or a reduction in the negative nature of the contact. One means of controlling the nature of this contact may be through the careful selection and training of stockpeople. The objectives of this chapter are to identify the effects of human–animal interactions on animal welfare, the principles involved, and opportunities to improve welfare through management of these human–animal interactions. In reporting on the effects of human–animal interactions on experimental chickens, Gross and Siegel (1979) stated that:

> Providing only for their physical needs does not necessarily result in superior experimental animals. Also important factors in the outcome of experiments will be gentle care and familiarity with the animal handlers and experimental procedures.

More recent recognition of the importance of human–animal interactions for animals is found in a series of reviews on the consequences of human–animal interactions for experimental animals (Davis and Balfour, 1992). In introducing these reviews, which also have obvious implications for farm and zoo animals, Davis and Balfour remarked that:

> Only recently have we acknowledged the bond that frequently, perhaps inevitably, develops between subject (experimental animal) and researcher. Whatever the qualities of this relationship, an increasing body of evidence suggests that it may result in profound behavioural and physiological changes in the animal.

14.2. Human Contact and its Effects on Fear of Humans, Productivity and Welfare

Studies, particularly with pigs and poultry, have shown that the level of fear of humans varies considerably among animals and farms. A considerable proportion of this variation may be attributed to the nature of handling that these animals have received. Handling which induces a high level of fear may adversely affect the productivity and welfare of the animals. The threat to welfare of these fearful animals arises because of injuries that they may sustain in trying to avoid humans during routine inspections and handling, the fact that these animals are likely to experience a chronic stress response and, finally, the effects of this chronic stress response on immunosuppression (Hemsworth *et al.*, 1993), which in turn may have serious consequences on the health of the animals. The detrimental effects of fear on animals demonstrate both the seriousness of high fear levels in farm animals and the need to reduce fear levels.

A series of studies with pigs has shown that handling treatments which result in high levels of fear of humans may markedly reduce the growth and reproductive performance of pigs (Hemsworth *et al.*, 1993). The mechanism involved in which fear may affect productivity appears to be a chronic stress response, because in a number of these experiments, pigs which were highly fearful of humans had a sustained elevation of free corticosteroid concentrations in the absence of humans with consequent adverse effects on nitrogen balance and reproduction. The practical implications of these results are demonstrated by the findings of studies in the industry which reveal significant negative relationships, based on farm averages, between the level of fear of humans and the productivity of commercial pigs (Hemsworth *et al.*, 1993). The results of handling studies and the improvement in productivity arising from successfully reducing fear in commercial pigs (Hemsworth *et al.*, 1994a) provide evidence that this fear–productivity relationship in the industry is a cause and effect relationship. As found with pigs, studies conducted on poultry indicate that high levels of fear of humans may limit the productivity of commercial birds. Significant negative relationships between the level of fear of humans and the productivity of commercial broiler chickens and laying hens have been found in the industry (Hemsworth *et al.*, 1993, 1994b). Similar relationships have recently been found in the dairy industry (Hemsworth *et al.*, 1995).

Not all handling appears to be negative in nature. Gross and Siegel (1979, 1980) found that birds that received frequent human contact, apparently of a positive nature, from an early age had improved growth rates and feed efficiency and were more resistant to infection than either birds that received minimal human contact or birds which had been deliberately scared. Although the behavioural response of the birds to humans was not quantified, the authors stated that the handled birds were easier to handle during weighing and blood sampling than the other birds. The results of a number of other studies with poultry support the proposition that handling of a positive nature is associated with increased productivity relative to handling involving either minimal human contact or contact of a negative nature (see Chapter 6 and Hemsworth *et al.*, 1993).

There is also evidence of positive effects of handling on rodents. The extensive literature on the effects of early experience with humans on rodents basically consists of two types of studies: those termed 'handling studies', which involve brief removal of pre-weaned animals from their home cages, and those termed 'gentling studies', which involve brief stroking of post-weaned animals. Although the results have often been contradictory, these treatments at times have produced increased growth and accelerated development, reduced activity and defecation in an open-field test, improved performance in learning tasks and more appropriate endocrine responses to subsequent stressors (Dewsbury, 1992). However, an acute stress response produced in the young animal at the time of handling has been implicated in these effects on subsequent behaviour and physiology.

Thus, the interactions of humans with animals may be either positive or negative. It is important to know the characteristics of these interactions which determine their effect. These characteristics may be based on the stimuli involved, the timing of the interactions and genetic and experiential contributions.

14.3. Behavioural Basis for the Response to Handling

An understanding of the human factors that influence the fear responses of animals to humans may enable fear responses to be reduced in order to improve welfare and productivity. Animals may respond to tactile, visual, olfactory, gustatory and auditory stimuli from humans and these interactions may influence the immediate fear responses of the animals, as well as the subsequent fear responses of the animals to humans. Studies conducted on pigs and dairy cattle under laboratory and commercial conditions indicate that fear of humans is particularly affected by tactile interactions from stockpeople.

Pigs are very sensitive to brief tactile interactions from humans. Negative tactile interactions imposed briefly but regularly will produce high levels of fear of humans. For example, aversive handling treatments, involving brief shocks with a battery-operated prodder or brief slaps whenever the animal approached or failed to avoid an experimenter, imposed for only 15 to 30 seconds daily, consistently resulted in high levels of fear of humans by pigs (Hemsworth *et al.*, 1993). In contrast, positive handling treatments, involving pats or strokes whenever pigs approached an experimenter, resulted in low fear levels. Studies conducted in the pig industry to identify the human behavioural patterns regulating the commercial pig's fear of humans have indicated that the nature of the human tactile interactions is a major factor. The percentage of negative tactile interactions to the total tactile interactions was found to be highly predictive of the level of fear of humans by pigs (Hemsworth *et al.*, 1993). Negative tactile interactions included moderate to forceful slaps, hits, kicks and pushes, while positive tactile interactions included pats, strokes and the hand resting on the pig's back. Surprisingly, high levels of fear of humans were best predicted at commercial farms when the classification of negative behaviours included not only forceful kicks, hits, slaps and pushes, but also the less intuitively obvious negative behaviours such as moderate slaps and pushes. Thus it appears that conditioned approach–avoidance responses develop in pigs as a consequence of associations between the stockperson and the aversive and rewarding elements of the handling bouts. It is the proportion of these negative tactile interactions to the total tactile interactions that predominantly determine the commercial pig's fear of humans.

Recent research in the dairy industry examining the relationships between human and animal factors indicates that similar behavioural patterns by stockpeople regulate the fear responses of commercial dairy cows to humans. The percentage of forceful negative tactile interactions was highly predictive of the level of fear of humans by cows (Hemsworth *et al.*, 1995). The main negative interactions were pushes, slaps and hits while moving cows in and out of the milking shed and into position for milking, while the main positive interactions were pats, strokes and the hand on the cow's flank or leg during milking.

Handling studies on cattle, sheep and goats which have attempted to reduce levels of fear of humans have often involved the imposition of positive tactile interactions. These studies have generally found that handled animals displayed less avoidance of humans in a range of testing situations designed to assess the behavioural response to humans (Hemsworth *et al.*, 1993). In addition to effects on the behavioural response to humans, handled animals in some of these studies had lower heart rate and plasma cortisol responses in a range of situations involving varying amounts of human contact than those that had received less human contact. In addition to presumably positive tactile interactions such as pats, strokes and fondling, some of these studies involved either the experimenter quietly speaking to the animals or the experimenter providing food to attract the animals at the time of handling. Therefore, the reduced fear responses to humans in some of these studies may have been associated with the reward of food rather than handling *per se*.

Thus for many farm animals, the tactile interactions by humans are important determinants of the animal's fear of humans. However, there is evidence that other forms of human contact may affect the behavioural responses of farm animals to humans. Studies, particularly with poultry, indicate that visual contact with humans may affect the animal's fear of humans. Jones (1993) found that regular treatments involving an experimenter placing his hand either on or in the chicken's cage and allowing birds to observe other birds being handled resulted in reductions in the subsequent avoidance behaviour of young chickens to humans. Furthermore, the treatment involving the experimenter's hand in the chicken's cage was more effective than regular handling, which involved picking up and stroking the bird. It is possible that the latter treatment, which involves active tactile interaction by the experimenter, may contain some aversive elements for the bird such as picking the bird up or stroking the bird. Barnett *et al.* (1994b) also found that regular visual contact, involving positive elements such as slow and deliberate movements, reduced the subsequent avoidance behaviour of mature laying hens in comparison to minimal human contact. Thus, while tactile interactions by humans are important determinants of fear responses to humans in many farm animals, poultry appear to be particularly sensitive to visual contact with humans and indeed positive visual contact may be more effective in reducing levels of fear of humans than human tactile contact. Relatively little is known of the negative visual interactions from humans that may elevate fear levels in farm animals. Cransberg and Hemsworth (1995) in studying the behaviour of stockpeople at broiler (meat) chicken farms found that the speed of movement of the stockperson was positively associated with fear levels of birds at the farm. There have been few studies involving auditory or olfactory stimuli, but there is evidence that odours may affect the initial approach behaviour of pigs to humans (Hemsworth *et al.*, 1986b).

Differences in the avoidance responses of animals to humans may reflect either a general fear of unfamiliar stimuli (neophobia), or a specific response to humans. Selection against neophobia is considered a characteristic of domestication, and should result in a reduction in the initial response of naïve animals to all novel stimuli, including humans (Price, 1984). Thus, although genetic selection may have reduced the initial avoidance responses of animals to novel stimuli, there is the opportunity for experienced animals to develop a response to humans that is stimulus-specific, based on their previous experiences with humans. Subsequent changes in these human–animal interactions that involve novel elements, such as a new location, unfamiliar clothing or unfamiliar behaviour by the stockperson, are likely to introduce a component of neophobia in the animal's response. Murphy and Duncan (1978) studied two stocks of chickens, termed 'flighty' and 'docile' on the basis of their responses to humans. They found that early handling affected the behavioural responses of these two strains of birds to humans, with the docile birds showing a more rapid reduction in their withdrawal responses to humans than did flighty birds. Murphy (1977) provided evidence that these strain differences may not be stimulus-specific with the observation that the behavioural responses of these docile and flighty birds to novel stimuli did not necessarily reflect their responses to humans.

Evidence that handling effects on the behavioural response of animals to humans may sometimes be stimulus-specific, and not generalized to a range of fear-provoking stimuli, comes from a series of studies by Jones and colleagues (Jones *et al.*, 1991; Jones and Waddington, 1992). These scientists examined the effects of regular handling on the behavioural responses of quail and domestic chickens to novel stimuli and humans and found that handling predominantly affected the responses of birds to humans, rather than to novelty. These data indicate that experience with humans results in stimulus-specific effects rather than effects on general fearfulness. In contrast, Lyons (1989) reported that early human contact not only affected the behavioural responses of goats to humans but also their behavioural responses to a range of novel stimuli. In comparison to dam-reared goats, those reared by humans showed increased approach to and less avoidance of a number of stimuli including humans. However, considerable human exposure was involved in testing the responses of these goats to novel stimuli and thus their response to humans at the time of testing may have influenced their responses to novel stimuli. Furthermore, early weaning of the human-reared goats may have affected the animals' development, including their response to novelty, as observed in a number of the early handling studies on rodents.

The concept of critical or sensitive periods affecting social attachments traces back to studies of imprinting in precocial birds. Extensive studies on dogs (Scott, 1992), on the effects of early human contact on socialization to humans, demonstrate the long-term effects of such early interaction. Human contact from the age of 3 to 8 weeks of age, involving as little as a few minutes of daily visual contact or just two 20-minute periods of visual contact, has profound effects on the subsequent behavioural responses of dogs to humans. Dogs receiving this amount of human contact early in life show reduced fear responses to humans in adulthood compared to control animals that have received minimal early contact. The sensitive periods in chickens and dogs appear to be associated with a period in the animals' lives when interaction with conspecifics would be more common than with members of other species. Extending this concept of times of social encounters or attachment, Hemsworth *et al.* (1987b, 1989) reported that dairy heifers, exposed to humans while giving birth, are less fearful of humans for several weeks thereafter. On the other hand, handling young pigs prior to weaning had little effect on their responses to humans later in life (Hemsworth *et al.*, 1986a).

The fact that both positive and negative handling of farm animals is possible raises the issue of offsetting one with the other. Pigs handled inconsistently, with a set ratio of positive and negative encounters, were more similar to those consistently handled in a negative manner than those handled positively (Hemsworth *et al.*, 1987a). However, in commercial situations, the proportion of negative to the total tactile interactions predominantly determines the commercial pig's fear of humans (Hemsworth *et al.*, 1993). Associating positive rewards with otherwise negative handling may be a useful means of reducing the aversiveness of the procedure. Sheep provided with feed after being handled aversively were less hesitant to repeat the procedure than those not fed (Hutson, 1985). The ability to utilize human–animal interactions to manipulate the behaviour of animals is well illustrated by some of the techniques used by horse trainers. Many techniques have been devised to manipulate the behaviour of horses in a desirable manner and Waring (1983) has reviewed a number of the common ones. Training of horses often builds on existing stimulus–response relationships. For instance, a swift and focused response towards an inexperienced horse generally initiates flight while a slower and indirect approach generally results in less avoidance. As repeated approaches occur with no adverse effect on the animal, a reduced avoidance response will occur through habituation. Providing human contact early in life can be useful in developing a desirable relationship and Waring (1983) describes the results of a number of studies in which early human contact resulted in improved ease of handling of foals. Horse training also utilizes opportunities to provide a mixture of reinforcement (both positive and negative) and punishment, and again Waring (1983) has described a number of techniques that utilize classical and instrumental conditioning. A reassuring voice and gentle stroking are considered examples of positive reinforcement, while a harsh voice and the harsh use of a bit or whip are suitable as a punishment or in a programme of negative reinforcement. These examples are typical of training procedures often used to train other companion animals.

14.4. The Necessity of Human–Animal Interactions

Conventional animal management involves frequent interactions between humans and animals. The nature of these interactions differs in degree of contact or control by humans. Some interactions are restricted to observation, perhaps without entering the animals' pen. Others involve directed movement of the animals, with or without actual contact between animals and the stockperson. Interactions having the greatest potential to affect the welfare of animals are those which require restraint of the animal in order to perform management or veterinary procedures, or tactile contact used by a stockperson to move an animal, such as the use of an electric prod or slap. All interactions contribute to the overall relationship that animals have with humans, and determine whether that relationship is positive, neutral, or negative. Because of the potential for negative interactions, it is appropriate to ask how necessary interactions between humans and animals are. Is it possible to eliminate some interactions which contribute to a poor relationship between humans and animals?

Careful observation of animals under one's care is considered an essential part of good stockmanship. Although not necessarily a legal requirement, codes of practice for farm, zoo and laboratory animals state that daily observation of animals in confined conditions is considered essential. Humans must also interact with animals when they inspect equipment such as feeders and waterers in animal pens. As a result of these inspections, animals interact with humans hundreds of times during their lifetime. Although these observations do not necessarily involve contact with the animals, we must question whether such interactions are potentially stressful. Studies with poultry have shown that visual contact with humans can indeed affect the fear responses to humans (Chapter 6; Barnett *et al.*, 1994b).

A second level of human interaction with animals involves moving animals but without the use of restraint. Such handling occurs only a few times in the life of some animals. Range animals are herded between pastures as part of the seasonal grass management. Pigs are moved from pen to pen in order to provide accommodation suitable to their stage of life. Other animals are moved much more frequently. Dairy cows, except those which are milked in place, are moved to milking facilities twice daily for most of their lives. Herding of animals may be stressful, particularly if the handling facilities are poorly designed or the stockperson does not use proper equipment (Grandin, 1993b). In addition to the problem of poor equipment or facilities, there is also the human factor of how carefully the stockperson uses these aids. A major factor contributing to lameness in dairy herds is the impatience of the stockperson in moving cows to the milking shed (Chesterton *et al.*, 1989).

Human–animal interactions also include those times when animals must be restrained and subjected to management or health procedures. Some animals may never be restrained during their lives while others are restrained on a regular basis. Some sort of restraint is used for weighing, milking, vaccinating and blood sampling. Animals are handled and restrained for procedures that are probably painful such as castration, branding, ear-tagging and dehorning. When humans handle animals in an unpleasant or inconsistent manner the animals develop a fear of humans (Hemsworth *et al.*, 1987a). It may be possible to reduce or eliminate some of these procedures. Branding has been eliminated in many countries but remains a legal requirement in some jurisdictions. Other procedures, such as vaccinations and blood sampling for diagnosis, are intended to improve the overall welfare of the animals through improved health even if they involve some degree of discomfort or pain. Procedures such as milking and shearing are directly related to the reason the animals are kept, and could only be eliminated if the industry were closed. Weighing, ear-tagging, castration and dehorning are justified by facilitating management, improving product quality or reducing the possibility of injury to animals or humans. Although some reduction in these procedures may be possible, it is likely that they will remain part of animal care and production for some time. The association of fear and pain from these procedures with humans performing them will increase the fear of humans which animals exhibit in other situations, such as during routine inspections. The effect these procedures have on the human–animal relationship relates both to the stressfulness of the procedure and the association of people with that stress. The critical questions then are whether the aversiveness of the procedure can be reduced and whether the procedure can be performed without the presence of humans. Rewarding experiences, such as provision of a preferred feed or even positive handling, around the time of the procedure, may ameliorate the aversiveness of the procedure (Hutson, 1985; Hemsworth *et al.*, 1996).

Is it possible to accomplish the necessary inspection, handling and manipulation of animals without human interactions? If so, will this reduce the stressfulness of the procedure itself or the response of animals to humans when interaction is unavoidable? The reduction or elimination of human involvement in animal management has been the focus of several labour efficiency projects. Examples include robotic shearing of sheep, robotic milking of cows and automated handling facilities for sheep (Syme *et al.*, 1981) and pigs (Barton Gade *et al.*, 1992). The effect of removing humans from such handling procedures on animal responses is best illustrated by research on mechanical harvesting of broiler chickens (Duncan *et al.*, 1986). Birds were caught either by hand or by a specially designed machine. The maximum heart rates of birds caught by either method were similar, but remained high for longer in manually caught animals. In tonic immobility tests, manually caught birds showed a longer response, possibly indicative of greater fear. These results indicate that the stressfulness of some procedures may be reduced by eliminating humans from the procedure. Similar research on management and health procedures should be conducted to determine the effects of the component of the procedure involving human contact on the animals' responses. In situations where the human contact component is highly aversive to the animal, procedures that eliminate human involvement or changes in the behaviour of the human should be sought. For instance, since the method of catching laying hens in cages affects the incidence of bird injuries (Gregory *et al.*, 1993), those techniques which minimize injury should be identified.

14.5. Human Factors Affecting the Behaviour of Stockpeople Towards Farm Animals

It is important to identify those attributes of human behaviour which affect the performance and welfare of farm animals and also the origins of those attributes. Considerable research into the role of the stockperson's attitude and behaviour on the behaviour, productivity and welfare of commercial pigs has been conducted (Hemsworth *et al.*, 1993; Coleman *et al.*, 1997). The theoretical underpinning for this research has its origins in Ajzen and Fishbein's theory of reasoned action (Ajzen and Fishbein, 1980). In brief, this theory holds that:

> As a general rule, we intend to behave in favourable ways with respect to things and people we like and to display unfavourable behaviours towards things and people we dislike. And, barring unforeseen events, we translate our plans into actions.

The research conducted on pigs and, to a lesser extent, that conducted on dairy cows and poultry has clearly demonstrated that the attitude and behaviour of the stockperson have important implications for intensively managed farm animals. Because stockpeople's behaviour toward animals is largely under their control, this behaviour is strongly influenced by the attitudes that they hold about the animals. These attitudes and consequent behaviours predominantly affect the animal's fear of humans which, in turn, affects the animal's performance and welfare. In general, the studies in the pig industry indicate that in comparison to stockpeople with a poor attitude, stockpeople with a good attitude towards handling pigs exhibited less negative or aversive behaviours towards pigs and consequently their pigs were less fearful of humans and had higher productivity (Hemsworth *et al.*, 1993).

While empirical support for the theory of reasoned action is abundant (Ajzen and Fishbein, 1980), it is evident that it may represent an over-simplification of the determinants of intentional behaviour. Eagly and Chaiken (1993) have reviewed the literature extensively and argued the case for several additional facts which may be relevant to predicting behaviour. Aspects of the person which have been omitted from the theory of reasoned action and which may add to the prediction of behaviour include self-identity (e.g. personal beliefs about what being a stockperson entails), personal moral beliefs (i.e. beliefs about right and wrong) and past experience (e.g. habits).

Some authors have highlighted the importance of other stockperson characteristics such as empathy and personality variables (Seabrook, 1972a,b, 1991; English, 1991). For example, Seabrook (1972a,b) reported that the stockperson's personality was related to behaviour of the cows and milk yield of the herd. In 28 one-person herds, the highest-yielding herds were those where the stockpeople were introverted and confident and where the cows were most willing to enter the milking parlour and were less restless in the presence of the stockperson. However, the strongest predictors of the stockperson's behaviour (and thus animal fear and productivity) have been found to be the stockperson's attitudes. Variables such as confidence, introversion and empathy may modulate the manner in which a stockperson's beliefs, behaviour and their consequences are established (Ajzen and Fishbein, 1980). For example, personality may affect the way in which the stockperson responds to handling problems with animals, and may therefore modify the stockperson's beliefs about the animals. Coleman *et al.* (1997) reported significant relationships in the pig industry between stockperson attitudes and empathy. Nevertheless, it has yet to be determined whether such variables as personality and empathy would independently contribute to fear, welfare and productivity in farm animals or would act by modulating attitudes and beliefs as Ajzen and Fishbein (1980) have proposed.

It is also possible that the stockperson's attitudes may influence other important human factors affecting their work performance. For example, the attitude of the stockperson towards the animal may affect such job-related characteristics as work ethic, motivation to learn new skills and knowledge about the animal and job satisfaction, which in turn may affect work performance. If the stockperson's attitude towards the animal is poor, the stockperson's commitment to the surveillance of, and the attendance to, production and welfare problems facing the animal is likely to deteriorate. Thus, the attitudinal and behavioural profiles of the stockperson may have marked effects on animal productivity and welfare both via fear of humans by the animal and via work performance of the stockperson. In fact, some recent research in the Australian pig industry (Coleman *et al.*, 1997) has indicated important relationships between the stockperson's attitudes and job-related variables. In particular, the willingness of stockpeople to attend training sessions in their own time was correlated with attitudes. Job enjoyment and opinions about working conditions showed similar relationships with attitudes. Thus, the stock-person's attitudes may indeed be related to aspects of work apart from handling of pigs. In order to manipulate these human–animal relationships it is obviously important to improve our understanding of the interrelationships between the stockperson's attitude, stockperson's behaviour and other variables including job-related variables.

14.6. Opportunities to Manipulate the Behaviour of Stockpeople to Improve the Welfare and Productivity of Farm Animals

The strong stockperson attitude–behaviour relationships found in the pig industry (Hemsworth et al., 1993; Coleman et al., 1997) demonstrate the potential to improve the attitudinal and behavioural profiles of stockpeople in order to improve the productivity and welfare of intensively managed animals. Training stockpeople to improve their attitudinal and behavioural profiles towards pigs and selecting stockpeople for employment on the basis of their attitudinal profile are likely candidates in this regard.

The opportunity for, and the potential of, training stockpeople in terms of their attitude and behaviour towards farm animals are demonstrated by a recent study. Hemsworth et al. (1994a) successfully used a training procedure to improve the attitude and behaviour of stockpeople in the pig industry with consequent positive effects on the fear and productivity of their pigs. Because of the reciprocal relationship between the attitudes and behaviour of the stockperson and the equally strong relationships between the stockperson's attitude and behaviour and the fear and productivity and welfare of pigs, this behavioural modification procedure targeted both the attitudes and behaviour of stockpeople for improvement.

Therefore, since the attitude and behaviour of stockpeople towards pigs appear to be integral components in the pathway(s) which affect the productivity and welfare of pigs, there appears to be considerable opportunity for the pig industry to improve the performance and welfare of pigs by training stockpeople. Similar opportunities may exist in other animal industries but research is required to confirm whether similar human attitude and behaviour, and animal behaviour, productivity and welfare relationships exist and whether or not there is opportunity to manipulate these human factors to improve animal welfare and productivity. Recent and current work in the dairy and poultry industries indicate some exciting opportunities (Barnett et al., 1992; Hemsworth et al., 1993, 1994b, 1995; Cransberg and Hemsworth, 1995).

The development of selection procedures for stockpeople also offers potential to improve animal welfare and productivity. The attitude questionnaires that have been used as a research tool in the pig, poultry and dairy industries, and which have been shown to be predictive of stockperson behaviour and level of fear and productivity of animals, show considerable potential to form the basis of a selection aid for experienced stockpeople. However, their potential use is presently limited to experienced stockpeople because the questions which are most predictive of the stockperson's behaviour generally target the stockperson's beliefs about handling animals and their own behaviour toward animals. Since inexperienced stockpeople do not have reliable attitudes towards farm animals, because attitudes are a product of past beliefs and experiences, the value of this questionnaire to predict the subsequent performance of the stockperson is questionable. Recent observations in the pig industry indicate relationships between attitudes and job-related variables, such as job satisfaction and motivation to learn, and empathy (Coleman *et al.*, 1997) and these observations indicate the opportunities that may exist through the development of selection procedures targeting other personal and job-related variables.

It is likely that developments of this type, which assist in establishing farm animal husbandry as a job with a recognized skill base, will have substantial implications for the welfare and productivity of commercial animals.

14.7. Conclusions

- Human–animal interactions have profound effects on the behaviour and physiology of farm animals. Our knowledge of human–animal interactions is still limited, but several avenues for improving animal welfare exist.
- Tactile interactions by humans may be either positive or negative in nature and it is important not only to make all interactions as positive as possible, but to ensure that the proportion of negative interactions is kept low.
- If negative interactions are necessary, their effect may be reduced by manipulation of the animals, by genetic selection for more docile animals or by positive handling; the latter may be done earlier (at sensitive periods of the animals' lives) or on a regular basis, or at the time of the negative interaction.
- Selection and training procedures which target the attitude and behaviour of stockpeople offer considerable opportunity to improve animal welfare.

CHAPTER 15
Genetic selection

Andrew D. Mills (INRA, France), Rolf G. Beilharz
(University of Melbourne, Australia) and Paul M. Hocking
(Roslin Institute, UK)

Abstract

Production diseases and mismatches between behaviour and artificial husbandry conditions are the source of welfare problems in many domesticated
species. Such problems have arisen because of rapid changes in intensive
animal housing systems, selection for economic traits which has not taken
account of secondary traits related to the animals' welfare, or a combination of
these factors. This chapter reviews the potential role of genetic improvement
programmes as a means of promoting animal welfare. Considerable evidence
exists that there is genetic variation in traits relevant to welfare, so it should be
possible to select for such traits. The major problems associated with such genetic improvement programmes are the need to develop measures of welfare
which are compatible with selection on a commercial scale, and potential competition between selection for production- and welfare-related traits. The relative advantages and disadvantages of both quantitative and molecular genetic
approaches to the improvement of welfare are considered. It is concluded that
whatever the genetic approach adopted, selection for traits, such as fearfulness
or sociality, which are common to various types of husbandry systems is likely
to be of greater long-term value than selection for traits which result in
adaptation to specific husbandry systems.

15.1. Introduction

Modern day domestic animals are the product of thousands of generations of
selective breeding, as Bowman (1974) noted:

> Animal breeding is not a new activity. From the time of man's early attempts
> at domestication of reindeer, pigs, goats and other farm species in the Neolithic
> period (around 7000 BC) he has been controlling the mating and reproductive
> opportunities of these and other species. Throughout man has attempted to
> change the behaviour, anatomy and morphology of domesticated species to
> suit his own requirements.

Indeed, Darwin (1875) recognized that the behaviour and physiology of
domestic animals had been modified during domestication and Zeuner (1963)
noted that selective breeding programmes had been changed during the
history of many domesticated species. An example of the diverse selection
pressures exerted during domestication is found in the domestic fowl which

was originally selected for 'song', then aggression and only more recently for meat and egg production (Wood-Gush, 1959).

Until recently, humans practised artificial selection by retaining individuals that they felt exhibited more desirable traits and culling those with less desirable traits (Siegel and Dunnington, 1990). Such selection was performed in the absence of knowledge of the laws of genetics and was based on appraisal of each individual for a wide variety of traits (Faure, 1981). However, within the last century animal breeding and husbandry have undergone radical changes. Rediscovery of Gregor Mendel's 'fundamental laws of inheritance' in 1900 (Strickberger, 1976) and subsequent development of quantitative genetics by Fisher, Haldane, Lush and Wright allowed the application of these principles to animal breeding (Lush, 1945; Lerner, 1951). This allowed selection on the basis of breeding values for particular traits rather than overall assessment of temperament, performance or productivity (Faure, 1980). At the same time there was considerable progress in the fields of animal nutrition, veterinary science and design of housing systems which, by permitting animals to express their genetic potential better, further contributed to genetic gain in those production traits subject to selection.

Unfortunately gains in productivity have brought negative side effects. Selection has frequently been concentrated on economic characters confounding several biological processes, such as body weight at a given age, without taking account of 'secondary' but related characteristics. So selection for production traits has often had negative effects on the general adaptation of the animals to their environment and on their welfare (Sørensen, 1989). One aspect of this has been the occurrence of what have been called production diseases (Blood and Studdert, 1988):

> Production diseases are defined as diseases caused by systems of management, especially feeding and breeding of high producing strains of animals and birds, in which production exceeds dietary and thermal input.

Broiler chickens, which have been selected for rapid growth rate, provide examples of this type of disorder. Today, broiler chickens reach a body weight of 1.6 kg in half the time they did in 1945 and consume one-third less food in so doing (Hartmann, 1989). However, selection for body weight has been accompanied by the appearance of leg weakness, higher mortality and increased appetite (Sørensen, 1989). In breeding birds, severe food restriction to control body weight is necessary to promote adequate fertility and egg production (Hocking et al., 1987; Hocking, 1990). This in turn leads to hunger and behaviour which is characteristic of undernourishment and frustration of feeding behaviour (hyperactivity and polydipsia: Savory et al., 1993).

In fact environmental limitation is the norm in wild and most domestic animals (Beilharz et al., 1993). As such, selection of production traits is only possible if fitness and other traits fall below their optima, unless there is continuing increase in environmental resources. In the normal, limited situation, raising production traits may increase the mismatch between available resources and demands of phenotypic development. Recognition of environmental limitation in animal production should alert us to the possibility of genetic–

environmental mismatches and allow us to avoid unnecessary welfare problems by choosing only obtainable breeding goals.

In many species, gains in animal production have been accompanied by a rapid movement towards artificial, intensive and highly standardized rearing conditions. Although adaptation to these conditions has occurred and will continue to occur through natural selection, in many cases the rate of environmental change has been such that there has been insufficient time for adaptation through natural selection to occur (Czako and Santha, 1978) – as has been noted by Faure (1980):

> If the actual conditions of present day accommodation were allowed to remain stable over the next few thousands of generations it is probable that the birds would again adapt.

Combined with artificial selection procedures which have already, to some degree, short-circuited the processes of adaptation by natural selection, this has also given rise to mismatches between the animals' behaviour and the environments in which they are kept. This situation has been further confounded by changes in behaviour due to random genetic drift or unconscious co-selection for behaviour when selecting for other traits (Mench, 1992; Newman, 1994). These mismatches are sometimes reflected in aspects of the animals' behaviour becoming apparently superfluous, maladaptive or even deleterious. Examples are tail-biting in pigs (Ewbank, 1973), feather-pecking in chickens (Hughes and Duncan, 1972) and the restless pacing behaviour shown by some strains of domestic hen in the period prior to laying in battery cages (Wood-Gush, 1972). Such mismatches are likely to become more frequent as selection techniques based on modern technology come into play, such as the estimation of breeding values by sophisticated computation (Henderson, 1984) or transgenesis (Bulfield, 1985).

On the other hand, genetic selection may be used to improve farm animal welfare. Mench (1992) has emphasized that 'Genetic selection may prove to be a powerful tool for decreasing the incidence of behaviors associated with welfare problems' and envisages *de novo* selection to 'modulate behavioural and physiological characteristics associated with welfare'. Sørensen and Leenstra (1986) take a different line in referring to 'repair of negative consequences of selection (for growth)'. They envisage use of selection to correct existing production diseases, an approach which Abplanalp (1982) suggested would require 'the same selection techniques that have brought about the initial changes causing them'.

If genetic selection is to be used to improve animal welfare a multidisciplinary approach will be needed. This will require links between animal producers who have tended to concentrate on economic return, geneticists who have until recently tended to concentrate on gene frequencies and animal behaviourists who have tended to assume a standard genotype but have perhaps been more aware of how severely environmental factors can constrain and limit welfare (Beilharz *et al.*, 1993). In the remainder of this chapter we will develop some of the problems and practicalities associated with putting such an approach into practice.

15.2. Feasibility of Selection for Traits Relevant to Welfare

The question of feasibility of selection to improve welfare was raised in relation to behavioural traits by Faure in 1980 – 'Is it possible to select for behaviours relevant to adaptation problems?' – and can be extended to selection against all kinds of production diseases. If selection is to be successful, there must be additive genetic variation in the trait or traits to be selected for. Evidence for such variation in at least some traits related to welfare comes from several sources.

First, there are breed or strain differences in the expression of many welfare-related traits in a wide range of species. Examples of such differences are the pre-laying behaviour of domestic hens in battery cages (Wood-Gush, 1972), avoidance and escape behaviour in White Leghorn chickens (Craig *et al.*, 1983), fear of humans in sheep (Le Neindre *et al.*, 1994) and aggressiveness in cattle (Boivin, 1991). Where such breed differences can be shown to exist in a common environment, they are, by definition, to some degree under genetic control and it should be possible to select for or against expression of these traits.

Second, quantitative genetic studies have generated moderate to high heritability estimates for traits as diverse as docility in cattle (Le Neindre *et al.*, 1994) and aspects of leg weakness in broiler chickens (Mercier and Hill, 1984). Such heritability estimates are direct evidence for additive genetic variance and imply that selection for, or against, such traits will be successful.

Third, it has already proved possible to select for a wide variety of traits related to welfare:

> Selection for or against such behaviours as aggressiveness, docility, response to stress and certain sexual behaviours in some livestock species has often been successful.
>
> (Newman, 1994)

Admittedly, most selection experiments have been of short duration (Siegel and Dunnington, 1990) but selection has been successfully applied to species and traits as diverse as dust-bathing behaviour in Japanese quail (Gerken and Petersen, 1987), aggressiveness in chickens (Guhl *et al.*, 1960), tameness in silver foxes (Belyaev, 1979) and leg weakness in broiler chickens (Leenstra *et al.*, 1984). There is, therefore, no apparent reason why selection should not be applied to these and other traits related to welfare.

Fourth, molecular genetic techniques have already been used to identify genes, or more precisely quantitative trait loci (QTL), related to welfare traits such as the porcine stress syndrome (Rempel *et al.*, 1993) and emotionality in laboratory mice (Flint *et al.*, 1995). Where differences in QTL exist there is scope for selection. There is circumstantial evidence that such loci exist for other traits related to welfare such as fearfulness in cattle (Holmes *et al.*, 1972).

15.3. Commercial Viability

However, the fact that it may be possible to select for traits relevant to welfare either in theory or under experimental conditions is not evidence in itself that such selection can be applied under commercial conditions. The application of selection under commercial conditions is dependent on economic factors (Faure, 1980) and on the limitations imposed by existing or future selection environments (Beilharz *et al.*, 1993). Selection in commercial conditions has limitations which are not encountered in laboratory studies. Commercially exploited domestic animals are already subjected to selection for multiple economic traits. In addition, commercial population sizes tend to be much larger than those found in laboratory studies.

The first of these limitations is a practical problem. When animals are subjected to simultaneous selection for multiple traits, the selection pressure that can be applied on a given trait is limited. The extent of this limitation depends on two interrelated factors: the relevant economic importance of the traits considered and, perhaps to a lesser degree, the genetic correlation between the traits to be selected. If the correlation is high then genetic gain is likely to be rapid for all parameters and economic considerations will not compete markedly with selection for traits relevant to welfare. If the genetic correlation between economic and welfare traits is low or negative, then traits will compete with each other and overall genetic gain will be achieved only slowly. In the absence of knowledge about such correlation, commercial breeders will concentrate selection on those traits which are most closely related to economic performance. Hence, as Faure (1980) points out, if 'welfare is not defined in terms of production, we cannot expect that welfare problems will be taken into account in breeding plans'.

It is possible that selection for welfare-related traits might be 'consumer driven' in that if suitable breeding programmes are not developed then consumers may reject the end product. However, this is to some degree speculative and the relationships between productivity and traits relevant to welfare remain largely unknown. Further, the limited experimental findings concerning such relationships have often been contradictory. Newman (1994) states that in many cases 'negative relationships have been demonstrated between production traits and behaviors associated with welfare'. However Gerken *et al.* (1988) found no relationship between inherent fearfulness, egg production and egg shell quality in Japanese quail. Mills *et al.* (1991) found that high fearfulness was associated with poor egg shell quality in domestic hens and Remignon *et al.* (1996) found that pre-mortem stress had greater negative effects on meat quality in quail selected for high levels of fearfulness than in quail selected for low levels of fearfulness.

The second problem associated with selection for traits relevant to welfare is the number of animals that must be scored for multiple traits. Even if there is willingness to select for traits relevant to welfare, scoring sufficient animals to allow selection on a commercial basis may prove problematic. Depending on the species considered, estimates of breeding values require that hundreds or even thousands of individuals be assessed for one or more traits. This has inherent but not insurmountable problems. To date, most studies relating to the behaviour of domestic species have used measures which would not be viable for the numbers of animals found in commercial breeding stock. For example, in Wood-Gush's (1972) study of strain differences in pre-laying behaviour in battery cages, already mentioned, observations were commenced 'more than one hour before [the hen] laid' and in Ortman and Craig's (1968) study of social dominance, observation of individual birds frequently took as long as one hour. However, Faure (1981) has emphasized that it is possible, within certain limitations, to develop measures of welfare traits which are compatible with selection on a commercial scale.

Faure suggests that behavioural traits relevant to welfare can be assigned to five categories depending on their suitability for incorporation into commercial breeding programmes. These are, in order from most to least suitable:

1. Behaviour patterns which leave permanent traces. These can be used as direct measures for selection. Examples are tail-biting in pigs (Ewbank, 1973) and feather-pecking in chickens (Cuthbertson, 1980).

2. Behaviour which can be measured automatically. Automatic recording is usually cheaper and less ambiguous than measures obtained from direct observation by a human being. An example is general activity either in the home cage (Bessei and Bessei, 1974) or in tests of emotionality such as the open-field test (Faure and Folmer, 1975).

3. Behaviour which is expressed over long periods of time. The incidence of such behaviour can be measured in large numbers of individuals by simple scanning techniques. Broodiness has virtually been eliminated from modern commercial strains of laying hens (Faure, 1980) and provides an example of the application of such selection on a commercial scale. Perching behaviour in domestic hens would also lend itself to selection by this method (Faure and Jones, 1982).

4. Behaviour which is easily induced. Aggression (Guhl et al., 1960) and sexual behaviour (Siegel, 1975) in chickens fall into this category. Faure (1981) considers that it would be difficult to incorporate selection for such traits into commercial breeding programmes because of the time required to test each individual. However, Le Neindre et al. (1994) suggest that it should be possible to select for reduced aggressiveness in cattle using short-term reactions to a human as the measure of selection.

5. Traits which are difficult or impossible to induce or predict. Faure (1980) cites pre-laying behaviour in domestic birds as an example of such a trait and considers that behaviour of this type will be impossible to select for 'because one observer can measure no more than a few birds'. However, Mills (1983) suggested that selection for certain types of pre-laying behaviour would be possible using scanning techniques because the majority of birds lay within a relatively short period of time.

This classification omits one problem associated with selection for any trait, whether related to welfare or not. Measures for selection must be repeatable because repeatability is closely related to heritability (Falconer, 1977). Repeatability is not a problem when traits such as weight or presence or absence of some physiological abnormality are considered but can be a major problem with behavioural traits. Methods for the estimation of repeatability are given elsewhere (Falconer, 1977) but it is clear that if it is low then each animal must be scored several times before even its true phenotype can be assessed, to say nothing of its breeding value. Where such problems occur, the use of full- or half-sib analyses (Falconer, 1977) may be appropriate.

In reality, most welfare-related traits are intermediate on Faure's (1981) scale of classification and although some traits may respond to selection more readily than others, increasing knowledge of behaviour and physiology should allow the development of short-term measures of welfare-related traits which are viable and unambiguous predictors of the trait or traits to be selected. However, as Beilharz (1994) cautions, great care must be used in defining the traits to be selected because 'what you select is precisely what you get'. Artificial selection is a very powerful tool and selection for a trait in early life in a given environment may not be reflected in adult or even in juvenile behaviour in other environments (but see also Launay *et al.*, 1993). However, to summarize, published selection experiments, the development of short-term measures of behaviour and recent developments in quantitative and molecular genetics imply that it should be possible to select for traits relevant to welfare on a commercial scale.

15.4. Biotechnology and Animal Well-being

Recent progress in molecular genetics also provides evidence that it may be possible to develop new measures for selection of traits relevant to welfare. Developments in molecular biology provide tools for understanding the genetic basis of complex polygenic traits and for changing gene frequencies directly.

> There have been remarkable developments in the field of molecular biology. These allow the opportunity to identify animals of superior genetic merit by direct analysis of DNA and the ability to make precise copies and transfers of genetic material within and across species boundaries.
>
> (Newman, 1994)

This means that it may be possible to apply selection for genetic markers of genes or even for genes themselves rather than attempting to change gene frequencies through selection on phenotypic information. The technology behind such selection is based on the discovery of sections of DNA showing short tandem repeat (STR) base sequences or microsatellites. These are numerous, highly polymorphic and uniformly distributed throughout the genome. Standard molecular biology methods (Ziegler *et al.*, 1992) make it possible to use STR base sequences to automate the genotyping of large numbers of animals for many genetic markers.

The power of such new technology can be illustrated by an example of the application of QTL analysis to the determination of fearfulness or emotionality in mice. Flint *et al.* (1995) used two lines of mice selected for high and low open-field activity. In addition, the high line showed less defecation in the open field than the low line and it was also possible to distinguish between the lines using three other tests of fearfulness. Flint and colleagues crossed these lines and produced nearly 900 F_2 progeny which were individually evaluated for each of the five traits. The top and bottom ranking 10% of mice for open-field activity were genotyped with 84 markers covering the entire genome. Analysis of QTL markers revealed that there were six loci involved in determination of open-field activity. The scientists then went on to genotype another 10% of the animals to include the top and bottom ranking mice for all five traits and found that there were three common loci. The six quantitative trait loci for open-field activity accounted for a very similar proportion of the genetic variance as the heritability of the trait. The results suggested that few loci affected the trait and that they acted in an independent and additive manner. Furthermore, there was direct evidence that three of the loci affected other measures of fear.

These results and evidence that behavioural traits respond readily to selection suggest that there may be relatively few genes controlling behavioural traits of importance to the welfare of farm animals. Whilst conventional selection would be effective in altering behaviour (see above), there are benefits of marker-assisted selection (selection on a DNA marker) which may make such indirect methods attractive. First, the problems of measuring the trait(s) in selection candidates are removed. This is valuable if the trait is difficult or expensive to measure, is sex limited, or requires the animal to be killed. Second, selection on a marker may be more efficient (higher effective heritabilities). Third, the search for candidate markers will be made easier because of the conserved synteny that exists between different species. For example, a locus in poultry could be evaluated as a candidate gene in pigs. Fourth, the genetic basis of the trait may be known in advance of selection for it.

However, the effectiveness of marker-assisted selection is still unproven and the problems of multiple selection objectives and genetic progress in the major selection criteria remain. Genotyping at present is expensive but so are standard selection methods and it seems likely that the costs of genotyping will become more affordable in the near future. Problems of identifying marker loci also exist: currently a cross of two widely divergent lines must be made and lines of commercial animals tend not to differ greatly for behavioural and welfare-related traits. However, experimental lines divergent for traits relevant to welfare exist and could be used to identify loci of importance.

As an experimental tool, the use of markers is potentially very powerful as the paper by Flint et al. (1995) demonstrates. Nevertheless, the search for a gene and the study of gene action is at present a long and tedious procedure. Against this, the similarity of genetic architecture in different species means that selecting candidate genes from more extensively studied species such as humans or mice will become increasingly feasible. Additionally, marker-assisted selection only requires that the flanking loci are reasonably closely linked to the gene or genes of interest.

The use of molecular genetics in the improvement of animal welfare also raises the question of the creation of transgenic animals, because if genes related to welfare can be isolated then the technology exists for inserting them into mammals and birds. However, at least at present the development of transgenic animals has been largely experimental and no welfare-related transgenes have been identified. However, Newman (1994) suggests that the development of transgenic animals may lead to the elimination of genetic defects from animal populations, more efficient production leading to the use of fewer animals and a better understanding of animal welfare. Therefore it is possible that, with increasing knowledge, molecular genetic techniques will play an increasing role in the genetic control of welfare traits.

15.5. Choice of Traits

As there is clear evidence that it is possible to select animals for traits relevant to welfare, the question arises as to which traits should be selected for:

> Various studies have shown that it is possible to select for or against traits, related to welfare problems which are particular to specific husbandry systems. However, it is also possible to select for welfare related traits which are common to different types of husbandry systems. Which type of selection is preferable?
>
> (adapted and translated from Mills *et al.*, 1994)

Examples of selection for or against specific traits in given environments include pre-laying restlessness (Mills *et al.*, 1985a), dust-bathing (Gerken and Petersen, 1987) and perching in laying hens (Faure and Jones, 1982). However, at least with respect to behavioural traits, such selection has inherent disadvantages.

First, selection for 'environment specific traits' runs the risk of adapting animals to a particular husbandry system. Such selection is appropriate only if husbandry systems do not change in the future. This is unlikely both for commercial reasons and because most research into animal welfare has advocated changes in husbandry systems rather than genetic change in the animals (Appleby and Hughes, 1993). Faure (1980) summarized the extremes of this problem in his paper, 'To adapt the environment to the bird or the bird to the environment'.

Studies of pacing during the pre-laying period by domestic hens kept in battery cages provide an example of the potential problems associated with selection for environment specific traits. Wood-Gush (1972) studied the pre-laying behaviour of domestic hens kept in battery cages. He suggested that modifying battery cages to incorporate environmental factors likely to release sitting behaviour would decrease the expression of stereotyped pacing in the pre-laying period and increase time spent sitting, and tested this hypothesis (Wood-Gush, 1975) by reducing the slope of the floors of battery cages and providing the birds with nesting material. The result of these environmental modifications were as he had predicted. However, Mills *et al.* (1985a) were able to produce similar reductions in pre-laying pacing by selection on the basis of time spent sitting in the ten minutes prior to oviposition. Mills *et al.* (1985b) then went on to demonstrate that the birds which showed sitting behaviour before laying had lower heart rates than those that showed restless pacing.

This was taken to imply that selection for increased sitting time had reduced frustration attributable to the absence of nesting material in the battery cages and thereby reduced the expression of pre-laying restlessness. Therefore, both genetic and environmental change could be used to modify pre-laying behaviour in battery cages but each obviated the need for the other. Hence, although most laying hens are presently housed in battery cages, a switch to the housing of birds in alternative systems such as aviaries, deep-litter systems or modified cages, where the environmental stimuli necessary for nest-seeking and nest-building behaviour are present, would make costly selection against pre-laying restlessness redundant.

Second, some animals such as dairy cattle experience more than one set of environmental conditions within their lifetime. This situation led Beilharz and Zeeb (1981) to suggest that:

> While a case can be made for adapting animals genetically to intensive housing if they are to be always indoors, another approach must be used for animals which spend most of their time outside. Most dairy cows spend at least six months each year on pasture, performing all the typical outdoor behaviours. It would be unreasonable to house them in winter under conditions in which they could not perform their 'natural' behaviour.

Under such conditions selection for greater phenotypic plasticity or adaptability might be appropriate. The value of such an approach is discussed below.

Third, the same breed or strain of animal may be kept under a range of different husbandry systems as is already the case for laying hens which are kept in systems as diverse as outdoor runs and battery cages, and some strains of broiler chickens which may be housed either in outdoor runs or deep-litter houses. In such cases adaptation to one environment is unlikely to be matched by adaptation to the other ones. An example of a problem of this type is selection for egg production in pheasants reared in aviaries or battery cages. Birds reared in cages produce poorly in aviaries and vice versa (Faure *et al.*, 1992). Similar results have been reported for chickens selected for egg production in colony cages or individual cages. It has been suggested that, at least in pheasants, shuttle selection for egg production, whereby successive generations are selected alternately in each environment, maintains production in both environments. Similar selection for other traits might reduce the incidence of problems associated with keeping animals of the same strain in differing environments (Faure *et al.*, 1992). However, set against this is Muir's (1996) argument concerning genotype–environment interactions which suggests that there may be 'specific adaptation of each genotype to each environment, which implies not only a lack of adaptation to the other environment, but a maladaptation'. For example, if there were negative genetic correlations between traits adaptive to each environment, then responses to shuttle selection would be slow or mutually negating.

Fourth, breeding stock may be kept under different conditions than their progeny. Such a situation exists in layer hens where selection is performed in single-bird cages and progeny are kept in multiple-bird cages or in open housing. There is experimental evidence that selection in these conditions results in aggressive birds with a tendency to cannibalism (Muir, 1996). On the other hand, selection of progeny would not necessarily be accompanied by increased welfare or adaptation of breeding stock (see also Beilharz, 1982).

Selection for 'environment specific traits' does not, therefore, seem to be a viable long-term approach to the improvement of animal welfare. However, many traits which are common to virtually all husbandry systems exist and we argue that it is in the selection for (or against) such traits that the greatest potential for the improvement of animal welfare is to be found. Fear, aggression and social stress are obvious candidates. It is difficult to imagine any husbandry system where the animals are not exposed to frightening stimuli (contact with humans or machinery), competition (restricted feeding or limited access to feeders) or housing in groups with abnormal social composition (many animals of the same sex and age). Environmental change is unlikely to correct problems of this type.

Fear and its correlates, panic and hysteria, have negative effects on welfare and production (Chapter 6). Furthermore, many husbandry systems involve practices which disrupt established social relationships. For example, when animals are housed in single sex and same age groups, anomalies in social behaviour may occur because of the disruption of the normal social structure (Duncan, 1981a). Mixing of groups of animals for practical reasons can also lead to aggression during the establishment of new hierarchies.

Breed and strain differences have already been demonstrated in fear responses and social behaviour in domesticated species as diverse as sheep, cattle and domestic fowl (Bouissou et al., 1994; Le Neindre et al., 1994; Mills and Faure, 1990). Therefore, as has been suggested earlier, it ought to be possible to reduce the negative aspects of these traits through genetic manipulation. Selection against fear and for sociability in Japanese quail provide examples of the application of such an approach.

Mills and Faure (1991) attempted to reduce fearfulness in Japanese quail by selecting for reduced duration of the tonic immobility (TI) response (see Jones, 1986, for a review of this measure as an indicator of fear). They selected animals on the basis of TI in a test, with a maximum duration of five minutes, when the birds were only ten to eleven days of age. The response to selection was rapid and subsequent studies showed not only that the selected lines differed in TI throughout their lives but also that differences in fear responses were present in a wide variety of behavioural and physiological measures under different experimental conditions (Mills et al., 1994).

Mills and Faure (1991) also selected for high or low levels of social reinstatement in Japanese quail chicks. Social reinstatement was assessed by measuring the distance the animals were prepared to run to rejoin a group of conspecifics, in a five-minute treadmill test. Again the response to selection was rapid. Subsequent research indicated that the effects of selection persisted throughout the life of the animals and were reflected in differences in interindividual distances, responses to social deprivation and the social facilitation of feeding behaviour (Launay et al., 1993; Mills et al., 1993a,b, 1994).

Therefore it is possible to select for traits which are not environment specific and lead to improved welfare irrespective of the husbandry system imposed on the animals.

15.6. Discussion

Genetic manipulation has sometimes been downplayed as a means of improving animal welfare. For example, a workshop reported by Appleby and Hughes (1993) suggested that:

> Both genetic selection and genetic manipulation pose problems for applied ethology. In genetic selection we can rarely identify precisely the genes which have been selected, while genetic manipulation techniques (e.g. transgenics) are still uncertain . . . In some cases this research is driven as much by commercial as by scientific considerations.

However, breed differences in traits related to welfare already exist and the judicious choice of strains or breeds according to the husbandry system used could already lead to improvements in welfare. Selection of animals for desirable traits does not require that the genes implicated in the trait or traits be identified and mapped on the genome. If this were the case then there would have been no progress in animal breeding before, or after, the development and application of the theories underlying quantitative genetics. Conversely, transgenic change does require the identification of particular genes but, as we have argued, the identification of genes involved in welfare traits is increasingly feasible and the dissemination of such genes can be practised. Two examples can be used to illustrate these points.

Leenstra et al. (1984) demonstrated that combined selection for reduced incidence of twisted legs and body weight in broiler chickens achieved decreased incidence of twisted legs, with no noticeable effect on body weight relative to a strain selected only for body weight. This experiment was carried out in the absence of any knowledge of the genes underlying body weight, leg weakness or their interactions.

Mérat (1984) identified a sex-linked recessive gene of fowl which led to a dwarf phenotype in homozygous recessive males or hemizygous recessive females. This gene resulted in a reduction of body weight of approximately one-third in females. Mérat showed that introduction of the 'dwarfing gene' to broiler breeder stock could be used to improve both welfare and economic return. Crossing females to males homozygous for the dominant allele of the gene produced normal offspring. However, dwarf breeder females do not require as severe food restriction as normal broiler breeder females and showed lower incidences of leg weakness than their normal-size counterparts.

The workshop reported by Appleby and Hughes (1993) further suggested that animal welfare will be better served by environmental change than by genetic adaptation to existing environments, at least in the short term: 'Husbandry conditions should be improved, rather than relying too heavily on animals adapted through genetic selection.' However, another workshop at the same conference (Appleby and Hughes, 1993) stated that 'there is a requirement for more basic knowledge of the biology of domestic animals and for increased precision in establishing their needs'. In other words, it is not possible to develop new husbandry systems without taking into account variation in animals' behaviour relative to that of their ancestors. Furthermore, since the behaviour of domestic animals varies within species, the design of housing systems must take into account genetic variability in traits relevant to welfare. If environmental change is applied without due consideration of these factors then animals which are phenotypically unable to adapt may suffer (Beilharz, 1982). Furthermore, under such circumstances, any adaptation which does occur will be through natural selection and as many studies of free-living species show (e.g. Mock *et al.*, 1987) such selection is often far from welfare friendly.

15.7. Conclusions

- Selection for traits relevant to animal welfare is possible, although certain practical problems associated with exact methods of selection remain to be overcome.
- Compared to other methods for the improvement of welfare, selection has the disadvantage of being long term (several generations) but is probably the most effective solution to certain types of problems.
- With certain exceptions, selection for traits related to adaptability is likely to be more appropriate than selection for environment specific characteristics.
- Selection and environmental modification are not mutually exclusive approaches to the improvement of welfare. In fact, a combination of genetic manipulation (or even the judicious use of existing line and breed differences) and environmental modification is likely to prove a powerful method for the improvement of welfare and productivity.

Part V
Implementation

The objective of all those working in the field of welfare is improvement of quality of life for animals and success will be measured by how effectively such efforts are implemented. Many of the solutions covered in Part IV will have economic costs and it is important to consider those costs. However, economics – the subject of Chapter 16 – is not just about the cost of implementing changes suggested by other approaches. It is also about how our attitudes to issues such as animal welfare are reflected in our behaviour. Similarly, legislation (Chapter 17) is not just a 'fire extinguisher' to cope with a problem once it has started – it is one approach among others, bound up with public attitudes and other influences on how we treat animals. So Part V continues the emphasis of the rest of the book on the practical nature of the matters under discussion. Certainly if animal welfare is to be safeguarded and improved, then economics and legislation will be central to those aims.

CHAPTER 16
Economics

Richard M. Bennett (University of Reading, UK)

Abstract

This chapter discusses the relevance of economics to the study of animal welfare and considers the relationship between ethics and economics. It presents a number of techniques of economic analysis, together with some assessment of their use, and includes a case-study relating to cage egg production. It considers the relevance of economics to policy decisions about animal welfare. Economic considerations are central to the animal welfare debate and are integral (and inescapable) aspects of issues concerning the use of animals and of any interdisciplinary inquiry into animal welfare, alongside ethics and animal science.

16.1. Introduction

Although the ethical and scientific aspects of animal welfare and animal rights have been extensively debated over the last thirty years (Harrison, 1964; Singer, 1975, 1980; Regan, 1982, 1984), the relevance of economic considerations has received relatively little attention. The assumption may have been that animal welfare and how humans treat animals are moral issues, which need scientific information to help determine what is good or bad for the welfare of animals but where economic considerations are secondary or perhaps even largely irrelevant. Indeed, many may find distasteful the thought that money should be a consideration at all. After all, how can we put a price on animal suffering?

However, economics is not concerned with money *per se*, although it often finds money a useful measuring rod. Economics is concerned with how we in society make decisions about using resources to achieve the things that we want. The central problem for economics (and for society) is that we all want a multitude of different things but the resources that we have to achieve those wants are limited. We cannot therefore all have everything we want. This leaves us with three important interrelated decisions. For what should we use these scarce resources (i.e. what do we want)? How should we best use them? And who in society gets the benefits? Economics has evolved (out of the study of ethics) as a discipline to address these very questions.

Alfred Marshall, a notable Victorian economist, wrote (in 1890) that:

> Economics is a study of mankind in the ordinary business of life; it examines that part of individual and social action which is most closely connected with the attainment and with the use of the material requisites of wellbeing . . . Money is

a means towards ends . . . and is sought as a means to all kinds of ends, high as well as low, spiritual as well as material . . . Thus though it is true that 'money' or 'general purchasing power' or 'command over material wealth', is the centre around which economic science clusters; this is so, not because money or material wealth is regarded as the main aim of human effort, nor even as affording the main subject matter for the study of the economist, but because in this world of ours it is the one convenient means of measuring human motive on a large scale . . . But with careful precautions money affords a fairly good measure of the moving force of a great part of the motives by which men's lives are fashioned . . . Economics has a great and an increasing concern in motives connected with . . . the collective pursuit of important aims. Economics has then as its purpose . . . to throw light on practical issues.

(Marshall, 1947, pp. 1, 22, 39)

Amongst these practical issues Marshall raises that of 'those who suffer the evil, but do not reap the good' and poses the question 'how far is it right that they should suffer for the benefit of others?' Although Marshall was referring to human society, this question is surely central to the study of animal welfare.

16.2. Economic Perspective of Animal Welfare

In the context of animal welfare, what constitute acceptable or unacceptable uses of animals are matters of social choice, made by collective and individual decisions, rather than scientific assessment. From an economic perspective, animals may be seen merely as resources to be used to benefit people (Fig. 16.1). In his economic perspective of animal welfare McInerney (1994, pp. 13–14) wrote that:

Animal welfare is therefore just a subset of man's perception of his own welfare, and only indirectly to do with what is good for animals. There should be no surprise, therefore, that the welfare standards a society pursues are a coincidental outcome of its primary concern – the pursuit of human welfare . . . In economic terms animals are no more than resources employed in economic processes which generate benefits for people.

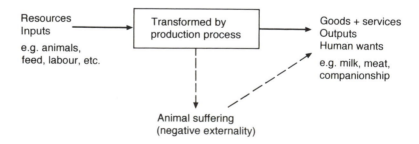

Fig. 16.1. Economic perspective of animals as inputs.

This view is in accordance with Jeremy Bentham's assertion that animals 'stand degraded into the class of things' (Bentham, 1789). From this perspective, the fact that animals may suffer in the process of producing goods and services for humans becomes a (regrettable) side-effect of the production system. Economists often refer to such indirect effects as 'externalities' (environmental pollution is another example of such an externality). Within this framework, animal welfare matters only because of human sensibilities toward animal suffering which affect human welfare. Thus the perception that animals are unnecessarily suffering may be a source of disutility for some people which reduces their (human) welfare and so imposes a very real cost on them and hence on society as a whole.

Arguably, concerns over poor animal welfare are determined entirely by people's perceptions of animal suffering and how they interpret what they see or measure in terms of animal behaviour, changes in physiological processes, etc. People's perceptions are likely, therefore, to depend on the degree of anthropomorphism or reference to human suffering (Sandøe and Simonsen, 1992; Mason and Mendl, 1993). Perceptions are related to what people consider to be necessary or unnecessary, acceptable or unacceptable uses of animals which depend, in turn, on the perceived feasible alternatives (alternative production systems, products, etc.) available. For example, many people may feel that the slaughter of farm animals is necessary and acceptable (although they may recognize that 'some' animal suffering will be involved even with 'humane' methods) because they see no other alternative if they are to continue to eat meat. However, these same individuals may consider cage egg production unacceptable because they see a more acceptable alternative in the form of 'free-range' systems. Others may feel that all farm animal production systems are unacceptable and find acceptable non-animal alternative products to consume. It is clear that these perceptions are influenced by a host of factors ranging from cultural practices to aspects of lifestyle and revolve around people's awareness about current uses of animals and alternatives to them.

Clearly, the foregoing 'economic perspective' of animal welfare may be questioned from an ethical standpoint, and many people may feel that animal welfare is important in its own right regardless of the sensibilities of humans. None the less, this simple economic perspective may still provide a useful framework for the consideration of animal welfare issues in society.

16.3. Cost-Benefit Analysis

16.3.1. Basics

One way of addressing animal welfare issues is through the principle of cost-benefit analysis. Cost-benefit analysis is a corner-stone of economics, and has been described as the 'economic ethic' (Boulding, 1969). This is an approach for analysing and assessing the advantages and disadvantages *to society* associated with a policy. It involves weighing benefits to society against costs in terms of a common monetary unit and then assessing whether a policy appears worthwhile or not. The presumption is that any policy should result in a net benefit to society to be worth implementing. Anything that we do not want resulting from a policy is regarded as a *cost* and something that we do want as a *benefit*. Thus, in the context of animal production in agriculture, products such as milk, meat, etc. are benefits and the use of resources to produce these products such as human labour, land, natural resources and physical capital incur costs. Animal suffering may be an additional cost (but, if the McInerney perspective is accepted, only if at least some people care about it). Cost-benefit analysis aims to consider *all* benefits (advantages) and costs (disadvantages) associated with a resource-allocation decision affecting society. Clearly, in practice, this can prove very difficult given the often wide-ranging and far-reaching effects of policy. It is also recognized that not everything readily lends itself to having a monetary measure attached to it. The central problems of cost-benefit analysis revolve around how benefits and costs are defined and how they are measured. An important aspect of the social cost-benefit analysis approach is that it also identifies the distributional effects associated with any policy. This means that it tries to assess who in society gets the benefits and who loses out or suffers some cost as a result of a particular policy. The definition of what constitutes 'society' in any assessment may also be problematic. In the context of animal welfare, it may be argued that 'society' should also include non-human animal species and that cost-benefit analyses should explicitly account for the needs and wants of animals.

The following sections consider the nature of costs and benefits and how they might be measured in the context of animal welfare issues.

16.3.2. The concept of value

Economic theory usually assumes that people make choices according to their preferences or 'wants' in such a way that they seek to maximize their own satisfaction or 'utility' (Mill, 1848; Marshall, 1947). Welfare economics is based on the utilitarian principle that value is derived from the utility that individuals derive from satisfying their own wants and this is often measured in terms of people's willingness to pay. Thus an individual's willingness to pay for something is used as a measure of the utility that he/she derives from the entity in question and hence a measure of benefit and of the value of the entity to the individual. Welfare economics then aggregates individuals' willingness to pay measures of benefit to produce an aggregate measure of benefit for society. There is a substantial literature questioning the use of the utility concept as a measure of value and whether this can be captured by people's willingness to pay (e.g. Sen, 1987). The inadequacies and problems associated with aggregating such measures into a measure of societal benefit have long been recognized and debated by economists (for example, it is unreasonable to assume that £1 spent by a wealthy man on a flower for his buttonhole has the equivalent value/benefit to society as £1 spent on food by a starving man). The idea that people seek to maximize their own utility/benefit has also been criticized. Clearly, people are not solely motivated by a desire selfishly to maximize their own well-being. The needs and wants of others (including other species) may also be important considerations, linked to moral values of responsibility, justice, etc. Indeed, the utilitarian principle can take account of the plurality of people's motivations including the 'satisfaction' of moral principles. This was recognized by Adam Smith (1790), the 'father' of modern economics, in 1759, and later by Bentham in 1789 who included human benevolence and sympathy to animals amongst his categorization of 'pleasures' and refers to the 'pleasures of the moral sanction'. In theory, the utilitarian principle can even take explicit account of the 'wants' and needs of non-human animal species by incorporating animal utility functions alongside human ones when assessing societal well-being. For example, Blackorby and Donaldson (1992) specify a social value function based on the individual utility functions of more than one species within a critical level utilitarian framework. They state (pp. 1345, 1363, 1366) that:

> It is possible to produce an 'ethics' of animal exploitation by noting that humans care about animal suffering, and themselves are made worse off by it. This argument takes account of human sentiment for animal well-being. Thus animal well-being appears in the value function through human utility functions. We have no objection to this formulation of human utilities, but suggest that it is not a valid substitute for the recognition of the moral standing of all sentient creatures, regardless of whether they are liked or disliked by humans . . . We combine an explicit ethical view that accords all sentient creatures moral standing with simple models of animal food production and animal research . . . The well-being of each individual, human or not, is given equal weight, thus satisfying Singer's axiom of 'equal consideration of interests'.

Their analysis is a thought-provoking one. The two authors acknowledge the simplistic nature of their economic models and that they have omitted consideration of several important aspects of the ethical problem. Neither have they addressed the practicalities of trying to apply these models to the real world, for example to help guide policy. Amongst the many difficulties are questions concerning the nature and weighting (and hence the trade-offs) of animals' utility functions between different species and within species (including humans). Notwithstanding these, there is the practical problem of how to gauge non-human animal preferences (see Chapter 11). For humans, economists use market information (i.e. how people spend their money) and where that is lacking they can at least ask people what they would be willing to pay for an entity.

Clearly, very real conceptual and practical problems remain with Blackorby and Donaldson's approach. However, it raises some interesting questions about the explicit consideration of animal welfare and the assignment of animal rights – for example, how an 'equal consideration of interests' (Singer, 1975) or the acquisition of 'those rights which never could have been withholden from them but by the hand of tyranny' (Bentham, 1789) might be incorporated into a social value function.

16.3.3. The nature of benefits

Benefits (in economics) represent the satisfaction of people's wants which is assumed to give rise to utility which is a measure of human well-being. A money measure of the value of benefits to the individual is their willingness to pay to obtain those benefits. The value of an egg produced from a free-range

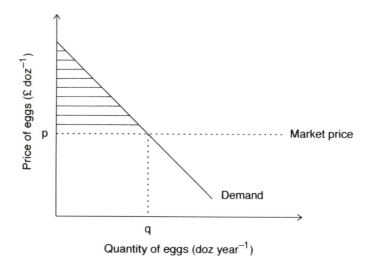

Fig. 16.2. Demand curve (for eggs).

hen is the money that someone would be willing (and able) to pay for that egg, rather than go without it. Economics uses demand functions to show how much of something people will want depending on its price. The demand curve shows the money value that people in society place on successive amounts of something, such as eggs in Fig. 16.2. Thus as people have more of something (e.g. eggs), they place a lower value on obtaining an additional unit of it.

A market demand curve results from all the purchasing decisions of individuals for the 'good' in question. People consume up to the point where the additional benefit (marginal benefit) that they get from consuming an extra unit of the commodity is equal to the marginal cost (i.e. price) of consuming that unit. At this point they maximize their net benefit from consumption. The net benefit to consumers from the good is represented by the shaded area in Fig. 16.2. It is the benefit over and above what people have to pay for the commodity in the market. Thus the lower the market price, the greater the net benefit to consumers from purchasing the product. It is clear from this that the prevailing market price for a good at any one time merely reflects the value that people place on an extra unit of the commodity (i.e. marginal benefit) and does not represent the value of the good in total (total benefit).

16.3.4. The nature of costs

The term 'cost' has a particular meaning in economics. Because resources are limited, devoting resources to one area of use necessarily deprives us of the benefits of their use in some other way – the 'opportunity cost' of using the resources. Thus the cost of producing livestock products such as milk, meat and eggs is considered in terms of the value of things that those resources could have produced if we had not used them to produce livestock products.

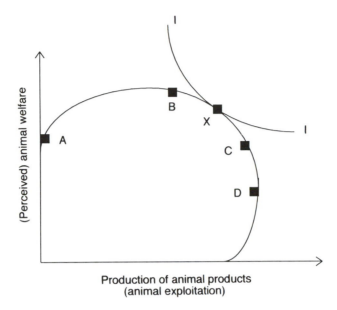

Fig. 16.3. The relationship between (perceived) animal welfare and the production of animal products.

This is shown in a simple way in Fig. 16.3 in terms of just two types of good – animal products and animal welfare. It makes more explicit the possible trade-offs between human welfare derived from animal products and the welfare of animals from which those products are derived.

The relationship in Fig. 16.3 assumes that up to a point (i.e. from A to B) animals and humans may derive mutual benefit from their association (although some may question this assumption – even for domesticated species). Thus point B marks a relationship of maximum welfare for animals with some important benefits for the human species. However, this does not maximize the output of animal products for human benefit. This would be achieved at point D but at a cost to the welfare of animals. If humans exploited animals beyond this point their welfare would be so affected that they would no longer be efficient producers of food and other products, and hence operating beyond D would be highly inefficient. The decision for society is where on the curve between B and D should we be? No doubt animals would prefer point B, whereas a human society uncaring about the welfare of animals (unless it affects production) would prefer point D. Arguably, within society at present, we might be operating at a point such as C. This implicitly gives a relative value to the welfare of animals, since it implies that, as a society, we would be unwilling to forego a unit of animal product to gain an additional unit of animals' welfare (or vice versa). This unit of animal product, say milk or eggs in the case of farm livestock, may be traded in markets and have a market price attached to it. Effectively then, society is placing an implicit (money) value on animal suffering.

However, we may feel that point C does not accurately reflect people's concerns for animal welfare and perhaps if we really knew society's preferences – shown by the function I – then we should rather be at point X (i.e. achieving a lower level of output of animal products but with higher levels of animal welfare). McInerney (1994, p. 18) wrote that:

> If economic analysis is to extend beyond the drawing of diagrams which set out the conceptual basis for decisions on animal welfare standards, the task of research is to identify the structure and relative weight of those preferences in society if our notion of a social optimum is to be pursued. On the other hand, imposing a welfare standard institutionally by the establishment and enforcement of particular codes raises the question as to *whose* value function it claims to reflect.

Economics uses supply functions to represent the costs associated with producing particular goods. Supply functions show the relationship between the market price of a good and how much of the good producers (in aggregate) are willing to supply. Figure 16.4 represents the supply function for the production of eggs. The higher the price, the more producers will supply. The supply function reflects the marginal costs incurred by producers to produce additional units of the good (i.e. the cost of additional resources used). The shaded area in Fig. 16.4 shows the net benefit that accrues to producers from their production (the difference between producer revenue and costs of production for a particular level of output).

The following section brings together a consideration of both costs and benefits, within a cost-benefit analysis framework, to explore the economic analysis of animal welfare issues.

16.3.5. Economic analysis and animal welfare – weighing costs and benefits

Economists use markets and market prices as a basis of values for both benefits and costs. However, they recognize that this can be problematic because

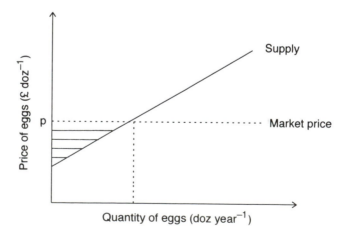

Fig. 16.4. Supply curve (for eggs).

markets do not necessarily reflect the true values of things to society. This is because: (i) market prices only reflect the value of things that are exchanged through those markets and only reflect the preferences of people participating in them, so there may be indirect costs and benefits ('externalities') which are not represented by market prices; (ii) market prices may be distorted in some way – for example, by government subsidies or taxation; and (iii) market prices reflect marginal values not total values. Thus, we cannot rely solely on market prices for information on the value that we place on something in society. This means that economists must sometimes use other means of valuing benefits and costs.

The negative animal welfare externalities (animal suffering) associated with the production of animal products and services do not explicitly feature in the markets for animal products and so remain as hidden costs. An important aspect of these externalities is that the preferences of people *not* buying goods in markets are not considered. For example, consider the market for veal produced by keeping calves in crates. The preferences of people that consume veal are recorded in terms of the quantity they are willing to buy and the price they are willing to pay. But there may be people in society who experience considerable disquiet about the use of calves in this way which reduces their (human) welfare and so imposes a cost on them (and hence, within a cost-benefit analysis framework, on society). These people have no way of expressing their wants through the market system. Even people who consume veal may not be entirely happy with how it is produced and would prefer that an alternative method were used, but they can only express their feelings by not buying veal, assuming they are not offered a more 'calf-friendly' alternative. Because markets only take account of the preferences of a subset (perhaps a minority) of people in society, they fail to allocate resources in a socially optimal way that maximizes the net benefit to society as a whole. Again, the economic argument is that the costs associated with such animal welfare externalities should be taken into account in making decisions about the use of animals. A formal economic analysis of how economics might address this issue is provided in Bennett (1995), and only the main argument of that analysis is presented here.

Providing that consumers are fully informed about the animal welfare implications of their purchasing decisions, the market will ensure that consumers purchase animal products which will maximize their individual net benefits from consumption. However, the market fails to take account of the costs arising from the negative externality of animal suffering, where some citizens in society experience a disutility because of other people's consumption of animal products and the animal suffering that they perceive to be associated with it. An analogy with the externality of 'passive smoking' in society is helpful to understand this concept. If this cost is fully accounted for, the real cost of animal exploitation to produce food and other products would be higher than that reflected by the market price for animal products. Net benefit to society would therefore be maximized at a lower level of animal use than at present. This means that unless we take account of the negative animal welfare externalities (considered in the analysis above solely in terms of human utility/disutility), then animals will be over-exploited and human welfare will be lower than it otherwise could be.

This has some important implications for policies toward animal welfare. The analysis poses two major questions: how can we estimate the optimum level of animal exploitation and how might we best ensure that this level of exploitation is actually achieved?

The first question can most readily be addressed by reference to estimating the social animal welfare costs associated with the production and consumption of animal products (i.e. animal exploitation). The benefits of consumption of animal products can be estimated from information about people's willingness to pay for those products in markets. The direct costs of production of animal products can also be estimated according to the value of resources needed to produce them. This then leaves the magnitude of the negative animal welfare externalities as the major unknown.

There are ways in which economists can estimate the values of non-market goods (Mitchell and Carson, 1989). One of the most obvious ways is to ask people what a good is worth to them. This is the basis of a valuation method called contingent valuation – a sophisticated survey technique which presents people with hypothetical market situations involving the good in question and then elicits their willingness to pay for the good. Such a technique could be used to obtain information from people on what they would be willing to pay for animals to be exploited at different levels (and so estimate their valuation of the associated animal welfare externalities) to determine the optimum level of animal exploitation for society.

16.4. Animal Welfare Policy Implications

The economic framework presented above may help to consider possible policy options for achieving an optimal level of animal exploitation. In relation to farm animals Bennett (1995, p. 58) wrote:

> There are three main policy options for trying to achieve a balance between the production of livestock products and farm animal welfare which optimizes the welfare of society. The first is to use the market mechanism and allow people to make an informed choice about the products they consume. For this to work, consumers need to be well-informed about the animal welfare characteristics of the products they purchase and about alternative production practices and products. This would no doubt require government intervention in the supply of information. However, even given such a high level of awareness on the part of consumers . . . the market mechanism would still fail to adequately capture the negative animal welfare externalities, particularly the public bad aspects of livestock product consumption. In order to try to address these aspects, government could intervene in two main ways. First, it could regulate the production of livestock products through legislation or codes of practice to ensure that the preferences of citizens for animal welfare friendly production practices are serviced. Secondly, it could tax those producing negative animal welfare externalities (the polluter pays principle) and/or subsidise those producing animal welfare goods, where those goods are not valued by the market.

If the market mechanism could be used, then the optimum level of animal exploitation could be achieved by pricing the exploitation of animals to produce goods at a higher level than current market prices. This could take the form of either a subsidy for producers/products which are perceived as resulting in good animal welfare or a tax on producers/products which are perceived as resulting in animal suffering. Clearly, if a tax or subsidy were applied, for instance, to egg production so that free-range eggs were the same price or cheaper than cage eggs in the shops, then relatively very few cage eggs would be sold or produced. Alternatively, government could intervene through legislation and ensure that only the optimum level of animal exploitation takes place. In practice, animal welfare policies have tended to take the latter approach – although some incentives have been paid to farmers, for example, for organic farming which has animal welfare benefits. Furthermore, data have not been available to enable an estimation of the optimum level of animal exploitation. Therefore, policy makers and others have rather put forward proposals concerning this level that they consider appropriate, based on scientific evidence, moral beliefs and the political process.

The next section presents a simplified case-study of an economic analysis of animal welfare policy. The case-study is intended to illustrate how economic analysis can be used to assess the likely impact on markets (and hence on consumers and producers) of policy and whether the benefits of policy outweigh the costs.

16.5. Case-study of Egg Production and Animal Welfare

Imagine a policy proposal for legislation to phase out the use of cages in egg production in the EU. Assume that policy makers would like some quantitative assessment of the costs and benefits of such a policy in the UK.

Let Fig. 16.5 represent the UK market for shell eggs. For simplicity, we assume no international trade in shell eggs and so UK producers supply UK demand. What then might be the impact of the legislation? Clearly, producers will have to change production systems to comply with the new legislation. There is evidence to suggest that input costs are likely to be significantly higher to produce eggs from non-battery systems, although costs depend on the exact nature of the production systems used and the economies of scale that can be achieved (Appleby *et al.*, 1992). For example, a comparison of input costs between battery and free-range producers from Roberts and Farrar (1993) shows that on average costs per dozen eggs produced were 26% (£0.14 per dozen) higher for the free-range producers than battery producers of a similar size. An assumed increase in production costs of £0.15 per dozen eggs following legislation to ban cages is shown in Fig. 16.5 by a shift in the egg supply curve from S to S^1. The figure assumes that the egg industry supply curve is relatively elastic compared with demand. The result of this cost increase is that the market price of eggs increases from p to p^1 and consumers buy fewer eggs. Note that most of the cost of production increase experienced by producers has actually been passed onto consumers in the form of a higher

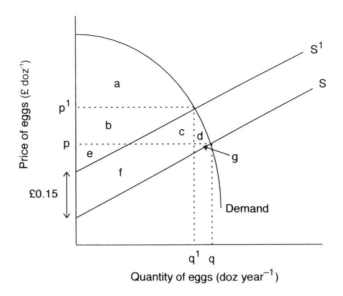

Fig. 16.5. Gains and losses to producers and consumers due to market effects of banning cages in the UK.

market price. At the same time, the purchase of eggs by consumers has fallen relatively very little. This is due to the 'inelastic' nature of demand for eggs. Because eggs have no close substitutes and because people's expenditure on them is a very small proportion of their food budget, people will still buy virtually the same amount of eggs even when the egg price increases. In fact, economists have estimated a 'price elasticity of demand' for shell eggs in the UK of around −0.08 (MAFF, 1994), which means that when the egg price increases by, say, 10%, on average people only buy 0.8% fewer eggs. This means that under the new legislation, people will actually spend more on eggs and producer revenue will be higher. Not all animal products are characterized in this way. For example, beef has an elasticity measure of around −1.2, so an increase in the price of beef will cause a correspondingly larger percentage fall in quantity demanded.

Figure 16.5 shows the gains and losses to producers and consumers as a result of changes in the egg market. Before the legislation, consumers had a net benefit from consuming eggs shown by the areas **a** + **b** + **c** + **d** (this is the difference between what consumers would have been willing to pay for eggs rather than not have them and the market price that they had to pay). After the legislation, consumers have a smaller net benefit equivalent to area **a**. Producers experience a net gain from producing eggs of areas **e** + **f** + **g** before the legislation, and areas **b** + **e** after the legislation. Thus, most of the increased costs of egg production from banning cages has been passed on to consumers in the form of higher egg prices. The net cost to society of changes to the egg market is represented by areas **c** + **d** + **f** + **g**. A quantitative estimate of these areas would require econometric estimations of the demand and supply functions for eggs.

The question now remains: are the benefits of better hen welfare worth these costs? One of the ways of assessing this is actually to ask people in society by using contingent valuation surveys (Bennett, 1996a). A contingent valuation survey of 2000 people in Great Britain (Bennett, 1996b) found that 79% of respondents supported the idea of legislation to ban the use of battery cages in the EU and were willing to pay an average of £0.43 per dozen increase in the price of eggs. This included respondents who were not willing to pay anything.

The magnitude of this estimate would suggest that the value people place on the greater welfare of hens by banning cages outweighs the additional costs of achieving that welfare. Note, however, that this simple analysis does not include the adjustment costs for the egg industry, administration costs associated with the legislation nor any effects on international trade, all of which would need to be taken into account in a full cost-benefit analysis.

16.6. Discussion

The foregoing analysis has been in terms of human preferences not (directly) animal ones. Furthermore, the extent of these human preferences (e.g. the value of better hen welfare to people) is measured only in terms of people's willingness to pay money (which is dependent on a host of factors, not least the disposable income available to people – because a wealthy person is willing to pay 10 times the money amount of the less-wealthy this does not mean that hen welfare is any more 'valuable' to the former than it is to the latter). Some may not accept the implicit ethical premise of some of the above economic analyses. It is because of such difficulties that important moral issues are often left to the political/democratic process. Nevertheless, some idea of the trade-offs between human and animal welfare are essential and these can be explored more rigorously by economic analysis.

Colin Spedding, the Chairman of the Farm Animal Welfare Council (FAWC), an independent advisory body to the UK government, wrote in 1993 (p. 116) that:

> The assessment of welfare by FAWC and the extent to which systems, practices and equipment improve or reduce welfare, is independent of economics. The Minister's responsibility includes consulting with those concerned with practice, and he or she has to take economic consequences into account in making political decisions . . . Since FAWC wishes to see real progress, however, it cannot totally ignore economic issues; but it must make clear how it assesses the welfare implications. In any case, practicability is very important.

The statement shows a desire to make judgements about the use of animals that are in the animals' best interests – a scientific assessment unadulterated by economic considerations. However, Spedding implicitly recognizes that there are inescapable trade-offs between animal and human welfare – which economics tries to make explicit – and hence economic considerations are inextricable to considerations about animal exploitation since they form the basis of judgements on 'practicability'. Otherwise it would merely be a question of how we can maximize the well-being of animals rather than optimize their use.

16.7. Conclusions

- Animal welfare and human welfare are inextricably linked. Economic analysis explicitly acknowledges this and considers the relationship between them.
- Economic considerations are central to the animal welfare debate and are integral, inescapable aspects of issues concerning the use of animals and of any interdisciplinary inquiry into animal welfare, alongside ethics and animal science.
- It is important that economics is perceived not merely as some financial accounting exercise, but as a discipline capable of incorporating different ethical considerations and using information from animal scientists which can help to make better decisions concerning human use of, and obligations to, animals.

CHAPTER 17

Legislation

Ute Knierim (Hanover School of Veterinary Medicine,
Germany) and William T. Jackson (Sussex, UK)

Abstract

An attempt is made to outline the main legal methods by which animal welfare
can be influenced, how the various measures evolved, their purpose and how
they relate to other mechanisms. Legislation relating to or influencing animal
welfare can be found on the national as well as on the supra- and international
level. Countries have differing legal and political systems and differing attitudes to
animals. Such variations tend to produce corresponding differences in national
law in reflection of this. However, from pressure of market forces and inter-
nationalization in general, an inter- and a supranational harmonization process
can and often does operate to affect welfare standards on a much wider base.

Space only permits the inclusion of some of the legal devices which have
been evolved or employed. Discussion of the effectiveness of the various measures has been included. Legal action in the field of animal welfare depends to
a large degree on public opinion but is also dependent on the input from any
experts able to provide solid scientific and practical information submitted on
the basis of a knowledge of the legal and political context of the measure.
Change of conditions relevant to animal welfare is often strongly resisted and
can frequently only be achieved by strict enforcement. At the same time,
however, measures encouraging dialogue and education are in the long term
indispensable to the promotion of animal welfare.

17.1. Introduction

When speaking about implementation of animal welfare in terms of legislation,
we have to be aware that this is not only about what is necessary on the basis
of scientific knowledge and established experience, but also about what is
politically and legally possible. This chapter seeks to highlight the two latter areas
by explaining some legal and political principles and outlining differences between
countries. Information and examples are given mainly from Europe. Readers
from elsewhere will compare these examples with what is in force locally.

There are a number of different ways by which animal welfare measures
can be implemented or influenced. The main legal methods are:

Intergovernmental agreements:
   Treaties
   Conventions

Animal Welfare (eds Michael C. Appleby and Barry O. Hughes)

National statute law:
    Statutes (Acts)
    Delegated legislation:
        Regulations made under national statute
        Statutory instruments or
        Welfare Codes
Supranational statute law:
    EC Directives implemented by national statute or
    EC Regulations made under European law
Case law:
    as authority in itself or
    used (especially in common law systems) to interpret statute law

After a short historical excursus we shall consider the different kinds of measures in more detail.

17.2. History

In the third century BC a Buddhist – Asoka, King of Maghada in north India, abolished sacrificial slaughter, banned the royal hunt and planted trees to give shade to man and beast (Brown, 1974, p. 5). Some 1800 years later the first positive attempts to improve the lot of animals in England and Wales (Scotland has a different legal system) came by way of cases brought before the courts. The earliest case was in AD 1592, The Case of Swannes (Swans, 1592) concerning cruelty to swans. As the public became aware of the need to protect animals from the various acts of omission and commission threatening their well-being, a body of case law gradually arose in various parts of the world.

Attempts at the establishment of statute law began in England and Wales only in April 1800. In that year a measure to prevent bull-baiting failed to become law. No progress came until 1822 when a law was passed which did much to establish the legal obligation to treat animals humanely. The law was 'to prevent the cruel and improper treatment of cattle'. It was followed by numerous pieces of statute all over the world, e.g. within the Saxonian criminal law of 1838, the French 'Loi Grammont' of 1850 or the 1866 New York Cruelty-to-Animals laws. However, in early times often it was only an offence to ill-treat animals in the presence of the public. It was believed that the public must be protected from the witnessing of cruel behaviour and thereby becoming brutal ('aesthetic animal protection'). Later on animals became legally protected for their own sake as sentient living beings ('ethical animal protection').

In former times the law was also used against animals. Numerous pigs, dogs and bullocks were prosecuted for crimes. Sometimes the accused animal was represented by Counsel. History does not record whether the animals were legally aided. Such cases went on until 1771 when a dog was tried and acquitted in Chichester, UK (Brown, 1974, p. 6).

17.3. Intergovernmental Agreements

Increasing worldwide trade and removal of borders have a considerable impact on the use of animals. Traffic in animals (farm animals for breeding or slaughter, wild animals for zoos and private owners in addition to experimental animals) expands, thereby increasing competition between farmers, industry and scientists of the different countries. Standards which impose restrictions on production or research and impair competitiveness will more readily be accepted and also be more effective if they must equally be observed by all competitors. Although it is often much easier to reach agreement only on the national level and progress can be considerably slowed down, for an effective protection of animals there is a need for international harmonization. The following examples illustrate possible levels of international influence on animal welfare legislation.

17.3.1. Treaties

A treaty is an agreement between nations. One example is the 'Treaty on European Union' which has important animal welfare implications.

During the process of European unification the 1957 'Treaties of Rome' establishing the European Communities (with the European Economic Community (EEC) being the most important, the others being Euratom and the European Coal and Steel Community) were repeatedly amended. The most comprehensive step was in 1992 with the treaty founding the European Union. The EU is based on the European Communities and on certain fields of joint policies and cooperation. The Union itself has no legislative powers, these remain within the European Community (EC, former EEC). Legal and political competences of the EC together with its objectives and the unified institutional framework are fixed within the 'Treaty establishing the European Community' (EC Treaty, former EEC Treaty which was amended by the 'Treaty on European Union').

Animal welfare is not embodied in the Treaty. The only basis for community legislation on animal welfare is Article 43 on Agriculture, quoted when the protection of farm animals is concerned, or Articles 100 and 100a on the Approximation of Laws, used in connection with the protection of experimental animals. In consequence the need for community legislation in the field of animal welfare is heavily debated, reference being made to the important principle of subsidiarity, which here means that any matter that can be regulated on a national level must be left to the member states. This argument certainly applies to the protection of pet animals and also to a Draft Directive on Zoo Animals which was withdrawn after long discussions and shall now only become a recommendation.

However, the political importance of animal welfare was emphasized by the Intergovernmental Conference at Maastricht in December 1991. In its Declaration No. 24 on the Protection of Animals, annexed to the final act of the Treaty on European Union:

> The Conference calls upon the European Parliament, the Council and the
> Commission, as well as the member states, when drafting and implementing

Community legislation on the common agricultural policy, transport, the internal market and research, to pay full regard to the welfare requirements of animals.

On the other hand, the EC Treaty imposes restrictions on possible national measures for animal protection, as an integral and most important part of the Treaty is to ensure freedom of trade and to prevent distortion of competition.

The removal of barriers to the free movement of goods, and the general rules of competition ensuring equal treatment of operators, are among the exclusive competences of the Community.

(Commission of the European Union, 1993)

By Articles 30 to 35 of the EC Treaty unilateral measures are forbidden which would hinder free trading between member states save for certain exceptions given in Article 36 which concern for instance the protection of public order, safety or health and life of humans, animals or plants. This exception is, however, generally interpreted in a very narrow sense.

Hence, a national ban on the importation of animals or animal products which have been treated or produced in a way which is not in accordance with national animal welfare provisions is in general against the Treaty. However, this does not prevent member states prohibiting certain treatments or production methods as long as it is only their own inhabitants who are saddled with the prohibition. An example is the production of foie gras which is prohibited in most EU-member states, but whose importation from (say) France or Belgium cannot be prohibited or limited. Another example is the importation of dogs with ears cropped or tails docked into countries which prohibit such practices. The principle applies to the vexed question of live animal transport. Any restriction on a national basis which would negatively affect foreign operators is almost certainly illegal.

17.3.2. Conventions

A Convention is in effect a special form of treaty between two or more sovereign states. The evolution of a Convention is a laborious and time-consuming process. It is possible to have a framework or outline treaty approach. Here the content of a Convention is limited to general undertakings or principles, with provisions made for a treaty body by which contracting parties tackle questions of detail.

Conventions dealing explicitly with animal welfare can be found within the Council of Europe, but other Conventions having different objectives may also considerably influence animal welfare; one activity of the Organization for Economic Cooperation and Development (OECD) is given below as an example.

Council of Europe

This intergovernmental organization must not be confused with the European Union (or the Council of the European Union). The Council of Europe has been in existence since 1949 with at present 39 member states and in particular undertakes action in the legal field with a view to harmonizing national laws. Additionally to its well-known work in the field of human rights and other activities it has set up five Animal Welfare Conventions (see Table 17.1).

Table 17.1. The five European Animal Welfare Conventions. States given in brackets have signed the Convention but not yet ratified.

European Convention	Contracting parties
1968 for the Protection of Animals during International Transport (supplemented by a Protocol of 1979 permitting, in particular, accession by the European Community)	The 15 EU-member states, Cyprus, Iceland, Norway, Romania, Russia, Switzerland, Turkey
1976 for the Protection of Animals Kept for Farming Purposes (supplemented by a Protocol of Amendment of 1992)	The 15 EU-member states, Bosnia Herzegovina, Croatia, Cyprus, Iceland, Macedonia, Malta, Norway, Slovenia, Switzerland, European Community
1979 for the Protection of Animals for Slaughter	(Belgium), Bosnia Herzegovina, Croatia, (Cyprus), Denmark, Finland, (France), Germany, Greece, Ireland, Italy, Luxembourg, Macedonia, Netherlands, Norway, Portugal, Slovenia, Sweden, Switzerland, (United Kingdom, European Community)
1986 for the Protection of Vertebrate Animals Used for Experimental and Other Scientific Purposes	Belgium, Cyprus, (Denmark), Finland, (France), Germany, Greece, (Ireland, Netherlands), Norway, Spain, Sweden, Switzerland, (Turkey, United Kingdom, European Community)
1987 for the Protection of Pet Animals	Belgium, Cyprus, Denmark, Finland, Germany, Greece, (Italy), Luxembourg, (Netherlands), Norway, Portugal, Sweden, Switzerland

The five Conventions are based on ethical concepts common to all the participating countries and aim to avoid unnecessary suffering or injury to animals, and to provide conditions in accordance with the animals' specific physiological and behavioural needs.

Only the 'Convention for the Protection of Animals kept for Farming Purposes' is an explicit framework Convention with provision for a Standing Committee responsible for the elaboration and adoption of recommendations for the keeping of different types of farm animals. Within the other Conventions further recommendations can be elaborated by multilateral consultations of the parties laid before the Committee of Ministers for adoption. Recommendations concerning the transport of horses (1987), pigs (1988), cattle, sheep, goats and poultry (all 1990) as well as on the slaughter of animals (1991) in the form of codes of conduct have already been adopted by the Committee of Ministers. They are not directly linked to the Conventions from a legal point of view, but provide very detailed further information on the principles of the

Conventions and are useful to people engaged in transporting or slaughtering animals and for competent authorities in a practical situation.

The Standing Committee of the 'Convention for the Protection of Animals kept for Farming Purposes' consists of representatives sent by the contracting parties, mainly veterinarians working in government administrations. Observers from member states not being a contracting party as well as from invited non-member states (e.g. Australia, New Zealand or the USA) and from invited bodies such as the European Confederation of Agriculture, the Federation of Veterinarians of Europe, the International Society for Applied Ethology and the World Society for the Protection of Animals are also allowed to attend the meetings.

Recommendations can only be adopted unanimously. Recommendations for the keeping of laying hens (1986, became part of a Recommendation concerning domestic fowl in 1995 which also covers broilers and parent stock), pigs (1986), cattle (1988), fur animals (1990), sheep and goats (1992) have been adopted so far.

Covering an even wider range of countries with differing attitudes towards animal welfare from that of the European Union, wordings of the Recommendations and Conventions have perforce to be very general and rather vague. Furthermore, the rules of international law allow contracting parties to bring rules in line with the Conventions through legislation or administrative practice according to their own interpretation. Instruments of control and strict enforcement are lacking. Thus the obligation is largely a moral and political one. An example of differing interpretations of Convention provisions is provided by Article 6 of the 'Convention for the Protection of Animals kept for Farming Purposes':

> No animal shall be provided with food or liquid in a manner, nor shall such food or liquid contain any substance, which may cause unnecessary suffering or injury.

Whereas it is many contracting parties' interpretation that force feeding of ducks or geese (to produce foie gras) must be forbidden, in other countries this practice is still continued, the parties claiming that the treatment does not cause the animals any suffering or injury.

Despite the weakness of enforcement, Conventions are important not only in themselves but also for the promotion of the idea of animal welfare in countries which have as yet minimal animal welfare legislation or none. For instance the Eastern European countries are showing great interest and some governments have already asked the Council of Europe for advice on the introduction of animal welfare measures in their countries. At the same time there are strong links to the European Union, and EC Directives on animal welfare are to a large extent based on Conventions and Recommendations of the Council of Europe.

Organization for Economic Cooperation and Development (OECD)

Another example of a Convention affecting animal welfare – here with regard to animal testing – is the one by which the OECD was founded in 1961. The organization has at present 25 member states (the 15 EU member states,

Australia, Canada, Iceland, Japan, Mexico, New Zealand, Norway, Switzerland, Turkey and the USA). Among its different very broad activities the OECD has adopted guidelines on the testing of chemical substances before they are brought on the market. The guidelines on the one hand impose certain animal testing and, on the other hand, by ensuring that such tests will be acceptable in all OECD states, obviate the need for duplicate testing. The guidelines of 'Good Laboratory Practice' harmonize toxicological testing methods of industrial chemicals, pesticides, food and articles of everyday use.

17.4. National Statute Law

Before explaining legal measures on the national level it is necessary to discuss briefly two different systems of law so as to make differences between some countries easier to understand. The relationship between 'case law' and 'statute law' (as well as procedures) differs depending upon whether countries have 'common law' histories (the UK, USA and other countries which have historical links with England) or 'Romano-Germanic law' histories (most European countries and those historically linked with them).

Romano-Germanic law is bound up with the law of ancient Rome and was essentially developed by universities and jurists. Law was brought together in unified codes, a process called codification. The main weight is on legal texts which have more authority than cases.

Common law is largely based on unwritten but commonly agreed principles promulgated primarily by judges. It is still being developed further with judges deciding what the law is in a particular case. Sometimes people misinterpret this as changes to the law but that is not so. The judges merely apply well understood common-law rules to a new situation. Some very important criminal offences (e.g. murder) are common-law offences. Case law has considerable importance and can have effects on statute law, an example being the UK Dangerous Dogs Act 1991. Decided cases have resulted in a locked car parked on the road being defined as a 'public place' whilst a private garden to which the public have access is not a public place. Such decisions are binding in the UK if they are in a Crown Court or above, i.e. Queen's Bench Divisional Court, the Court of Appeal or the House of Lords sitting as a court with appellate jurisdiction.

17.4.1. Statutes

A 'statute' is an Act of Parliament. In the UK, it requires the consent of the Lords and the Commons. Many other jurisdictions have similar mechanisms involving Upper and Lower Houses, especially those countries with a federal structure. Here usually one house is the Federal Parliament, the other being the representative body of the federal states or regions. Examples are the US Congress consisting of the House of Representatives and the Senate, or the German Bundestag and Bundesrat.

Statutory provisions relating to animal welfare can be found in specific animal welfare Acts as they exist in several countries, or in 'Codes' or other measures covering a wider range of areas. Examples of the latter are found in France where animal welfare provisions are contained in the Code Pénal, Code Civil, Code Commune and Code Rural, and in the UK where the Protection of Animals Acts 1911–1988 provide specific cover but the Agriculture (Miscellaneous Provisions) Act 1968 contains among others some animal welfare provisions.

Statutes broadly either regulate or are 'enabling', i.e. they delegate powers to ministers. The latter method is used where matters are too technical to be decided there and then or the precise circumstances under which a need might arise are unpredictable. By this means the law can be made flexible and hence more effective. Statutes may be both regulatory and enabling.

17.4.2. Delegated legislation

Legislation enacted under an enabling Act is called delegated legislation. It can, for instance, be a Regulation, a Statutory Instrument, an Order in Council or a Welfare Code. Although this kind of legislation also passes through Parliamentary hands, the procedure is usually easier. For example, in Germany Regulations need the agreement of only the Bundesrat, or UK Statutory Rules and Orders only have to be placed in the library of the House of Commons for three weeks. If nobody objects they become law. However, UK Welfare Codes, prepared or revised after consultations, must be laid before both Houses of Parliament and approved by them.

Welfare Codes

Welfare Codes should not be confused with legal codes as used in European jurisdictions (see France – section 17.4.1 – for examples). Welfare Codes as used in countries including New Zealand or the UK are not mandatory. The UK Agriculture (Miscellaneous Provisions) Act 1968 provides that the breach of a Code provision, whilst not an offence in itself, can nevertheless be used in evidence as tending to establish the guilt of anyone accused of causing suffering under the Act (Section 3(4)). As an illustration the UK 'Highway Code' although established by law is not itself law. Although this is so, a failure to follow its provisions is normally difficult to justify. If, for example, a driver elects to drive on the wrong side of the road that is not illegal but if a head-on collision with another driver is the result of such an action, the highway code provision will assist the prosecution of any driver flouting that part of the code.

There are in practice many ways in which the welfare of animals can be safeguarded and it is for this reason that a more flexible attitude using the Codes has been adopted. Mandatory regulations enacted in advance of science could inhibit livestock husbandry development to the detriment of animal welfare. As time passes more knowledge is gained on animals' preferences and needs.

In the UK, the Codes issued concern cattle, sheep, pigs, domestic fowls, turkeys, ducks, rabbits, goats, farmed deer, animals in livestock markets, and horses, ponies and donkeys at markets, sales and fairs.

17.4.3. Statute law in different countries

Each of an increasing number of countries which have taken legal measures designed for the protection of animals has adopted its own approach. It is interesting to note correspondences and differences in substance going beyond the purely legal level of approach illustrated in outline above. From an increasingly comprehensive body of animal welfare legislation only a small subjective sample can be presented.

In many statutes reference is made to the biological needs of animals which must be supplied to spare the animals suffering or harm. A scientific basis is generally regarded as necessary to define such needs and thereby make sensible decisions on animal welfare.

The kind of animals which are protected differs between countries depending upon whether the animals are vertebrates or invertebrates, wild, feral or captive animals. In some countries legislation is mostly limited to pet animals, experimental and farm animals (e.g. Spain), in other countries it in general applies to all or most vertebrates and some specified invertebrates (e.g. Norway and Switzerland) or the whole animal kingdom (e.g. Germany). However, independently of the scope of application the majority of provisions refer to animals used as pet, farm or experimental animals.

In general, there are two ways to regulate, one is to allow anything not explicitly forbidden (a 'negative list' approach), the other is to forbid anything not explicitly allowed (a 'positive list' approach). Sometimes both are found in one Act. The positive list approach was largely adopted by the Netherlands in their Animal Health and Welfare Act of 1992. There, for instance, the keeping of animals or the killing of animals is generally forbidden unless permitted under Order in Council. There are good arguments for and against either approach. The evolvement of a positive list is time-consuming but there is the advantage that it has the effect of stimulating thorough debate. However, even in a positive list, expressions included to provide flexibility to allow for differing situations tend to leave the matter somewhat open to interpretation, and although a positive list might be more restrictive than a negative list, this need not necessarily be the case, depending on the generality of the terms used.

Some countries have identified certain areas as in need of special control and to this end have introduced the obligation to obtain official approval of matters in those areas. This sometimes applies to the keeping of wild animal species (e.g. Switzerland and the UK), the installation or reconstruction of farm animal holdings (e.g. Sweden and Norway), the commercial breeding and trading with certain animals or the running of riding establishments (e.g. Germany, Sweden and the UK) and to other areas. In Sweden and Switzerland and in future in the Netherlands new husbandry systems must be approved before they can be brought into use. With regard to animal testing most European countries have established procedures whereby experiments which may subject the animals to suffering may only be performed if authorized. The level of authorization differs between authorization of each experiment (e.g. Germany and Switzerland) and a general authorization with only the obligation to notify experiments to the competent authority (e.g. Belgium and the UK). Animal Welfare Acts in Belgium, Germany and Luxembourg also protect the animal's life itself. It is an offence to kill an animal without reasonable excuse, an important and much discussed provision especially regarding unwanted animals.

Measures to enforce legislation are as important as the content of the provisions themselves. Between countries, competent authorities differ in their organization as well as in the number and the qualifications of their personnel, however, usually at some point veterinarians are involved. For example, in Norway each local authority has an Animal Welfare Board consisting of three to five members, one being mandatorily a veterinarian. The board has powers of investigation and gives advice which if ignored is a criminal matter. Cyprus has recently adopted a similar approach. In Italy and Sweden provisions are made for Animal Welfare Inspectors who are not veterinarians but are specially trained to inspect and give advice. The entitlement of competent authorities to interfere during inspections with the personal rights of keepers or users of animals or persons who are suspected of having committed an offence varies between countries according to their constitution or legal principles.

Judicial Review, Administrative Courts

In the UK administrative decisions including those made by the government can be the subject of review by judges. The matter must be one involving the public and not just the person complaining. The courts have power to remit the matter to the administration requiring compliance with the law. A similar function is performed in other countries by the Administrative Courts. In such courts, however, there is no requirement for the matter to be one of public interest, each person can take his or her case to an Administrative Court.

17.5. Statute Law in the European Union

17.5.1. EC Directives

Directives are binding as to objectives only and require national legislation or administrative arrangements in each country to become effective. Explicitly or implicitly the form of a Directive says that 'Member States may, with due regard for the general rules of the Treaty, maintain or apply in their territory more stringent provisions than those contained in this Directive.' Thus, a Directive allows member states some flexibility in their decisions concerning national measures. All Community legislation directly providing protection of animals takes the form of a Directive (see Table 17.2).

The Directives also have an effect on third countries, i.e. countries outside the EU when they trade with EU countries. For example, the Directives on calves and pigs read:

> Animals imported from non-member countries must, with respect to the requirements for their welfare, whilst being reared, receive treatment at least equivalent to that guaranteed by this Directive to animals of Community origin. This requirement must be stated in a certificate issued by the competent authority of the non-member country concerned.

Comparable ideas are expressed in the Directives for transport and slaughter.

Table 17.2. The six EC Directives on Animal Welfare.

Subject	Number	Year
Animals Used for Experimental and Other Scientific Purposes	86/609/EEC	1986
Laying Hens Kept in Battery Cages	88/166/EEC	1988
Calves	91/629/EEC	1991
	and 97/2/EC	1997
Pigs	91/630/EEC	1991
Animals at the Time of Slaughter or Killing	93/119/EC	1993
Animals during Transport	91/628/EEC	1991
	& 95/29/EC	1995

Table 17.3. Two EC Regulations on Marketing Standards, fixing criteria for use of terms which indicate certain types of farming.

Subject	Terms	Number	Year
Eggs	'Free-range eggs' 'Semi-intensive eggs' 'Deep litter eggs' 'Perchery eggs (Barn eggs)'	1274/91	1991
Poultrymeat	'Extensive indoor (barn reared)' 'Free-range' 'Traditional free-range' 'Free-range – total freedom'	2891/93	1993

Hence, the influence of EC animal welfare legislation on countries outside the EU should not be underestimated.

17.5.2. EC Regulations

A Regulation is binding in its entirety and directly applicable in all member states. Regulations are used when it is especially important to safeguard a uniform implementation, e.g. marketing standards. Regulations on marketing standards may also indirectly influence husbandry methods and animal welfare (for examples, see Table 17.3). The more consumers try to exert influence by deliberate choices of products, e.g. by the purchase of free-range eggs, the more important it is to be certain of the requirements to which the labelling refers.

Other examples of areas which are regulated by EC Regulations and affect animal welfare are fishing with drift nets or the methods of trapping wild fur animals.

17.6. Case Law

17.6.1. *Case law as authority in itself: an historical example*

Waters v. *Braithwaite* (1913): On 12 June 1913 at 11.00 a.m. a cow owned
by Farmer Braithwaite arrived with her muzzled 12-day-old calf at Banbury
market after a walk of 5½ miles. The cow was in full milk and as a consequence
of her not having been milked for 19 hours had an inflamed distended udder
and great difficulty in walking. Five Justices of the Peace (Lower Court) had
dismissed a summons against Mr Braithwaite on the grounds that although
the cow suffered pain, it was an old established custom in the district to expose
cows for sale in an 'overstocked' (udder full of milk) condition. Three High
Court judges ruled he had committed an offence.

The case provided authority that such acts could not be justified on the
ground of old custom or commercial advantage.

17.6.2. *Interpretation of statute law*

Since it is in practice rarely possible to frame statute law in terms leaving no
room for argument, it is a basic task of courts to ascertain the intention of the
legislator.

Methods of interpretation vary between countries due in part to different
legal systems. The basic and common principle is, that legal provisions are
interpreted literally if possible. In common-law countries formerly the literal
method was applied even if it produced an absurd result. Nowadays an attempt
is made to modify the words so as to avoid this. However, if the wording is
ambiguous or appears to be against the statute read as a whole, other aspects
such as the history of the statute can be taken into account, i.e. what did it
replace? Asking what the provision was designed to combat can also be important. However, in the UK rules on the material aids to construction are very
strict. A reading of debates in Parliament was not permitted until 1992 when
the House of Lords (sitting as a court of law) decided that statements made by
a Minister would be allowed 'where such statements were sufficiently clear'
(*Pepper* v. *Hart*, 1992). Most continental countries adopt the opposite approach and encourage consultation of the parliamentary and political history
of the statute. These materials are known as 'travaux préparatoires' and are
an invaluable aid in discovering the intention of continental legislatures.

The Doctrine of Precedent

The interpretation of animal welfare statute law by the court concentrates on
a particular case. However, it can sometimes be very important for decisions
in similar cases. The significance of decisions differs between countries according to their legal system.

In common-law countries, the 'Doctrine of Precedent' applies, i.e. a court
is bound by decisions of a court above itself in the hierarchy and usually by a
court of equivalent standing. Decisions of foreign courts although not binding
can act as valuable persuasive authority. In the UK many cases in Commonwealth or former Commonwealth countries have been quoted and increasingly
cases from other European countries are being used. The precedent rules are

not applied with a sort of automatism; where necessary judges have always been adept at 'distinguishing' cases, i.e. finding slight differences of fact because it is only when facts are the same that cases are binding.

In contrast, in Romano-Germanic law systems, e.g. in Germany, courts are formally independent in their decisions from previously decided cases (an exception is decisions of the Federal Constitutional Court). Even though courts may make use of lines of reasoning in other courts they may well come to a different decision on the same set of facts.

Expert opinion

A major problem courts face with regard to animal welfare legislation is the controversial basis for decisions on the needs of animals and what constitutes suffering. Many countries make use of expert opinions on these matters. In some countries (e.g. the UK) the parties may appoint their own experts provided the court agrees, in other countries (e.g. Germany) parties may propose experts but the court appoints them and usually only one expert is appointed. Expert evidence sometimes differs but the court decides.

The expert's evidence should be the independent product of the expert concerning matters within his or her expertise uninfluenced by the needs of the client. Experts must assist the court and should give the full picture. If they are not sure of their opinion they should say so. If they later change their views they must tell the court. They should not attempt to argue the case; that is the role of the advocate (*National Justice Campagnia Navesia SA v. Prudential Assurance Co. The Ikarian Reefer*, 1993; *Early v. Newham H.A.*, 1994).

In Germany, expert opinions ('Gutachten') are also prepared independently of court cases on the appointment of the Federal Government when it regards certain questions on the interpretation of the Animal Welfare Act as of general importance. The aim behind such official expert opinions is to provide a kind of code of conduct. Courts may use them but are not obliged to do so. The responsible Minister appoints a group of experts ('Sachverständige'), usually scientists but also including people with practical experience on the issues in question and representatives from animal welfare organizations. Such opinions have included the keeping of fallow deer on farms, the keeping and killing of fur animals, the control of vertebrate pests, the keeping and training of circus animals and equestrian sports.

17.6.3. Community law

Community law, once made, is interpreted by the European Court of Justice whose decisions are binding on community institutions, national governments, companies and individuals.

17.7. Evolution and Implementation of Legal Measures – a General Remark on Effectiveness

17.7.1. Evolution

Animal welfare legislation is bound up with the whole legal system of a state or supra- or international body as well as with economics and politics. As a result there are constraints on legislation which can be disadvantageous in terms of animal protection, although there is sometimes good reason for this when the system is looked at as a whole.

In deciding whether there is a need for new legislation public opinion plays an invaluable part. It is difficult if not impossible to convince ministers of such need when there has been no public demand shown. However, the time-consuming procedure of law-making and the need to find widely accepted compromises make it almost impossible to fulfil any wish that 'something should be done now', because an action at that very instant is logically desirable. Moreover, legislation hurriedly enacted by public demand might be ill thought-out and is hard to remove.

Much statute law including Welfare Codes represents a compromise. During the procedure of its evolution, interest groups, such as animal welfare groups or representations of professional or hobby animal users, apply pressure for often opposing aims. When scientific knowledge exists, legislation based upon it is to be preferred. However, there is a regrettable but understandable tendency to base legislation on existing practices. Whilst keeping in mind the objects of the measure, efforts are made to offend as few people as possible. However, sometimes a compromise is to be preferred to losing the entire measure because it may be long before it can be presented again. Meanwhile the status quo continues.

Regarding cases which largely arise fortuitously, in countries with common-law systems much more could be done by the bringing of 'test cases' before the 'courts of record', i.e. the superior courts. Success binds subsequent cases in all the courts unless the case can be distinguished on the facts.

17.7.2. Implementation

The effectiveness of legal measures depends not only on the measure itself but to a great extent on the knowledge of animal users, competent authorities and jurists. Measures which encourage the building up of dialogue and the giving of advice are an important tool. However, certain goals will never be achieved without some pressure, i.e. an effective enforcement of animal welfare law.

Many people complain about the ineffectiveness of legal measures. Ruth Harrison (1987, p. 4) says about the UK Welfare Codes that 'the Codes have not been famous either for their uptake by farmers or for their impact'. Similar statements could be cited from any other country. Change is often strongly resisted. There is not only ignorance but also unreflected, outdated traditions and, possibly the strongest factor of all, economical forces. Much remains to be done. However, the question must be asked 'what would the situation be like without any legal measure in force?' In the animal's interest, nobody would like to be in that position.

17.8. Conclusions

- A remarkable body of animal welfare legislation has built up over the last 300 years, most of it during the twentieth century.
- Legislation reflects attitudes to animals as well as the legal and political systems of the different countries. These different, valid approaches must be seen in the context of their countries' history and present situation.
- Increasingly, international harmonization is taking place, to engender common ethical attitudes and to remove barriers to trade and distortion of competition.
- Knowledge of the legal and political context of animal welfare, as well as scientific and practical knowledge of animals' needs, is important.
- This information can exert an effective influence on legislators and enforcement authorities and help to promote the goal that many seek; improvement of animal welfare.

Legal Texts

Commission Regulation (EEC) No 1274/91 (1991) Commission Regulation of 15 May 1991 introducing detailed rules for implementing Regulation (EEC) No 1907/90 on certain marketing standards for eggs (OJ No L 121, 16.5.91, p. 11).

Commission Regulation (EEC) No 2891/93 (1993) Commission Regulation of 21 October 1993 amending Regulation (EEC) 1538/91 introducing detailed rules for implementing Regulation (EEC) No 1906/90 on certain marketing standards for poultry meat (OJ No L 263, 22.10.93, p. 12).

Council Directive 88/609/EEC (1986) Council Directive of 24 November 1986 on the Approximation of Laws, Regulations and Administrative Provisions of the member states regarding the Protection of Animals used for Experimental and other Scientific Purposes (OJ No L 358, 18.12.86, p. 1).

Council Directive 88/166/EEC (1988) Council Directive of 7 March 1988 complying with the judgement of the Court of Justice in Case 131/86 (annulment of Council Directive 86/113/EEC of 25 March 1986 laying down minimum standards for the protection of laying hens kept in battery cages) (OJ No L 74, 19.3.88, p. 83).

Council Directive 91/628/EEC (1991) Council Directive of 19 November 1991 on the Protection of Animals during Transport and amending Directives 90/425/EEC and 91/496/EEC (OJ No L 340, 11.12.91, p. 17).

Council Directive 91/629/EEC (1991) Council Directive of 19 November 1991 laying down Minimum Standards for the Protection of Calves (OJ No L 340, 11.12.91, p. 28).

Council Directive 91/630/EEC (1991) Council Directive of 19 November 1991 laying down Minimum Standards for the Protection of Pigs (OJ No L 340, 11.12.91, p. 33).

Council Directive 93/119/EC (1993) Council Directive of 22 December 1993 on the Protection of Animals at the time of Slaughter or Killing (OJ No L 340, 31.12.93, p. 21).

Council Directive 95/29/EC (1995) Council Directive of 29 June 1995 amending Directive 91/628/EEC on the Protection of Animals during Transport (OJ No L 148, 30.6.95, p. 52).

Council Directive 97/2/EC (1997) Council Directive of 20 January 1997 amending Directive 91/629/EEC laying down Minimum Standards for the Protection of Calves (OJ No L 25, 28.1.97, p. 24).

List of Cases

Early v. *Newham H.A.* (1994) 5 Med L.R. 214 Medical Law Reports.

National Justice Campagnia Navesia SA v. *Prudential Assurance Co. The Ikarian Reefer* (1993) 2 Lloyds Rep 68.81.

Pepper v. *Hart* (1992) 3 W.L.R. 1033 H.L. Weekly Law Reports.

Swans (1592) Coke's Report p. 17b.

Waters v. *Braithwaite* (1913) 78 J.P. 421 Justice of the Peace Reports.

Discussion

Michael C. Appleby (University of Edinburgh, UK) and
Barry O. Hughes (Roslin Institute, UK)

Recent years have brought a considerable increase in our understanding of animal welfare and of the factors which affect it – as shown by the high proportion of work covered in the preceding chapters which was published within the last decade. This understanding has been partly associated with rejection of mechanistic views of animals such as behaviourism: it has become recognized that reductionist approaches to animal biology are inadequate to explain its complexities. This is not to say, of course, that there has been uncritical adoption of approaches at the opposite extreme such as anthropomorphism. Animals are not 'little humans' and a cow's perception of being branded, for example, will not be the same in all respects as a human's perception of undergoing the same procedure (although there will be aspects in common). However, we do use our human minds in interpreting the world around us, including the perceptions and minds of non-human animals.

It is clear that an area of increasing importance in future research will be aspects of cognition such as feelings. This is a field which is already receiving attention in books such as Griffin's 'Animal Minds' (1992) and Dawkins' 'Through Our Eyes Only? The Search for Animal Consciousness' (1993), although there are some dissenting voices such as Kennedy's 'The New Anthropomorphism' (1992). It is clear that the burgeoning philosophical and scientific interest in all aspects of consciousness has major implications for non-human animals (Dennett, 1991; Gallup et al., 1995). Understanding of animal cognition has obvious consequences for how we treat animals. De Waal (1996, pp. 214, 216) makes this point in relation to his studies on primates and to experimentation on animals; it also applies more generally:

> Recent studies of animal behaviour, mine included, provide ample reason to reconsider the way animals are used for science, entertainment, food, education and other purposes. We need to re-evaluate traditional attitudes developed over a long history without realistic alternatives and without awareness of the sensibilities and cognitive abilities of animals. This process is well under way at zoos and research institutions and in society at large . . . How much do we care and what can we afford? There are excellent reasons to insist on respect and concern for animals that serve the human cause. Apes do warrant special consideration. We should either phase out experiments on certain species altogether, or if humanity cannot forgo the benefits derived from them, we must at least enrich and enhance their lives in captivity and reduce their suffering.

It is also apparent, from the chapters in Part IV of this book, that research on systems and on details of husbandry will continue to be needed. Work on welfare will continue to be applied to practical situations. Such application, though, will be in the context of other pressures from society: people interested in welfare are increasingly aware that they are not working on 'facts' independent of values but on a variety of approaches (of which the scientific approach is only one) to value-laden areas – as emphasized in Part I.

How important are these other pressures? It sometimes seems that although much has been said about welfare over the last thirty years there has not been much actual improvement: most laboratory rats are still in barren cages and most laying hens are also still in battery systems. However, this impression is misleading. First, and perhaps most important, there has been a change in the attitude of the majority of people involved with animals. This will have led to many improvements in how animals are kept or handled: in other words, to improvements in husbandry, which is crucial to welfare. Second, there have been innumerable changes which are relatively inconspicuous but nevertheless important: stronger enforcement of legislation, improved structure of cages, reductions in numbers of experimental animals used, phasing out of harmful procedures, development of alternatives for animal use in school, college and university teaching. Third, there have been some major changes. Animal experimentation in many countries is now regulated by institutional animal care committees, and carried out with the '3 Rs' (reduction, refinement, replacement) in mind. Zoos have radically changed their approach to housing, driven by public attitudes which at one time seemed to threaten the very existence of these institutions. The conditions in which farm animals are kept are increasingly affected by welfare reports and codes of recommendations, and some are now kept in completely different systems partly because of welfare perceptions: for example, about 30% of pigs in the UK are now kept outdoors. Indeed, a major justification for intensive agricultural systems was control of disease, but consensus may now have begun to swing towards the belief that extensive conditions are better for immunocompetence as well as for behavioural expression (Hartung, 1994; Lawrence and Appleby, 1996).

There are setbacks for animal welfare as well as advances. Breeding of animals for maximum output in minimum time has increased morbidity in animals such as broiler chickens and dairy cattle, while certain work on genetic modification involves suffering for an increasing number of laboratory animals (Day, 1995; Appleby, 1998). However, advances will continue because social values are changing. Thus Hurnik (1995, p. 561) suggests that: 'The strong social interest in welfare is the most outstanding ethical development affecting twentieth century agriculture.' Bernard Rollin (1995, pp. 146, 148, 157) goes further:

> What is essentially happening in society regarding animals is a growing dissatisfaction with the venerable ethic that underlies the laws I have been discussing, the ethic of kindness and cruelty . . . Society is groping for a new ethic for animals in an inchoate way and the direction in which it is moving is both rational and inevitable . . . Clearly some message important to current social thought is being carried by the notion that animals have rights.

Future changes will partly continue existing trends, for example in legislation. However, one reason for the relatively limited changes which have occurred so far is the negative nature of most relevant legislation: our laws define what we may not do to animals not what we should do, and new laws of this proscriptive sort are difficult to frame. Some argue that there should be a shift towards positive provision for animals (Everton, 1989) and in some countries this has already occurred, at least with regard to farm animals. In Switzerland, all new equipment has to be checked by government research institutions before implementation. Rollin (1995, p. 158) points out that:

> Sweden has passed a law for agricultural animals that mandates that all systems of keeping farm animals must first and foremost accommodate the animals' natures. For example, the law grants cattle 'the right to graze' in perpetuity.

One area in which such an approach would be particularly effective is in use of public funds, as we have argued previously (Appleby *et al.*, 1992, p. 209):

> The possibility that the costs of legislation on animal housing should be met partly by subsidy from public funds has been less considered than other options. It could be argued that if society is concerned with the conditions in which animals are kept, society should be willing to contribute to the costs of their upkeep. Use of public funds in this way would spread those costs more widely than insisting that producers and purchasers should pay the whole cost. It could also usefully be associated with existing or expanded programmes of farm inspection, so that such inspection could result in reward rather than just punishment as at present.

Webster (1995, p. 162) makes concrete proposals along these lines in relation to farm animals:

> All attempts, such as those within the Council of Europe, to devise legislation to improve the welfare of the laying hen have, so far, been obsessed with the need to define minimum standards for cage design. There is, however, a much more attractive way to achieve the same objective, namely improved living standards for the laying hen. This is to devise financial incentives and penalties designed to shift the economic balance in favour of alternative systems such as a subsidy for producers who kept birds on free range with flock sizes no larger than 200 birds. There need be no limit to the number of flocks maintained on any one farm. The standard response of Eurogovernments to such a suggestion is that legislation by financial incentive is impossible since there is no new money. That objection can be easily dismissed. There is no need for new money. In 1993, 42% of income to farmers within the European Union came from government grants and subsidies using taxpayers' money. At present many subsidies, such as those for extensification and set-aside, are dictated almost entirely by the need to avoid overproduction. There is some emphasis on the maintenance of environmental quality and living standards for the small farmer but, at present, no example of subsidy directly designed to maintain the quality of life on the land, and this should imply quality of life for both farmers and their animals. I suggest most strongly that matters of animal welfare should be central to any discussion as to the best use of agricultural subsidy.

However, in view of the other changes outlined above, such as those in attitudes, new legislation will not be the only major influence on the management and husbandry of animals and may not even be the most important one. As discussed in Chapter 16, market forces will play an increasing role in future. As one example, supermarkets buying farm animal products have considerable influence on the conditions in which those animals are kept. One supermarket chain in the UK has recently adopted the Freedom Food label of the Royal Society for Prevention of Cruelty to Animals and started to market eggs laid by hens in barn systems at the same price as those from cages, despite the fact that this results in less profit to both the producer and the supermarket (Anonymous, 1996). This is a response to pressure from their customers, pressure that will probably be expressed increasingly by various sectors of the general public in future.

We started this book by noting that concern for animal welfare has increased in many nations. We must recognize, of course, that priorities differ between nations and that while some of these priorities have positive effects on welfare others have negative effects. For example, Norway has legislation to limit farm size, because it regards rural employment as important, and this limitation probably has some benefits for welfare. France puts emphasis on food quality, with some positive effects (free-range, slower-growing broilers are common) and some negative (force-feeding of geese is controversial). Other countries understandably put emphasis on food availability, and it is not the intention of this book to tell less developed countries that they ought to be more interested in animal welfare. Indeed, some cost-benefit analyses of animal use are now attempting to incorporate other concerns such as effect on less developed countries and the environment as well as impact on welfare (Mepham, 1993). Nevertheless, the material in this book supports that initial impression of a worldwide growth in interest in this area. We note, indeed, that the quotation with which we began, expressing the moral imperative of such growth, came from the leader of a less developed country with plenty of other problems, Mahatma Gandhi.

REFERENCES

Abplanalp, H. (1982) Contribution of genetics to the solution of problems requiring multi-disciplinary approaches. *World's Poultry Science Journal* 38, 59–60.

Ajzen, I. and Fishbein, M. (1980) *Understanding Attitudes and Predicting Social Behaviour.* Prentice Hall, New Jersey.

Alberts, A.C. (1994) Dominance hierarchies in male lizards: implications for zoo management programs. *Zoo Biology* 13, 479–490.

Algers, B. and Jensen, P. (1991) Teat stimulation and milk production during early lactation in sows: effects of continuous noise. *Canadian Journal of Animal Science* 71, 51–60.

Al-Rawi, B. and Craig, J.V. (1975) Agonistic behaviour of caged chickens related to group size and area per bird. *Applied Animal Ethology* 2, 69–80.

Animal Welfare Advisory Committee (1994) *Annual Report.* Ministry of Agriculture and Fisheries, Wellington, New Zealand.

Anonymous (1989) How Astrid Lindgren achieved enactment of the 1988 law protecting animals in Sweden: a selection of articles and letters published in Expressen, Stockholm, 1985–1989. Animal Welfare Institute, Washington, USA.

Anonymous (1992) NFU responds to EC paper on hen welfare. *Poultry Forum* July, 4.

Anonymous (1996) Freedom barn match cage eggs on price. *Poultry World*, August, 2.

Appleby, M.C. (1993) Should cages for laying hens be banned or modified? *Animal Welfare* 2, 67–80.

Appleby, M.C. (1996) Can we extrapolate from intensive to extensive conditions? *Applied Animal Behaviour Science* 49, 23–28.

Appleby, M.C. (1997) Life in a variable world: behaviour, welfare and environmental design. *Applied Animal Behaviour Science* (in press).

Appleby, M.C. (1998) Genetic engineering, welfare and accountability. *Journal of Applied Animal Welfare Science* (in press).

Appleby, M.C. and Hughes, B.O. (1993) The future of applied animal ethology. *Applied Animal Behaviour Science* 35, 389–395.

Appleby, M.C. and Hughes, B.O. (1995) The Edinburgh Modified Cage for laying hens. *British Poultry Science* 36, 707–718.

Appleby, M.C. and Lawrence, A.B. (1987) Food restriction as a cause of stereotypic behaviour in tethered gilts. *Animal Production* 45, 103–111.

Appleby, M.C., Hughes, B.O. and Elson, H.A. (1992) *Poultry Production Systems: Behaviour, Management and Welfare.* CAB International, Wallingford, UK, 238 pp.

Archer, J. (1976) The organization of aggression and fear in vertebrates. In: Bateson, P.P.G. and Klopfer, P.H. (eds) *Perspectives in Ethology.* Plenum Press, New York, pp. 231–298.

Archer, J. (1979) Behavioural aspects of fear. In: Sluckin, W. (ed.) *Fear in Animals and Man*, Van Nostrand Reinhold, New York, pp. 56–85.

Arey, D.S. (1992) Straw and food as reinforcers for prepartal sows. *Applied Animal Behaviour Science* 33, 217–226.

Arey, D.S., Petchey, A.M. and Fowler, V.R. (1991) The preparturient behaviour of sows in enriched pens and the effect of pre-formed nests. *Applied Animal Behaviour Science* 31, 61–68.

Arnsten, A.F.T., Berridge, C. and Segal, D.S. (1985) Stress produces opioid-like effects on investigatory behavior. *Pharmacology, Biochemistry and Behavior* 22, 803–809.

Association of Veterinary Teachers and Research Workers (1986) Guidelines for the recognition and assessment of pain in animals. *Veterinary Record* 118, 334–338.

Baldwin, B.A. and Ingram, D.L. (1967) Behavioural thermoregulation in pigs. *Physiology & Behavior* 2, 15–21.

Baldwin, B.A. and Start, I.B. (1985) Illumination preferences of pigs. *Applied Animal Behaviour Science* 14, 233–243.

Banks, E.M. (1982) Behavioral research to answer questions about animal welfare. *Journal of Animal Science* 54, 434–436.

Barber, J., Brooks, P.H. and Carpenter, J.L. (1989) The effects of water delivery rate on the voluntary food intake, water use and performance of early weaned pigs from 3 to 6 weeks of age. In: Forbes, J.M., Varley, M.A. and Lawrence, T.J.L. (eds) *The Voluntary Food Intake of Pigs.* Occasional Publication of British Society of Animal Production, No. 13, Edinburgh, pp. 103–104.

Barnett, J.L. (1993) A drug that reduces aggression in pigs – a welfare dilemma. In: Batterham, E.S. (ed.) *Manipulating Pig Production IV.* Australasian Pig Science Association, Attwood, Victoria, p.131.

Barnett, J.L. and Hemsworth, P.H. (1990) The validity of physiological and behavioural measures of animal welfare. *Applied Animal Behaviour Science* 20, 177–187.

Barnett, J.L., Hemsworth, P.H. and Newman, E.A. (1992) Fear of humans and its relationships with productivity in laying hens at commercial farms. *British Poultry Science* 33, 699–710.

Barnett, J.L., Cronin, G.M., McCallum, T.H. and Newman, E.A. (1993) Effects of 'chemical intervention' techniques on aggression and injuries when grouping unfamiliar adult pigs. *Applied Animal Behaviour Science* 36, 135–148.

Barnett, J.L., Cronin, G.M., McCallum, T.H. and Newman, E.A. (1994a) Effects of food and time of day on aggression when grouping unfamiliar adult pigs. *Applied Animal Behaviour Science* 39, 339–347.

Barnett, J.L., Hemsworth, P.H., Hennessy, D.P., McCallum, T.H. and Newman, E.A. (1994b) The effects of modifying the amount of human contact on behavioural, physiological and production responses of laying hens. *Applied Animal Behaviour Science* 41, 87–100.

Barnett, S.A. and McEwan, I.M. (1973) Movements of virgin, pregnant and lactating mice in a residential maze. *Physiology & Behavior* 10, 741–746.

Barnett, S.A. and Smart, J.L. (1975) The movements of wild and domestic house mice in an artificial environment. *Behavioral Biology* 15, 85–93.

Barrett, L., Dunbar, R.I.M. and Dunbar, P. (1992) Environmental influences on play behaviour in immature gelada baboons. *Animal Behaviour* 44, 111–117.

Barton Gade, P., Blaabjerg, L. and Christensen, L. (1992) New lairage system for slaughter pigs – effects on behaviour and quality characteristics. *Proceedings 38th International Congress of Meat Science and Technology*, Vol II, pp. 161–164, Clermont Ferrand, France.

Bateson, P. (1991) Assessment of pain in animals. *Animal Behaviour* 42, 827–839.

Baxter, M.R. (1983) Ethology in environmental design. *Applied Animal Ethology* 9, 207–220.

Baxter, M.R. (1991) The 'Freedom' farrowing system. *Farm Progress* 104, 9–15.

Becker, B.A., Christenson, R.K., Ford, J.J., Manak, R., Nienaber, J.A., Hahn, G.L. and Deshazer, J.A. (1984) Serum cortisol concentrations in gilts and sows housed in tether stalls, gestation stalls and individual pens. *Annales de Recherches Vétérinaires* 15, 237–242.

Becker, B.A., Christenson, R.K., Ford, J.J., Nienaber, J.A., Deshazer, J.A. and Hahn, G.L. (1989) Adrenal and behavioral responses of swine restricted to varying degrees of mobility. *Physiology & Behavior* 45, 1171–1176.

Beilharz, R.G. (1982) Genetic adaptation in relation to animal welfare. *International Journal for the Study of Animal Problems* 3, 117–124.

Beilharz, R.G. (1994) Environmental limitation – Consequences for breeding programs. In: Smith, C., Gavora, J.S., Benkel, B., Chesnais, J., Fairfull, W., Gibson, J.P., Kennedy, E.B. and Burnside, E.B. (eds) *Proceedings of the 5th World Congress on Genetics Applied to Livestock Production*. Volume 18, University of Guelph, Guelph, Ontario, pp. 213–216.

Beilharz, R.G. and Zeeb, K. (1981) Applied ethology and animal welfare. *Applied Animal Ethology* 7, 3–10.

Beilharz, R.G., Luxford, B.G. and Wilkinson, J.L. (1993) Quantitative genetics and evolution: Is our understanding of genetics sufficient to explain evolution? *Journal of Animal Breeding and Genetics* 110, 161–170.

Belyaev, D.K. (1979) Destabilising selection as a factor in domestication. *Journal of Heredity* 70, 301–308.

Bennett, R.M. (1995) The value of farm animal welfare. *Journal of Agricultural Economics* 46, 46–60.

Bennett, R.M. (1996a) People's willingness to pay for farm animal welfare. *Animal Welfare* 5, 3–11.

Bennett, R.M. (1996b) Willingness-to-pay measures of public support for farm animal welfare legislation. *Veterinary Record* 139.

Bentham, J. (1789) *Introduction to the Principles of Morals and Legislation*. 1996 Imprint. Clarendon Press, Oxford.

Benus, R.F. (1988) Aggression and coping. PhD Thesis. University of Groningen, The Netherlands.

Berlyne, D.E. (1960) *Conflict, Arousal and Curiosity*. McGraw-Hill, New York.

Berman, C.M. (1990) Intergenerational transmission of maternal rejection rates among free-ranging rhesus monkeys. *Animal Behaviour* 39, 329–337.

Bernstein, I.S. (1991) Social housing of monkeys and apes: group formations. *Laboratory Animal Science* 41, 329–333.

Bessei, von H. and Bessei, H. (1974) Eine Messanlage zum Uberwachen der locomotorischen Aktivität von Hühnern in Bodenhaltung. *Archives für Geflügelkünde* 38, 94–98.

Beuving, G., Jones, R.B. and Blokhuis, H.J. (1989) Adrenocortical and heterophil/lymphocyte responses to challenge in hens showing short or long tonic immobility reactions. *British Poultry Science* 30, 175–184.

Beynen, A.C., Baumans, V., Bertens, A.P.M.G., Havenaar, R., Hesp, A.P.M. and van Zutphen, L.F.M. (1987) Assessment of discomfort in gallstone-bearing mice: a practical example of the problems encountered in an attempt to recognise discomfort in laboratory animals. *Laboratory Animals* 21, 35–42.

Blackorby, C. and Donaldson, D. (1992) Pigs and guinea pigs: a note on the ethics of animal exploitation. *The Economic Journal* 102, 1345–1369.

Blokhuis, H.J. (1989) The development and causation of feather pecking in the domestic fowl. PhD Thesis. The Agricultural University of Wageningen, The Netherlands.

Blom, H.J.M., van Vorstenbosch, C.J.A.H.V., Baumans, V., Hoogervorst, M.J.C., Beynen, A.C. and van Zutphen, L.F.M. (1992) Description and validation of a preference test system to evaluate housing conditions for laboratory mice. *Applied Animal Behaviour Science* 35, 67–82.

Blom, H.J.M., Baumans, V., van Vorstenbosch, C.J.A.H.V., van Zutphen, L.F.M. and Beynen, A.C. (1993) Preference tests with rodents to assess housing conditions. *Animal Welfare* 2, 81–87.

Blood, D.C. and Radostits, O.M. (1989) *Veterinary Medicine.* Seventh Edition. Ballière Tindall, London.

Blood, D.C. and Studdert, V.P. (1988) *Ballière's Comprehensive Veterinary Dictionary.* Ballière Tindall, London.

Bloom, S.R., Edwards, A.V., Hardy, R.M., Malinowska, K. and Silver, M. (1975) Cardiovascular and endocrine response to feeding in young calves. *Journal of Physiology* 253, 135–155.

Bohus, B., Benus, R.F., Fokkema, D.S., Koolhaas, J.M., Nyakas, C., Van Oortmerssen, G.A., Prins, A.J.A., De Ruiter, A.J.H., Scheurink, A.J.H. and Steffens, A.B. (1987) Neuroendocrine states and behavioral and physiological stress responses. In: De Kloet, E.R., Wiegant, V.M. and De Wied, D. (eds) *Progress in Brain Research.* Elsevier, Amsterdam, 72, 57–70.

Boissy, A. (1995) Fear and fearfulness in animals. *The Quarterly Review of Biology* 70, 165–191.

Boivin, X. (1991) Etude des facteurs experientiéls et génétiques de la relation des bovines domestiques (*Bos taurus L*) avec l'homme. Thèse de docteur en sciences de l'Université Rennes, France.

Bouissou, M.F., Vandenheede, M. and Romeyer, A. (1994) Les reactions de peur chez les ovins: quantification et facteurs de variation. In: Picard, M., Porter, R. and Signoret, J.P. (eds) *Un point sur comportement et bien-être animal.* Institut National de la Recherche Agronomique, Paris, pp. 109–125.

Boulding, K.E. (1969) Economics as a moral science. *The American Economic Review* 59, 1–12.

Bowman, J.C. (1974) *An Introduction to Animal Breeding.* The Institute of Biology's Studies in Biology no. 46. Edward Arnold (Publishers) Limited, London, 76pp.

Brake, J., Baker, M., Morgan, G.W. and Thaxton, P. (1982) Physiological changes in caged layers during a forced molt. 4. Leucocytes and packed cell volume. *Poultry Science* 61, 790–795.

Brambell Committee (1965) *Report of the Technical Committee to Enquire into the Welfare of Animals kept under Intensive Livestock Husbandry Systems.* Command Report 2836, Her Majesty's Stationery Office, London.

Breland, K. and Breland, M. (1961) The misbehavior of organisms. *American Psychologist* 16, 681–684.

Brochart, M. (1986) Foot lameness of the cow, a multifactorial disease. In: Wierenga, H.K. and Peterse, D.J. (eds) *Cattle Housing Systems, Lameness and Behaviour.* Martinus Nijhoff, The Hague, pp. 159–165.

Brooks, P.H. and Carpenter, J.L. (1990) The water requirement of growing-finishing pigs – theoretical and practical considerations. In: Haresign, W. and Cole, D.J.A. (eds) *Recent Advances in Animal Nutrition.* Butterworths, London, pp. 115–136.

Broom, D.M. (1987) Relationship between welfare and disease susceptibility in farm animals. In: Animal Disease – a Welfare Problem. *Proceedings of the 5th Symposium of the BVA Animal Welfare Foundation*, pp. 22–29.

Broom, D.M. (1996) Animal welfare defined in terms of attempt to cope with the environment. *Acta Agriculturæ Scandinavica*. Section A, Animal Science, Supplementation 27, 22–28.

Broom, D.M. and Johnson, K.G. (1993) *Stress and Animal Welfare*. Chapman and Hall, London.

Brown, A. (1974) *Who Cares for Animals?* Heinemann, London.

Brown, G.D. and Lynch, J.J. (1972) Some aspects of the water balance of sheep at pasture when deprived of drinking water. *Australian Journal of Agricultural Research* 23, 669–684.

Brown, K.I. and Nestor, K.E. (1974) Implications of selection for high and low adrenal response to stress. *Poultry Science* 53, 1297–1306.

Bruckberger, R.-L. (1971) *Saint François et le loup*. Editions G.-P., Paris, France.

Bryant, M.J. and Grant, J.W.A. (1995) Resource defence, monopolization and variation of fitness in groups of female Japanese medaka depend on the synchrony of food arrival. *Animal Behaviour* 49, 1469–1479.

Bryden, M.P. (1982) Lateralization of emotional processes. In: Bryden, M.P. (ed.) *Laterality: Functional Symmetries in the Intact Brain*. Academic Press, New York, p. 123.

Bulfield, G. (1985) The potential for improvement of commercial poultry by genetic engineering techniques. In: Hill, W.G. (ed.) *Poultry Genetics and Breeding*. British Poultry Science Ltd, Edinburgh, pp. 37–46.

Burghardt, G.M. (1995) Brain imaging, ethology, and the nonhuman mind. *Behavioral and Brain Sciences* 18, 339–340.

Cabanac, M. and Johnson, K.G. (1983) Analysis of a conflict between palatability and cold exposure in rats. *Physiology & Behavior* 31, 249–253.

Cabib, S. (1993) Neurobiological basis of stereotypies. In: Lawrence, A.B. and Rushen, J. (eds) *Stereotypic Animal Behaviour: Fundamentals and Applications to Welfare*. CAB International, Wallingford, UK, pp. 119–146.

Cannon, W.B. (1914) The emergency function of the adrenal medulla in pain and the major emotions. *American Journal of Physiology*, 33, 356–372.

Cannon, W.B. (1929) *Bodily Changes in Pain, Hunger, Fear and Rage*, 2nd edn. Appleton-Century Co., New York, USA.

Carlstead, K. (1986) Predictability of feeding: its effect on agonistic behaviour and growth in grower pigs. *Applied Animal Behaviour Science* 16, 25–38.

Carlstead, K., Seidensticker, J. and Baldwin, R. (1991) Environmental enrichment for zoo bears. *Zoo Biology* 10, 3–16.

Carlstead, K., Brown, J.L., Monfort, S.L., Killens, R. and Wildt, D.E. (1992) Urinary monitoring of adrenal responses to psychological stressors in domestic and non-domestic felids. *Zoo Biology* 11, 165–176.

Carlstead, K., Brown, J.L. and Seidensticker, J. (1993) Behavioral and adrenocortical responses to environmental changes in leopard cats (*Felis bengalensis*). *Zoo Biology*, 12, 321–331.

Chambers Dictionary (1983) *Chambers 20th Century Dictionary* (reprinted 1987).

Chamove, A.S. and Grimmer, B. (1993) Reduced visibility lowers bull aggression. *Proceedings of the New Zealand Society of Animal Production* 53, 207–208.

Chamove, A.S., Anderson, J.R., Morgan-Jones, S.C. and Jones, S.P. (1982) Deep woodchip litter: hygiene, feeding, and behavioural enhancement in eight primate species. *International Journal for the Study of Animal Problems* 3, 308–318.

Charles, D.R. (1989) Environmental responses of growing turkeys. In: Nixey, C. and Grey, T.C. (eds) *Recent Advances in Turkey Science*. Butterworths, London, pp. 201–214.

Charlton, D.B. (1990) Adrenal cortical innervation and glucocorticoid secretion. *Journal of Endocrinology* 126, 5–8.

Charvat, J., Dell, P. and Folkow, B. (1964) Mental factors and cardiovascular disorders. *Cardiologia* 44, 124–141.

Chesterton, R.N., Pfeiffer, D.U., Morris, R.S. and Tanner, C.M. (1989) Environmental and behavioural factors affecting the prevalence of foot lameness in New Zealand dairy herds – a case-control study. *New Zealand Veterinary Journal*, 37, 135–142.

Christison, G.I. and Farmer, C. (1983) Physical characteristics of perforated floors for young pigs. *Canadian Agricultural Engineering* 25, 75–80.

Clarkson, M.J. and others (1993) An epidemiological study to determine the risk factors of lameness in dairy cows. Unpublished Report, Liverpool University.

Coleman, G.J., Hemsworth, P.H., Hay, M. and Cox, M. (1997) Predicting stockperson behaviour towards pigs from attitudinal and job-related variables and empathy. *Applied Animal Behaviour Science* (in press).

Colpaert, F.C. (1987) Evidence that adjuvant arthritis in the rat is associated with chronic pain. *Pain* 28, 201–222.

Commission of the European Union (1993) Communication from the Commission to the Council and the European Parliament on the Protection of Animals. Com (93) 384 final, Brussels, 22 July 1993.

Cooper, J.J. and Nicol, C. (1994) Neighbour effects on the development of locomotor stereotypies in bank voles, *Clethrionomys glareolus*. *Animal Behaviour* 47, 214–216.

Cooper, J.J., Emmans, G.C. and Friggens, N.C. (1994) Effect of diet on behaviour of individually penned lambs. *Animal Production* 58, 441.

Cooper, J.J., Ödberg, F. and Nicol, C. (1996) Limitations on the effectiveness of environmental enrichment in reducing stereotypic behaviour in bank voles (*Clethrionomys glareolus*). *Applied Animal Behaviour Science* 48, 237–248.

Coppinger, T.R., Minton, J.E., Reddy, P.G. and Blecha, F. (1991) Repeated restraint and isolation stress in lambs increases pituitary-adrenal secretions and reduces cell-mediated immunity. *Journal of Animal Science* 69, 2808–2814.

Cowan, P.E. (1977) Systematic patrolling and orderly behaviour of rats during recovery from deprivation. *Animal Behaviour* 25, 171–184.

Cowan, P.E. (1983) Exploration in small mammals: ethology and ecology. In: Archer, J. and Birke, L.I.A. (eds) *Exploration in Animals and Humans*. Van Nostrand Reinhold Inc., London, pp. 147–176.

Craig, J.V. and Muir, W.M. (1993) Selection for reduced beak-inflicted injuries among caged hens. *Poultry Science* 72, 411–420.

Craig, J.V. and Swanson, J.C. (1994) Review: welfare perspectives on hens kept for egg production. *Poultry Science* 73, 921–938.

Craig, J.V., Craig, T.P. and Dayton, A.D. (1983) Fearful behavior by caged hens of two genetic stocks. *Applied Animal Ethology* 10, 263–273.

Cransberg, P.H. and Hemsworth, P.H. (1995) Human factors affecting the behavioural response and productivity of commercial broiler chickens. *Queensland Poultry Science Symposium* 4, 1–8.

Cronin, G.M., Wiepkema, P.R. and Hofstede, G.J. (1984) The development of stereotypies in tethered sows. In: Unshelm, J., van Putten, G. and Zeeb, K. (eds) *Proceedings of the International Congress on Applied Ethology in Farm Animals*. KTBL, Dalmstadt, pp. 97–100.

Cronin, G.M., Wiepkema, P.R. and van Ree, J.M. (1985) Endogenous opioids are involved in abnormal stereotyped behaviours of tethered sows. *Neuropeptides* 6, 527–530.

Curtis, P. (1990) *A Handbook of Poultry and Game Bird Diseases*. Liverpool University Press, Liverpool.

Curtis, S.E. (1983) *Environmental Management in Animal Agriculture*. Iowa State University Press, Ames.

Curtis, S.E. (1987) Animal well-being and animal care. *Veterinary Clinics of North America: Food Animal Practice* 3, 369–382.

Cuthbertson, G. (1980) Genetic variation in feather pecking behaviour. *British Poultry Science* 21, 447–450.

Czako, J. and Santha, T. (1978) Data on the technological tolerance of cattle of various genotypes. *Acta Agronomic Academy of Science Hungary* 27, 9–15.

Daan, S., Beersma, D.G.M. and Borbély, A.A. (1984) Timing of human sleep: recovery process gated by a circadian pacemaker. *American Journal of Physiology* 246, R161–R178.

Dallman, M.F. and Jones, M.T. (1973) Corticosteroid feedback control of ACTH secretion: effort of stress induced corticosterone secretion on subsequent stress response in the rat. *Endocrinology* 92, 1367–1375.

Danish National Committee for Pig Breeding and Production (1986) *Svinearl og-Production*. The National Committee for Pig Breeding, Health and Production, Copenhagen.

Dantzer, R. (1986) Behavioral, physiological, and functional aspects of stereotyped behavior: a review and a re-interpretation. *Journal of Animal Science* 62, 1776–1786.

Dantzer, R. (1990) Animal suffering: The practical way forward. *Behavioral and Brain Sciences* 13, 17–18.

Dantzer, R. and Mormède, P. (1983) Stress in farm animals: A need for reevaluation. *Journal of Animal Science* 57, 6–18.

Dantzer, R., Arnone, M. and Mormède, P. (1980) Effects of frustration on behaviour and plasma corticosteroid levels in pigs. *Physiology & Behavior* 24, 1–4.

Dantzer, R., Terlouw, C., Mormède, P. and Le Moal, M. (1988) Schedule-induced polydipsia experience decreases plasma corticosterone levels but increases plasma prolactin levels. *Physiology & Behavior* 43, 275–279.

Darwin, C. (1875) *The Variation of Animals and Plants under Domestication*, 2nd edn. John Murray, London.

Davis, H. and Balfour, A.D. (1992) The inevitable bond. In: Davis, H. and Balfour, A.D. (eds) *The Inevitable Bond: Examining Scientist–Animal Interactions*. Cambridge University Press, Cambridge, pp. 27–43.

Davis, L.E. and Donnelly, E.J. (1968) Analgesic drugs in the cat. *Journal of the American Veterinary Medical Association* 153, 1161–1167.

Dawkins, M.S. (1977) Do hens suffer in battery cages? Environmental preferences and welfare. *Animal Behaviour* 25, 1034–1046.

Dawkins, M.S. (1980) *Animal Suffering: The Science of Animal Welfare*. Chapman and Hall, London, UK.

Dawkins, M.S. (1983a) Battery hens name their price: consumer demand theory and the measurement of ethological 'needs'. *Animal Behaviour* 31, 1195–1205.

Dawkins, M.S. (1983b) The current status of preference tests in the assessment of animal welfare. In: Baxter, S.H., Baxter, M.R. and MacCormack, J.A.D. (eds) *Farm Animal Housing and Welfare*. Martinus Nijhoff Publishers, The Hague, The Netherlands, pp. 20–26.

Dawkins, M.S. (1988) Behavioural deprivation: a central problem in animal welfare. *Applied Animal Behaviour Science* 20, 209–225.

Dawkins, M.S. (1989) Time budgets in Red Junglefowl as a baseline for the assessment of welfare in domestic fowl. *Applied Animal Behaviour Science* 24, 77–80.

Dawkins, M.S. (1990) From an animal's point of view: motivation, fitness, and animal welfare. *Behavioral and Brain Sciences* 13, 1–9 and 54–61.

Dawkins, M.S. (1993) *Through Our Eyes Only? The Search for Animal Consciousness*. W.H. Freeman, Oxford.

Dawkins, M.S. and Beardsley, T. (1986) Reinforcing properties of access to litter in hens. *Applied Animal Behaviour Science* 15, 351–364.

Day, J.E.L., Kyriazakis, I. and Lawrence, A.B. (1995) The use of a second order schedule to measure feeding motivation in the pig. *Applied Animal Behaviour Science* 50, 15–31.

Day, S. (1995) Invasion of the shapechangers. *New Scientist* 28th October, 30–35.

de Boer, S.F., Koopmans, S.J., Slangen, J.L. and Van der Gugten, J. (1990) Plasma catecholamine, corticosterone and glucose responses to repeated stress in rats: effect of interstressor interval length. *Physiology & Behavior* 47, 1117–1124.

Delbende, C., Delarue, C., Lefebre, H., Tranchand-Brunel, D., Szafarczyk, A., Mocaër, E., Kamoun, A., Jégou, S. and Vaudry, H. (1992) Glucocorticosteroids, transmitters and stress. *British Journal of Psychology* 160, 24–34.

Dellmeier, G.R. (1989) Motivation in relation to the welfare of enclosed livestock. *Applied Animal Behaviour Science* 22, 129–138.

Dember, W.N., Earl, R.W. and Paradise, N. (1957) Response by rats to differential stimulus complexity. *Journal of Comparative and Physiological Psychology* 50, 514–518.

Denenberg, V.H. (1962) The effects of early experience. In: Hafez, E.S.E. (ed.) *The Behaviour of Domestic Animals*. Baillière, Tindall and Cox, London, pp. 109–138.

Dennett, D.C. (1991) *Consciousness Explained*. Little, Brown & Co., USA.

de Passillé, A.M.B., Christopherson, R.J. and Rushen, J. (1993) Nonnutritive sucking and postprandial secretion of insulin, CCK and gastrin by the calf. *Physiology & Behavior* 54, 1069–1073.

Deutsch, J.A., Moore, B.O. and Heinrichs, S.C. (1989) Unlearned specific appetite for protein. *Physiology & Behavior* 46, 619–624.

de Waal, F. (1996) *Good Natured: the Origins of Right and Wrong in Humans and Other Animals*. Harvard University Press, Cambridge, Mass.

de Wilt, J.G. (1985) Behaviour and welfare of veal calves in relation to husbandry systems. PhD thesis, The Agricultural University, Wageningen, The Netherlands.

Dewsbury, D.A. (1992) Studies of rodent–human interactions in animal psychology. In: Davis, H. and Balfour, A.D. (eds) *The Inevitable Bond: Examining Scientist–Animal Interactions*, Cambridge University Press, Cambridge, pp. 27–43.

Dobson, H. and Smith, R.F. (1995) Stress and reproduction in farm animals. *Journal of Reproduction and Fertility Suppl.* 49, 451–461.

Dohoo, S.E. and Dohoo, I.R. (1996) Factors influencing the postoperative use of analgesics in dogs and cats by Canadian veterinarians. *Canadian Veterinary Journal*, 37, 552–556.

Dubreuil, P., Couture, Y., Tremblay, A. and Martineau, G.P. (1990) Effects of experimenters and different blood sampling procedures on blood metabolite values in growing pigs. *Canadian Journal of Veterinary Research* 54, 379–382.

Dubreuil, P., Farmer, C., Couture, Y. and Petitclerc, D. (1993) Hematological and biochemical changes follwing an acute stress in control and somatostatin-immunized pigs. *Canadian Journal of Animal Science* 73, 241–252.

Duff, S.R.I. and Hocking, P.M. (1986) Chronic orthopaedic disease in adult male broiler breeding fowls. *Research in Veterinary Science* 41, 340–348.

Duncan, I.J.H. (1978a) The interpretation of preference tests in animal behaviour. *Applied Animal Ethology* 4, 197–200.

Duncan, I.J.H. (1978b) Overall assessment of poultry welfare. In: Sørensen, Y. (ed.) *First Danish Seminar on Poultry Welfare in Egglaying Cages*. National Committee for Poultry and Eggs, Copenhagen, pp. 79–88.

Duncan, I.J.H. (1981a) Animal behaviour and welfare. In: Clark, J.A. (ed.) *Environmental Aspects of Housing for Animal Production*. Butterworths, London, pp. 455–470.

Duncan, I.J.H. (1981b) Animal rights – animal welfare: A scientist's assessment. *Poultry Science* 60, 489–499.

Duncan, I.J.H. (1987) The welfare of farm animals: an ethological approach. *Science Progress, Oxford* 71, 317–326.

Duncan, I.J.H. (1990) Reactions of poultry to human beings. In: Zayan, R. and Dantzer, R. (eds) *Social Stress in Domestic Animals*. Kluwer Academic Publishers, Dordrecht, pp. 121–131.

Duncan, I.J.H. (1992a) Measuring preferences and the strength of preferences. *Poultry Science* 71, 658–663.

Duncan, I.J.H. (1992b) Designing environments for animals – not for public perceptions. *British Veterinary Journal* 148, 475–477.

Duncan, I.J.H. (1993) Welfare is to do with what animals feel. *Journal of Agricultural and Environmental Ethics* 6 (Supplement 2), 8–14.

Duncan, I.J.H. (1996) Animal welfare defined in terms of feelings. *Acta Agriculturæ Scandinavica*, Section A, Animal Science, Supplementum 27, 29–35.

Duncan, I.J.H. and Dawkins, M.S. (1983) The problem of assessing 'well-being' and 'suffering' in farm animals. In: Smidt D. (ed.) *Indicators Relevant to Farm Animal Welfare*. Martinus Nijhoff, The Hague, The Netherlands, pp. 13–24.

Duncan, I.J.H. and Hughes, B.O. (1972) Free and operant feeding in domestic fowls. *Animal Behaviour* 20, 775–777.

Duncan, I.J.H. and Hughes, B.O. (1988) Can the welfare needs of poultry be measured? In: Hardcastle, J. (ed.) *Science and the Poultry Industry*. Agricultural and Food Research Council, London, UK, pp. 24–25.

Duncan, I.J.H. and Molony, V. (eds) (1986) *Assessing Pain in Farm Animals*. Commission of the European Communities, Luxembourg.

Duncan, I.J.H. and Petherick, J.C. (1991) The implications of cognitive processes for animal welfare. *Journal of Animal Science* 69, 5071–5022.

Duncan, I.J.H. and Wood-Gush, D.G.M. (1971) Frustration and aggression in the domestic fowl. *Animal Behaviour* 19, 500–504.

Duncan, I.J.H. and Wood-Gush, D.G.M. (1972) An analysis of displacement preening in the domestic fowl. *Animal Behaviour* 20, 68–71.

Duncan, I.J.H., Slee, G.S., Kettlewell, P., Berry, P. and Carlisle, A.J. (1986) Comparison of the stressfulness of harvesting broiler chickens by machine and by hand. *British Poultry Science* 27, 109–114.

Duncan, I.J.H., Slee, G.S., Seawright, E. and Breward, J. (1989) Behavioural consequences of partial beak amputation (beak trimming) in poultry. *British Poultry Science* 30, 479–488.

Eagly, A.H. and Chaiken, S. (1993) *The Psychology of Attitudes*. Harcourt Brace Jovanovitch College Publishers, Fort Worth, Texas.

Edwards, S.A. and Mauchline, S. (1993) Designing pens to minimise aggression when sows are mixed. *Farm Buildings Progress* 113, 20–23.

Ehnert, K. and Moberg, G.P. (1991) Disruption of estrous behavior in ewes by dexamethasone or management-related stress. *Journal of Animal Science* 69, 2988–2994.

Ekesbo, I. (1966) Disease incidence in tied and loose housed dairy cattle and causes of this incidence: variation with particular reference to the cowshed type. *Acta Agriculturæ Scandinavica*, Supplementum 15, 1–74.

Ekesbo, I. (1981) Some aspects of sow health and housing. In: Sybesma, W. (ed.) *The Welfare of Pigs*. Martinus Nijhoff, The Hague, pp. 250–264.

Ekkel, E.D., van Doorn, C.E.A., Hessing, M.J.C. and Tielen, M.J.M. (1995) The specific-stress-free system has positive effects on productivity, health and welfare of pigs. *Journal of Animal Science* 73, 1544–1551.

English, P.R. (1991) Stockmanship, empathy and pig behaviour. *Pig Veterinary Journal* 26, 56–66.

Engström, B. and Schaller, G. (1993) Experimental studies of the health of laying hens in relation to housing system. In: Savory, C.J. and Hughes, B.O. (eds) *Proceedings of the Fourth European Symposium on Poultry Welfare*, Universities Federation for Animal Welfare, Potters Bar, UK, pp. 87–96.

Enquist, M. and Leimar, O. (1983) Evolution of fighting behaviour: decision rules and assessment of relative strength. *Journal of Theoretical Biology* 102, 387–410.

Erwin, J., Anderson, B., Erwin, N., Lewis, L. and Flynn, D. (1976) Aggression in captive pigtail monkey groups: effects of provision of cover. *Perceptual and Motor Skills* 42, 319–324.

Estevez, I., Newberry, R.C. and Arias de Reyna, L. (1997) Broiler chickens – a tolerant social system? *Etologia* (in press).

Everton, A. (1989) The legal protection of farm livestock: avoidance of 'unnecessary suffering' and the positive promotion of welfare. In: Blackman, D.E., Humphries, P.N. and Todd, P. (eds) *Animal Welfare and the Law*. Cambridge University Press, Cambridge, UK.

Ewbank, R. (1973) Abnormal behaviour and pig production. An unsuccessful attempt to reduce tail biting by feeding a high energy low fibre vegetable protein ration. *British Veterinary Journal* 129, 366–369.

Ewbank, R. (1987) Opening address. In: Animal Disease – a Welfare Problem. *Proceedings of the 5th Symposium of the BVA Animal Welfare Foundation*, pp. 4–6.

Fagen, R. (1982) Evolutionary issues in the development of behavioural flexibility. In: Bateson, P.P.G. and Klopfer, P.H. (eds) *Perspectives in Ethology*, Vol. 5. Plenum Press, New York.

Falconer, D.S. (1977) *An Introduction to Quantitative Genetics* (8th reprinted edn). Longman Group Limited, London, 365 pp.

Falk, J.L. (1961) Production of polydipsia in normal rats by intermittent food schedule. *Science* 133, 195–196.

Farm Animal Welfare Council (1992) FAWC updates the five freedoms. *Veterinary Record* 131, 357.

Farm Animal Welfare Council (1993) *Report on Priorities for Animal Welfare Research and Development*. Farm Animal Welfare Council, Surbiton. 26 pp.

Farmer, C. and Christison, G.I. (1982) Selection of perforated floors by newborn and weanling pigs. *Canadian Journal of Animal Science* 62, 1229–1236.

Faure, J.M. (1980) To adapt the environment to the bird or the bird to the environment. In: Moss, R. (ed.) *The Laying Hen and its Environment*. Current Topics in Veterinary Medicine and Animal Science. Volume 8. Martinus Nijhoff Publishers, The Hague – Boston – London, pp. 19–42.

Faure, J.M. (1981) Behavioural measures for selection. In: Sørensen, Y. (ed.) *Report of proceedings of the first European symposium on poultry welfare*. Danish Branch of the World's Poultry Science Association, Slagelsetryk, Slaglelse,pp. 37–41.

Faure, J.M. and Folmer, J.C. (1975) Etude génétique de l'activité précoce en open-field du jeune poussin. *Annales de Génétique et Sélection Animale* 7, 123–132.

Faure, J.M. and Jones, R.B. (1982) Effect of age, access and time of day on perching behaviour in the domestic fowl. *Applied Animal Ethology* 8, 357–364.

Faure, J.M., Melin, J.M. and Mills, A.D. (1992) Selection for behavioural traits in relation to poultry welfare. In: *Proceedings of the 19th World's Poultry Conference*. World's Poultry Science Association, Ponsen and Looijen, Wageningen, The Netherlands, pp. 405–408.

Feh, C. and de Mazieres, J. (1993) Grooming at a preferred grooming site reduces heart rate in horses. *Animal Behaviour* 46, 1191–1194.

FELASA (1994) Pain and distress in laboratory rodents and lagomorphs: report of the Federation of European Laboratory Animal Science Associations (FELASA) Working Group on Pain and Distress. *Laboratory Animals* 28, 97–112.

Ferchmin, P.A. and Eterovic, V.A. (1977) Brain plasticity and environmental complexity: role of motor skills. *Physiology & Behaviour* 18, 455–461.

Ferchmin, P.A., Bennett, E.L. and Rosenzweig M.R. (1975) Direct contact with enriched environment is required to alter cerebral weights in rats. *Journal of Comparative and Physiological Psychology* 88, 360–367.

Festing, M. (1992) Discussion. In: Botting, J.H. (ed.) *Animal Experimentation and the Future of Medical Research*. Portland Press, London.

Flecknell, P.A. (1984) The relief of pain in laboratory animals. *Laboratory Animals* 18, 147–160.

Flecknell, P.A. (1994) Advances in the assessment and alleviation of pain in laboratory and domestic animals. *Journal of Veterinary Anaesthesia* 21, 98–105.

Flecknell, P.A., Kirk, A.J.B., Liles, J.H., Hayes, P.H. and Dark, J.H. (1991) Postoperative analgesia following thoracotomy in the dog: an evaluation of the effects of bupivacaine intercostal nerve block and nalbuphine on respiratory function. *Laboratory Animals* 25, 319–324.

Flint, J., Corley, T., DeFries, J.C., Fulker, D.W., Gray, J.A. and Miller, S. (1995) A simple genetic basis for a complex psychological trait in laboratory mice. *Science* 269, 1432–1435.

Forbes, J.M. (1995) *Voluntary Food Intake and Diet Selection in Farm Animals*. CAB International, Wallingford, UK.

Forbes, J.M., Johnson, C.L. and Jackson, D.A. (1991) The drinking behaviour of lactating cows offered silage ad lib. *Proceedings of the Nutrition Society* 50, 97A.

Fordyce, G., Goddard, M.E. and Seifert, G.W. (1982) The measurement of temperament in cattle and the effect of experience and genotype. In: *Proceedings of the Australian Society for Animal Production* 14, 329–332.

Fordyce, G., Wythes, J.R., Shorthose, W.R., Underwood, D.W. and Shepherd, R.K. (1988) Cattle temperaments in extensive beef herds in northern Queensland 2. Effect of temperament on carcass and meat quality. *Australian Journal of Experimental Agriculture* 28, 689–693.

Fowler, H. (1965) *Curiosity and Exploratory Behaviour*. MacMillan, New York.

Fox, M. (1990) Transgenic animals: ethical and animal welfare concerns. In: Wheale, P. and McNally, R. (eds) *The Bio-Revolution: Cornucopia or Pandora's Box?* Pluto Press, London, pp. 31–45.

Fox, M.W. (1965) Environmental factors influencing stereotyped and allelomimetic behavior in animals. *Laboratory Animal Care* 15, 363–370.

Franzmann, A.W. (1986) Wildlife Medicine. In: Fowler, M.E. (ed.) *Zoo and Wild Animal Medicine*. Second Edition. Saunders, Philadelphia.

Fraser, A.F. (1989) Welfare and well-being. *Veterinary Record* 125, 332–333.

Fraser, A.F. (1992) *The Behaviour of the Horse*. CAB International, Wallingford, UK, pp. 226–263.

Fraser, A.F. and Broom, D.M. (1990) *Farm Animal Behaviour and Welfare*, 3rd edn. Baillière Tindall, London, UK. (Reprinted 1996, CAB International.)

Fraser, D. (1985) Selection of bedded and unbedded areas by pigs in relation to environmental temperature and behaviour. *Applied Animal Behaviour Science* 14, 117–126.

Fraser, D. (1987) Attraction to blood as a factor in tail-biting by pigs. *Applied Animal Behaviour Science* 17, 61–68.

Fraser, D. (1992) Role of ethology in determining farm animal well-being. In: Guttman, H.N., Mench, J.A. and Simmonds, R.C. (eds) *Science and Animals: Addressing Contemporary Issues*. Scientists Center for Animal Welfare, Bethesda, Maryland, pp. 95–102.

Fraser, D. (1993) Assessing animal well-being: Common sense, uncommon science. In: *Food Animal Well-Being*. Purdue University Office of Agricultural Research Programs, West Lafayette, USA, pp. 37–54.

Fraser, D. (1995) Science, values and animal welfare: Exploring the 'inextricable connection'. *Animal Welfare* 4, 103–117.

Fraser, D. (1996) Preference and motivational testing to improve animal well-being. *Lab Animal* 25, 27–31.

Fraser, D. and Rushen, J. (1987) Aggressive behavior. In: Price, E.O. (ed.) *Farm Animal Behavior. Veterinary Clinics of North America: Food Animal Practice,* 3, pp. 285–305.

Fraser, D., Ritchie, J.S.D. and Fraser, A.F. (1975) The term 'stress' in a veterinary context. *British Veterinary Journal* 131, 653–662.

Fraser, D., Patience, J.F., Phillips, P.A. and McLeese, J.M. (1990) Water for piglets and lactating sows: quantity, quality and quandaries. In: Haresign, W. and Cole, D.J.A. (eds) *Recent Advances in Animal Nutrition*. Butterworths, London, pp. 137–160.

Fraser, D., Phillips, P.A., Thompson, B.K. and Tennessen, T. (1991) Effect of straw on the behaviour of growing pigs. *Applied Animal Behaviour Science* 30, 307–318.

Fraser, D., Phillips, P.A. and Thompson, B.K. (1993) Environmental preference testing to assess the well-being of animals – An evolving paradigm. *Journal of Agricultural and Environmental Ethics* 6 (Suppl. 2), 104–114.

Fraser, D., Weary, D.M., Pajor, E.A. and Milligan, B.M. (1997) A scientific conception of animal welfare that reflects ethical value. *Animal Welfare* (in press).

Furness, R.W. and Monaghan, P. (1987) *Seabird Ecology*. Blackie, Glasgow, UK.

Galef, B.G. (1993) Functions of social learning about food: a causal analysis of effects of diet novelty on preference transmission. *Animal Behaviour* 46, 257–265.

Gallup, G.G., Povinelli, D.J., Suarez, S.D., Anderson, J.R., Lethmate, J. and Menzel, E.W. (1995) Further reflections on self-recognition in primates. *Animal Behaviour* 50, 1525–1532.

Gentle, M.J. (1986) Beak trimming in poultry. *World's Poultry Science Journal* 42, 268–275.

Gentle, M.J. (1992) Pain in birds. *Animal Welfare* 1, 235–247.

Gerken, M. and Petersen, J. (1987) Bi-directional selection for dustbathing activity in Japanese quail. *British Poultry Science* 28, 23–27.

Gerken, M., Bamburg, H. and Petersen, J. (1988) Studies of the relationship between fear-related responses and production traits in Japanese quail (*Coturnix coturnix japonica*) bidirectionally selected for dustbathing activity. *Poultry Science* 67, 1363–1371.

Giattina, J.D. and Garton, R.R. (1983) A review of the preference-avoidance responses of fishes to aquatic contaminants. *Residue Reviews* 87, 43–90.

Gibbons, A. (1992) Chimps: more diverse than a barrel of monkeys. *Science* 255, 287–288.

Glanzer, M. (1958) Curiosity, exploratory drive and stimulus satiation. *Psychological Bulletin* 55, 302–315.

Goddard, M.E. and Beilharz, R.G. (1984) A factor analysis of fearfulness in potential guide dogs. *Applied Animal Behaviour Science* 12, 253–265.

Gold, K.C. and Maple, T.L. (1994) Personality assessment in the gorilla and its utility as a management tool. *Zoo Biology* 13, 509–522.

Goldstein, S., Halbreich, U., Asnis, G., Endicott, J. and Alvir, J. (1987) The hypothalamic–pituitary–adrenal system in panic disorder. *American Journal of Psychiatry* 144, 1320–1323.

Gonyou, H.W. (1993a) Animal welfare: Definitions and assessment. *Journal of Agricultural and Environmental Ethics* 6 (Supplement 2), 37–43.

Gonyou, H.W. (1993b) Behavioural principles of animal handling and transport. In: Grandin, T. (ed.) *Livestock Handling and Transport*. CAB International, Wallingford, UK, pp. 11–20.

Gonyou, H.W. (1993c) The social environment and swine growth. In: Hollis, G.R. (ed.) *Growth of the Pig*. CAB International, Wallingford, UK, pp. 107–118.

Gonyou, H.W., Rohde-Parfet, K.A., Anderson, D.B. and Olson, R.D. (1988) Effects of amperozide and azaperone on aggression and productivity of growing-finishing pigs. *Journal of Animal Science* 66, 2856–2864.

Grandin, T. (1991) Handling problems caused by excitable pigs. In: *Proceedings of the International Congress of Meat Science and Technology*, Volume 1. Kulmbach, Germany.

Grandin, T. (ed.) (1993a) *Livestock Handling and Transport*. CAB International, Wallingford, UK.

Grandin, T. (1993b) Introduction: management and economic factors of handling and transport. In: Grandin, T. (ed.) *Livestock Handling and Transport*. CAB International, Wallingford, UK, pp. 1–9.

Grandin, T., Curtis, S.E. and Taylor, I.A. (1987) Toys, mingling and driving reduce excitability in pigs. *Journal of Animal Science* 65, suppl. 1, 230.

Gray, J.A. (1971) *The Psychology of Fear and Stress*. Weidenfeld and Nicolson, London, 256 pp.

Gray, J.A. (1979) Emotionality in male and female rodents: A reply to Archer. *British Journal of Psychology* 70, 425–440.

Gray, S. and Hurst, J.L. (1995) The effects of cage cleaning on aggression within groups of male laboratory mice. *Animal Behaviour* 49, 821–826.

Gregory, N.G., Wilkins, L.J., Alvey, D.M. and Tucker, S.A. (1993) Effect of catching method and lighting intensity on the prevalence of broken bones and on the ease of handling of end of lay hens. *Veterinary Record* 132, 127–129.

Griffin, D.R. (1992) *Animal Minds*. University of Chicago Press, Chicago.

Grigor, P.N. (1993) Use of space by laying hens: social and environmental implications for free-range systems. PhD thesis. University of Edinburgh.

Gross, W.B. and Siegel, P.B. (1979) Adaptation of chickens to their handlers and experimental results. *Avian Diseases* 23, 708–714.

Gross, W.B. and Siegel, P.B. (1980) Effects of early environmental stresses on chicken body weight, antibody response to RBC antigens, feed efficiency and response to fasting. *Avian Diseases* 24, 549–579.

Gross, W.B. and Siegel, P.B. (1985) Selective breeding of chickens for corticosterone response to social stress. *Poultry Science* 64, 2230–2233.

Guhl, A.M., Craig, J.V. and Mueller, C.D. (1960) Selective breeding for aggressiveness in chickens. *Poultry Science* 39, 970–980.

Harrison, R. (1964) *Animal Machines*. Vincent Stuart Ltd, London, 186 pp.

Harrison, R. (1987) *Farm animal welfare: what, if any, progress?* UFAW, London.

Hart, B.L. (1988) Biological basis of the behavior of sick animals. *Neuroscience and Biobehavioral Reviews* 12, 123–137.

Hartmann, W. (1989) From Mendel to multi-national in poultry breeding. *World's Poultry Science Journal* 45, 5–26.

Hartung, J. (1994) Environment and animal health. In: Wathes, C.M. and Charles, D.R. (eds) *Livestock Housing*. CAB International, Wallingford, UK, pp. 25–48.

Hartwell, S.I., Jin, J.H., Cherry, D.S. and Cairns, J. (1989) Toxicity versus avoidance response of golden shiner, *Notemigonus crysoleucas*, to five metals. *Journal of Fish Biology* 35, 447–456.

Hassall, S.A., Ward, W.R. and Murray, R.D. (1993) Effects of lameness on the behaviour of cows during the summer. *Veterinary Record* 132, 578–580.

Hebb, D.O. (1955) Drives and the C.N.S. (Conceptual nervous system). *Psychological Review* 62, 243–254.

Hediger, H. (1950) *Wild Animals in Captivity*. Butterworth, London.

Hemsworth, P.H. and Barnett, J.L. (1989) Relationships between fear of humans, productivity and cage position of laying hens. *British Poultry Science* 30, 505–518.

Hemsworth, P.H., Barnett, J.L., Hansen, C. and Gonyou, H.W. (1986a) The influence of early contact with humans on subsequent behavioural response of pigs to humans. *Applied Animal Behaviour Science*, 15, 55–63.

Hemsworth, P.H., Gonyou, H.W. and Dzuik, P.J. (1986b) Human communication with pigs: The behavioural response of pigs to specific human signals. *Applied Animal Behaviour Science* 15, 45–54.

Hemsworth, P.H., Barnett, J.L. and Hansen, C. (1987a) The influence of inconsistent handling by humans on the behaviour, growth and corticosteroids of young pigs. *Applied Animal Behaviour Science* 17, 245–252.

Hemsworth, P.H., Hansen, C. and Barnett, J.L. (1987b) The effects of human presence at the time of calving of primiparous cows on their subsequent behavioural response to milking. *Applied Animal Behaviour Science* 18, 247–255.

Hemsworth, P.H., Barnett, J.L., Tilbrook, A.J. and Hansen, C. (1989) The effects of handling by humans at calving and during milking on the behaviour and milk cortisol concentrations of primiparous dairy cows. *Applied Animal Behaviour Science* 22, 313–326.

Hemsworth, P.H., Barnett, J.L. and Coleman, G.J. (1993) The human-animal relationship in agriculture and its consequences for the animal. *Animal Welfare* 2, 33–51.

Hemsworth, P.H., Coleman, G.J. and Barnett, J.L. (1994a) Improving the attitude and behaviour of stockpersons towards pigs and the consequences on the behaviour and reproductive performance of commercial pigs. *Applied Animal Behaviour Science* 39, 349–362.

Hemsworth, P.H., Coleman, G.J., Barnett, J.L. and Jones, R.B. (1994b) Behavioural responses to humans and the productivity of commercial broiler chickens. *Applied Animal Behaviour Science* 41, 101–114.

Hemsworth, P.H., Breuer, K., Barnett, J.L., Coleman, G.J. and Matthews, L.R. (1995) Behavioural response to humans and the productivity of commercial dairy cows. *Proceedings of 29th International Congress of the International Society of Applied Ethology* (Exeter, UK), 175–176.

Hemsworth, P.H., Verge, J. and Coleman, G.J. (1996) Conditioned approach avoidance responses to humans: The ability of pigs to associate feeding and aversive social experiences in the presence of humans with humans. *Applied Animal Behaviour Science* 50, 71–82.

Henderson, C.R. (1984) *Application of Linear Models in Animal Breeding.* University of Guelph, Guelph, Canada, 462 pp.

Hennessy, D.P., Stelmasiak, T., Johnston, N.E., Jackson, P.N. and Outch, K.H. (1988) Consistent capacity for adrenocortical response to ACTH administration in pigs. *American Journal of Veterinary Research* 49, 1276–1283.

Henry, J.P. and Stephens, P.M. (1977) *Stress, health and the social environment. A sociobiological approach to medicine.* Springer-Verlag, New York.

Hessing, M.J.C., Hagelso, A.M., Schouten, W.G.P., Wiepkema, P.R. and Van Beek, J.A.M. (1994a) Individual behavioural and physiological strategies in pigs. *Physiology & Behavior* 55, 39–46.

Hessing, M.J.C., Schouten, W.G.P., Wiepkema, P.R. and Tielen, M.J.M. (1994b) Implications of individual behavioural characteristics on performance in pigs. *Livestock Production Science* 40, 187–196.

Hinde, R.A. (1974) *Biological Bases of Human Social Behaviour.* McGraw-Hill, New York.

Hinde, R.A. and Stevenson-Hinde, J. (eds) (1973) *Constraints on Learning: Limitations and Predispositions.* Academic Press, London, UK.

Hocking, P.M. (1990) The relationship between dietary crude protein, body weight and fertility in naturally mated broiler breeder males. *British Poultry Science* 31, 743–757.

Hocking, P.M., Waddington, D., Walker, M.A. and Gilbert, A.B. (1987) Ovarian follicular structure of White Leghorns fed *ad libitum* and dwarf and normal broiler breeders fed *ad libitum* or restricted to point of lay. *British Poultry Science* 28, 493–506.

Hocking, P.M., Maxwell, M.H. and Mitchell, M.A. (1993) Welfare assessment of broiler breeder and layer females subjected to food restriction and limited access to water during rearing. *British Poultry Science* 34, 443–458.

Hogan, J.A. and van Boxel, F. (1993) Causal factors controlling dustbathing in Burmese Red junglefowl: some results and a model. *Animal Behaviour* 46, 627–635.

Hogan, J.A., Honrado, G.I. and Vestergaard, K. (1991) Development of a behavior system: dustbathing in the Burmese red junglefowl (*Gallus gallus spadiceus*). II. Internal factors. *Journal of Comparative Psychology* 105, 269–273.

Holmes, J.H.G., Robinson, D.W. and Ashmore, C.R. (1972) Blood lactic acid and behaviour in cattle with heredity muscular hypertrophy. *Journal of Animal Science* 35, 1011–1013.

Holmes, S.J. (1916) *Studies in Animal Behavior.* Richard G. Badger, Boston, USA.

Hopster, H. and Blokhuis, H.J. (1994) Validation of a heart rate monitor for measuring a stress response in dairy cows. *Canadian Journal of Animal Science* 74, 465–474.

Hughes, B.O. (1975) The concept of an optimal stocking density and its selection for egg production. In: Freeman, B.M. and Boorman, K.N. (eds) *Economic Factors Affecting Egg Production.* British Poultry Science Ltd., Edinburgh, UK. pp. 271–298.

Hughes, B.O. (1976a) Behaviour as an index of welfare. In: *Proceedings of the Fifth European Poultry Conference*, Malta, pp. 1005–1018.

Hughes, B.O. (1976b) Preference decisions of domestic hens for wire or litter floors. *Applied Animal Ethology* 2, 155–165.

Hughes, B.O. (1977) Selection of group size by individual laying hens. *British Poultry Science* 18, 9–18.

Hughes, B.O. (1978) Behaviour in different environments and its implications for welfare. In: Sørensen, Y. (ed.) First Danish Seminar on Poultry Welfare in Egg-laying Cages. National Committee for Poultry and Eggs, Copenhagen, pp. 21–27.

Hughes, B.O. and Black, A.J. (1973) The preference of domestic hens for different types of battery cage floor. *British Poultry Science* 14, 615–619.

Hughes, B.O. and Duncan, I.J.H. (1972) The influence of strain and environmental factors upon feather pecking and cannibalism in fowl. *British Poultry Science* 13, 525–547.

Hughes, B.O. and Duncan, I.J.H. (1988) The notion of ethological 'need', models of motivation, and animal welfare. *Animal Behaviour* 36, 1696–1707.

Hughes, B.O., Gilbert, A.B. and Brown, M.F. (1986) Categorisation and causes of abnormal egg shells: relationship with stress. *British Poultry Science* 27, 325–337.

Hughes, B.O., Duncan, I.J.H. and Brown, M.F. (1989) The performance of nest building by domestic hens: is it more important than the construction of a nest? *Animal Behaviour* 37, 210–214.

Hughes, M. (1983) Exploration and play in young children. In: Archer, J. and Birke, L.I.A. (eds) *Exploration in Animals and Humans*. Van Nostrand Reinhold Inc., London, pp. 230–242.

Humphrey, N.K. (1976) The social function of intellect. In: Bateson, P.P.G. and Hinde, R.A. (eds) *Growing Points in Ethology*. Cambridge University Press, Cambridge, pp. 303–317.

Hunter, L. and Houpt, K.A. (1989) Bedding material preferences of ponies. *Journal of Animal Science* 67, 1986–1991.

Hurnik, J.F. (1993) Ethics and animal agriculture. *Journal of Agricultural and Environmental Ethics* 6 (Supplement 1), 21–35.

Hurnik, J.F. (1995) Poultry welfare. In: Hunton, P. (ed.) *Poultry Production*. Elsevier, Amsterdam.

Hurnik, J.F. and Lehman, H. (1985) The philosophy of farm animal welfare: a contribution to the assessment of farm animal well-being. In: Wegner, R.-M. (ed.) *Second European Symposium on Poultry Welfare*. German Branch of the World's Poultry Science Association, Celle, Germany, pp. 255–266.

Hurnik, J.F. and Lehman, H. (1988) Ethics and farm animal welfare. *Journal of Agricultural Ethics* 1, 305–318.

Hurnik, J.F., Reinhart, B.S. and Hurnik, G.I. (1973) The effect of coloured nests on the frequency of floor eggs. *Poultry Science* 52, 389–391.

Hutchins, M., Hancocks, D. and Calip, C. (1978) Behavioural engineering in the zoo: a critique, part II. *International Zoo News* 25, 18–23.

Hutson, G.D. (1984) Animal welfare and consumer demand theory: Are preference tests a luxury we can't afford? *Animal Behaviour* 32, 1260–1261.

Hutson, G.D. (1985) The influence of barley food rewards on sheep movement through a handling system. *Applied Animal Behaviour Science* 14, 263–273.

Hutson, G.D. (1993) Behavioural principles of sheep handling. In: Grandin, T. (ed.) *Livestock Handling and Transport*. CAB International, Wallingford, UK, pp. 127–146.

Hutt, C. (1970) Specific and diversive exploration. In: Reese, H.W. and Lipsitt, L.P. (eds) *Advances in Child Development and Behavior*, Vol. 5. Academic Press, New York.

Illius, A.W. and Gordon, I.J. (1991) Prediction of intake and digestion in ruminants by a model of rumen kinetics integrating animal size and plant characteristics. *Journal of Agricultural Science*, Cambridge 116, 145–157.

Inglis, I.R. (1975) Enriched sensory experience in adulthood increases subsequent exploratory behaviour in the rat. *Animal Behaviour* 23, 932–940.

Inglis, I.R. (1983) Towards a cognitive theory of exploratory behaviour. In: Archer, J. and Birke, L.I.A. (eds) *Exploration in Animals and Humans*. Van Nostrand Reinhold Inc., London, pp. 72–117.

Inglis, I.R. and Ferguson, N.J.K. (1986) Starlings search for food rather than eat freely available, identical food. *Animal Behaviour* 34, 614–616.

Inglis, I.R. and Freeman, N.H. (1976) Reversible effects of ambient housing stimulation upon stimulation-seeking in rats. *Quarterly Journal of Experimental Psychology* 28, 409–417.

Inglis, I.R., Forkman, B. and Lazarus, J. (1997) Why do animals work for food in the presence of free food? A review, fuzzy model and functional explanation of contra-freeloading. *Animal Behaviour* 53 (in press).

IRAC (1985) US Government principles for utilization and care of vertebrate animals used in testing, research and training. In: *Guide for the Care and Use of Laboratory Animals*. NIH Publication No. 85–23 US Department of Health and Human Services, Washington DC, pp. 81–83.

Ixart, G., Barbanel, G., Conte-Devolx, B., Grin, M., Oliver, C. and Assenmacher, I. (1987) Evidence for basal and stress-induced release of corticotropin releasing factor in the push-pull cannulmated median emminence of conscious free-moving rats. *Neuroscience Letters* 74, 85–89.

Jackson, P.P.G. (1987) The assessment of welfare in diseased farm animals. In: Animal Disease – a Welfare Problem. *Proceedings of the 5th Symposium of the BVA Animal Welfare Foundation*, pp. 42–47.

Janssens, C.J.J.G., Helmond, F.A., Loyens, L.W.S., Schouten, W.G.P. and Wiegant, V.M. (1995) Chronic stress increases the opioid-mediated inhibition of the pituitary-adrenocortical response to acute stress in pigs. *Endocrinology* 136, 1468–1473.

Jensen, M.B., Kyriazakis, I. and Lawrence, A.B. (1993) The activity and straw directed behaviour of pigs offered foods with different crude protein content. *Applied Animal Behaviour Science* 37, 211–221.

Jensen, P. (1986) Observations on the maternal behaviour of free-ranging domestic pigs. *Applied Animal Behaviour Science* 16, 131–142.

Jensen, P. (1994) Fighting between unacquainted pigs – effects of age and of individual reaction pattern. *Applied Animal Behaviour Science* 41, 37–52.

Jensen, P. and Toates, F.M. (1993) Who needs 'behavioural needs'? Motivational aspects of the needs of animals. *Applied Animal Behaviour Science* 37, 161–181.

Job, R.F.S. (1987) Learned helplessness in chickens. *Animal Learning and Behavior* 15, 347–350.

Johnson, E. (1983) Life, death, and animals. In: Miller, H.B. and Williams, W.H. (eds) *Ethics and Animals*. Humana Press, Clifton New Jersey, pp. 123–133.

Johnson, E.O., Kamilaris, T.C., Chrousos, G.P. and Gold, P.W. (1992) Mechanisms of stress: A dynamic overview of hormonal and behavioral homeostasis. *Neuroscience and Biobehavioral Reviews* 16, 115–130.

Jones, R.B. (1986) The tonic immobility reaction of the domestic fowl: A review. *World's Poultry Science Journal* 42, 82–96.

Jones, R.B. (1987a) Fear and fear responses: a hypothetical consideration. *Medical Science Research* 15, 1287–1290.

Jones, R.B. (1987b) The assessment of fear in the domestic fowl. In: Zayan, R. and Duncan, I.J.H. (eds) *Cognitive Aspects of Social Behaviour in the Domestic Fowl*. Elsevier, Amsterdam, pp. 40–81.

Jones, R.B. (1993) Reduction of the domestic chick's fear of humans by regular handling and related treatments. *Animal Behaviour* 46, 991–998.

Jones, R.B. (1994) Regular handling and the domestic chick's fear of human beings: generalisation of response. *Applied Animal Behaviour Science* 42, 129–143.

Jones, R.B. (1995) Habituation to human beings via visual contact in docile and flighty strains of domestic chicks. *International Journal of Comparative Psychology* 8, 88–98.

Jones, R.B. (1996) Fear and adaptability in poultry: insights, implications and imperatives. *World's Poultry Science Journal* 52, 131–174.

Jones, R.B. and Harvey, S. (1987) Behavioural and adrenocortical responses of domestic chicks to systematic reductions in group size and to sequential disturbance of companions by the experimenter. *Behavioural Processes* 14, 291–303.

Jones, R.B. and Satterlee, D.G. (1996) Threat-induced behavioural inhibition in Japanese quail genetically selected for contrasting adrenocortical response to mechanical restraint. *British Poultry Science* 37, 465–470.

Jones, R.B. and Waddington, D. (1992) Modification of fear in domestic chicks, *Gallus gallus domesticus*, via regular handling and early environmental enrichment. *Animal Behaviour* 43, 1021–1033.

Jones, R.B., Beuving, G. and Blokhuis, H.J. (1988) Tonic immobility and heterophil/lymphocyte responses of the domestic fowl to corticosterone infusion. *Physiology & Behavior* 42, 249–253.

Jones, R.B., Mills, A.D. and Faure, J.M. (1991) Genetic and experiential manipulation of fear-related behaviour in Japanese quail chicks (*Coturnix coturnix japonica*). *Journal of Comparative Psychology* 105, 15–24.

Jones, R.B., Satterlee, D.G. and Ryder, F.H. (1992) Fear and distress in Japanese quail chicks of two lines genetically selected for low or high plasma corticosterone response to immobilization stress. *Hormones and Behavior* 26, 385–393.

Jones, R.B., Mills, A.D., Faure, J.M. and Williams, J.B. (1994a) Restraint, fear, and distress in Japanese quail genetically selected for long or short tonic immobility reactions. *Physiology & Behavior* 56, 529–534.

Jones, R.B., Satterlee, D.G. and Ryder, F.H. (1994b) Fear of humans in Japanese quail selected for low or high adrenocortical response. *Physiology & Behavior* 56, 379–383.

Jones, R.B., Blokhuis, H.J. and Beuving, G. (1995) Open-field and tonic immobility responses in domestic chicks of two genetic lines differing in their propensity to feather peck. *British Poultry Science* 36, 525–530.

Jones, R.B., Larkins, C. and Hughes, B.O. (1996) Approach/avoidance responses of domestic chicks to familiar and unfamiliar video images of biologically neutral stimuli. *Applied Animal Behaviour Science* 48, 81–98.

Jongebreur, A.A. (1983) Housing design and welfare in livestock production. In: Baxter, S.H., Baxter, M.R. and MacCormack, J.A.C. (eds) *Farm Animal Housing and Welfare*. Martinus Nijhoff, The Hague, pp. 265–269.

Kant, I. (1989) Duties in regard to animals. In: Regan, T. and Singer, P. (eds) *Animal Rights and Human Obligations*. Prentice Hall, Englewood Cliffs New Jersey, pp. 23–24.

Kant, G.J., Bunnell, B.N., Mougey, E.H., Pennington, L.L. and Meyerhoff, J.L. (1983) Effects of repeated stress on pituitary cyclic AMP and plasma prolactin, corticosterone and growth hormone in male rats. *Pharmacology, Biochemistry and Behavior* 18, 967–971.

Kastelein, R.A. and Wiepkema, P.R. (1989) A digging trough as occupational therapy for Pacific walruses (*Odobenus rosmarus divergens*) in human care. *Aquatic Mammals* 15, 9–17.

Keiper, R.R. (1969) Causal factors of stereotypies in caged birds. *Animal Behaviour* 17, 114–119.

Kendrick, K.M. (1992) Cognition. In: Phillips, C.J.C. and Piggins, D. (eds) *Farm Animals and their Environment*. CAB International, Wallingford, UK, pp. 209–231.

Kennedy, J.S. (1992) *The New Anthropomorphism*. Cambridge University Press, Cambridge, UK.

Kennedy, M.J. and Broom, D.M. (1994) A method of mixing gilts and sows which reduces aggression experienced by gilts. In: *Proceedings of the 28th International Congress of the ISAE*. National Institute of Animal Science, Foulum. P. 5.12.

Kennes, D., Ödberg, F.O., Bouquet, Y. and de Rycke, P.H. (1988) Changes in naloxone and haloperidol effects during the development of captivity-induced jumping stereotypy in bank voles. *European Journal of Pharmacology* 153, 19–24.

Kent, J.E., Molony, V. and Robertson, I.S. (1995) Comparison of the Burdizzo and rubber ring methods for castrating and tail docking lambs. *Veterinary Record* 136, 192–196.

Kent, S., Kelley, K.W. and Dantzer, R. (1993) Stress-induced hyperthermia is partially mediated by interleukin-1 (IL-1). *Society for Neuroscience Abstracts* 19, 226.

Kestin, S.C., Knowles, T.G., Tinch, A.E. and Gregory, N.G. (1992) Prevalence of leg weakness in broiler chickens and its relationship with genotype. *Veterinary Record* 131, 191–194.

Keverne, E.B., Martenz, N.D. and Tuite, B. (1989) Beta-endorphin concentrations in cerebrospinal fluid of monkeys are influenced by grooming relationships. *Psychoneuroendocrinology* 14, 155–161.

Kiley-Worthington, M. (1989) Ecological, ethological, and ethically sound environments for animals: Toward symbiosis. *Journal of Agricultural Ethics* 2, 323–347.

Kish, G.B. (1955) Learning when the onset of illumination is used as reinforcing stimulus. *Journal of Comparative and Physiological Psychology* 48, 261–264.

Klemcke, H.G., Nienaber, J.A. and Hahn, G.L. (1987) Stressor-associated alterations in porcine plasma prolactin. *Proceedings of the Society of Experimental Biological Medicine* 186, 333–343.

Kluger, M.J., O'Reilly, B., Shope, T.R. and Vander, A.J. (1987) Further evidence that stress hyperthermia is a fever. *Physiology & Behavior* 39, 763–766.

Knowles, T.G., Warriss, P.D., Brown, S.N. and Kestin, S.C. (1994) Long distance transport of export lambs. *The Veterinary Record* 29, 107–110.

Komai, T. and Guhl, A.M. (1960) Tameness and its relation to aggressiveness and productivity of the domestic chicken. *Poultry Science* 39, 817–823.

Komulainen, J., Takala, T.E.S. and Vihko, V. (1995) Does increased serum creatine kinase activity reflect exercise-induced muscle damage in rats? *International Journal of Sports Medicine* 16, 150–154.

Konarsky, M., Stewart, R.E. and McCarty, R. (1990) Predictability of chronic intermittent stress: effects of sympathetic adrenomedullary responses of laboratory rats. *Behavioural and Neural Biology* 53, 231–243.

Kostal, L., Savory, C.J. and Hughes, B.O. (1992) Diurnal and individual variation in behaviour of restricted-fed broiler breeders. *Applied Animal Behaviour Science* 32, 361–374.

Kvetnansky, R., Nemeth, S., Vegas, M., Oprsalova, Z. and Jurcovicova, J. (1984) Plasma catecholamines in rats during adaptation to intermittent exposure to different stress. In: Usdin, E., Kvetnansky, R. and Alexlrod, J. (eds) *Stress: The Role of Catecholamines and Other Neurotransmitters*. Gordon and Breach, New York, 537–562.

Kyriazakis, I. (1994) The voluntary food intake and diet selection of pigs. In: Wiseman, J., Cole, D.J.A. and Varley, M.A. (eds) *Principles of Pig Science*. Nottingham University Press, Nottingham, pp. 85–105.

Kyriazakis, I. and Emmans, G.C. (1992) The effects of varying protein and energy intakes on the growth and body composition of pigs. 2. The effects of varying both energy and protein intake. *British Journal of Nutrition* 68, 615–625.

Kyriazakis, I. and Emmans, G.C. (1995) The voluntary food intake of pigs given foods based on wheat bran, dried citrus pulp and grass meal, in relation to measurements of food bulk. *British Journal of Nutrition* 73, 191–207.

Kyriazakis, I., Emmans, G.C. and Whittemore, C.T. (1990) Diet selection in pigs: Choices made by growing pigs given foods of different protein concentrations. *Animal Production* 51, 189–199.

Kyriazakis, I., Emmans, G.C. and Whittemore, C.T. (1991) The ability of pigs to control their protein intake when fed in three different ways. *Physiology & Behavior* 50, 1197–1203.

Ladewig, J. and Matthews, L.R. (1996) The role of operant conditioning in animal welfare research. *Acta Agriculturae Scandinavica* section A: S27, 64–68.

Ladewig, J. and Smidt, D. (1989) Behavior, episodic secretion of cortisol, and adrenocortical reactivity in bulls subjected to tethering. *Hormones and Behavior* 23, 344–360.

Lagadic, H. (1989) Defining the domestic hen's requirement for space: Do operant conditioning techniques and physiological measures of stress agree? In: Faure, J.M. and Mills, A.D. (eds) *Proceedings of the Third European Symposium on Poultry Welfare*. French Branch of the World's Poultry Science Association, Tours, France, pp. 67–77.

Lagadic, H. and Faure, J.-M. (1987) Preferences of domestic hens for cage size and floor types as measured by operant conditioning. *Applied Animal Behaviour Science* 19, 147–155.

Lam, K., Rupniak, N.M.J. and Iversen, S.D. (1991) Use of a grooming and foraging substrate to reduce cage stereotypies in macaques. *Journal of Medical Primatology* 20, 104–109.

LASA (1990) The assessment and control of the severity of scientific procedures on laboratory animals. *Laboratory Animals* 24, 97–130.

Launay, F., Mills, A.D. and Faure, J.M. (1993) Effect of test age, line and sex on tonic immobility responses and social reinstatement behaviour in Japanese quail *Coturnix japonica*. *Behavioural Processes* 29, 1–16.

Lawrence, A.B. (1987) Consumer demand theory and the assessment of animal welfare. *Animal Behaviour* 35, 293–294.

Lawrence, A.B. and Appleby, M.C. (1996) Welfare of extensively farmed animals: principles and practice. *Applied Animal Behaviour Science* 49, 1–8.

Lawrence, A.B. and Rushen, J. (eds) (1993) *Stereotypic Animal Behaviour Fundamentals and Applications to Welfare*. CAB International, Wallingford, UK.

Lawrence, A.B., Terlouw, E.M.C. and Illius, A.W. (1991) Analysis of temperament in pigs exposed to non-social and social challenges. *Applied Animal Behaviour Science* 30, 73–86.

Lawrence, A.B., Terlouw, E.M.C. and Kyriazakis, I. (1993) The behavioural effects of undernutrition in farm animals. *Proceedings of the Nutrition Society* 52, 219–229.

Lay, D.C.,Jr, Friend, T.H., Randel, R.D., Bowers, C.L., Grissom, K.K. and Jenkins, O.C. (1992) Behavioral and physiological effects of freeze or hot-iron branding on crossbred cattle. *Journal of Animal Science* 70, 330–336.

Lea, S.E.G. (1978) The psychology and economics of demand. *Psychological Bulletin* 85, 441–466.

Lee, P.C. (1984) Ecological constraints on the social development of vervet monkeys. *Behaviour* 91, 245–263.

Leenstra, F.R., Van Voorst, A. and Haye, U. (1984) Genetic aspects of twisted legs in a broiler sire strain. *Annales Agriculturae Fennaie* 23, 261–270.

Lees, P. and Taylor, P.M. (1991) Pharmacodynamics and pharmacokinetics of flunixin in the cat. *British Veterinary Journal* 147, 298–305.

Leeson, S., Diaz, G. and Summers, J.D. (1995) *Poultry Metabolic Disorders and Mycotoxins*. University Books, Guelph, Ontario, Canada.

Le Magnen, J. (1985) *Hunger*. Cambridge University Press, Cambridge.

Le Neindre, P., Veissier, I., Boissy, A. and Boivin, X. (1992) Effects of early environment on behaviour. In: Phillips, C. and Piggins, D. (eds) *Farm Animals and the Environment*. CAB International, Wallingford, UK, pp. 307–322.

Le Neindre, P., Trillat, P., Chupin, P., Poindron, P., Boissy, A., Orgeur, P., Boivin, X., Bonnet, J.N., Bouix, J. and Bibé, B. (1994) Les ruminants et l'homme: un vieux lien qu'il faut entretenir. In: Picard, M., Porter, R. and Signoret, J.P. (eds) *Un point sur comportement et bien-être animal*. Institut National de la Recherche Agronomique, Paris, pp. 91–107.

Leng, R.A. (1990) Factors affecting the utilisation of 'poor quality' foragers by ruminants particularly under tropical conditions. *Nutrition Research Reviews* 3, 277–303.

Lerner, I.M. (1951) *Principals of commercial poultry breeding*. Manual 1, University of California College of Agriculture, Berkeley, 47 pp.

Leus, K. and Morgan, C.A. (1993) Analysis of diets fed to Babirusa (*Babyrousa babyrussa*) in captivity with respect to their nutritional requirements. *Proceedings 2nd International Symposium on Wild Boar* (Sus scrofa) *and on order Suiformis*, Turin.

Liles, J.H. (1994) The assessment and alleviation of pain in laboratory rats. PhD thesis, University of Newcastle.

Liles, J.H. and Flecknell, P.A. (1993) A comparison of the effects of buprenorphine, carprofen and flunixin following laparotomy in rats. *Journal of Veterinary Pharmacology and Therapeutics* 17, 284–290.

Lindberg, A.C. and Nicol, C.J. (1994) An evaluation of the effect of operant feeders on welfare of hens maintained on litter. *Applied Animal Behaviour Science* 41, 211–227.

Lindqvist, J.-O. (1974) Animal health and environment in the production of fattening pigs. *Acta Veterinaria Scandinavica*, Supplementum 51, 1–78.

Lockwood, M. (1979) Singer on killing and the preference for life. *Inquiry* 22, 157–170.

Loeffler, K. (1986) Assessing pain by studying posture, structure and function. In: Duncan, I.J.H. and Molony, V. (eds) *Assessing Pain in Farm Animals*. Commission of the European Communities, Luxembourg.

Lorenz, K. (1963) Do animals undergo subjective experience? In: Lorenz, K. *Studies in Animal and Human Behaviour*, Vol. 2. Methuen, London, UK, pp. 323–337.

Lorenz, K. (1981) *The Foundations of Ethology*. Springer, New York.

Love, J.A. and Hammond, K. (1991) Group housing rabbits. *Lab Animal* 20, 37–43.

Luescher, U.A., Friendship, R.M. and McKeown, D.B. (1990) Evaluation of methods to reduce fighting among regrouped gilts. *Canadian Journal of Animal Science* 70, 363–370.

Lumb, W.V. and Wynn Jones, E. (1973) *Veterinary Anesthesia*. Lea and Febiger, Philadelphia.

Lush, J.L. (1945) *Animal breeding plans*. 3rd edn. Iowa State College Press, Ames.

Lynch, J.J., Brown, G.D., May, P.F. and Donnelly, J.B. (1972) The effect of withholding drinking water on wool growth and lamb production of grazing Merino sheep in a temperate climate. *Australian Journal of Agricultural Research* 23, 659–668.

Lyons, D.M. (1989) Individual differences in temperament of dairy goats and the inhibition of milk ejection. *Applied Animal Behaviour Science* 22, 269–282.

Lyons, D.M. and Price, E.O. (1986) Relationships between heart rates and behaviour of goats in encounters with people. *Applied Animal Behaviour Science* 18, 363–369.

Lyons, D.M., Price, E.O. and Moberg, G.P. (1988) Individual differences in temperament of domestic dairy goats: Constancy and change. *Animal Behaviour* 36, 1323–1333.

Macdonald, D. (1992) *The Velvet Claw*. BBC Books, London.

Maestripieri, D., Schino, G., Aureli, F. and Troisi, A. (1992) A modest proposal: displacement activities as an indicator of emotions in primates. *Animal Behaviour* 44, 967–979.

MAFF (1994) *National Food Survey 1993*. HMSO, London, 110pp.

Marazziti, D., Di Muro, A. and Castrogiovanni, P. (1992) Psychological stress and body temperature changes in humans. *Physiology & Behavior* 52, 393–395.

Marshall, A. (1947) *Principles of economics*. Reprint of Eighth Edition. Macmillan and Co., Limited, London.

Martin, J.E. and Edwards, S.A. (1994) Feeding behaviour of outdoor sows: the effects of diet quantity and type. *Applied Animal Behaviour Science* 41, 63–74.

Marx, D. and Mertz, R. (1989) Ethologische Wahlversuche mit frühabgesetzten Ferkeln während der Haltung in Buchten mit unterschiedlicher Anwendung von Stroh. 1. Mitteilung: Auswirkungen verschiedener Anwendungen des Strohes und unterschiedlicher Bodenbeschaffenheit bei einheitlicher Flächengrösse. *Deutsche Tierärztliche Wochenschrift* 96, 20–26.

Mason, G.J. (1991a) Stereotypies and suffering. *Behavioural Processes* 25, 103–115.

Mason, G.J. (1991b) Stereotypies: a critical review. *Animal Behaviour* 41, 1015–1037.

Mason, G.J. (1993) Age and context affect the stereotypies of caged mink. *Behaviour* 127, 191–229.

Mason, G.J. and Mendl, M. (1993) Why is there no simple way of measuring animal welfare? *Animal Welfare* 2, 301–319.

Mason, G.J. and Mendl, M. (1997) Do the stereotypies of pigs, chickens and mink reflect adaptive species differences in the control of foraging? *Applied Animal Behaviour Science* (in press).

Mason, G.J. and Turner, M.A. (1993) Mechanisms involved in the development and control of stereotypies. In: Bateson, P.P.G., Klopfer, P.H. and Thompson, N. (eds) *Perspectives in Ethology 10: Behaviour and Evolution*. Plenum Press, New York, pp. 53–85.

Mason, J.W. (1974) Specificity in the organization of neuroendocrine response profiles. In: Seeman, P. and Brown, G. (eds) *Frontiers in Neurology and Neuroscience Research*. University of Toronto, pp. 68–80.

Mason, W.A. (1991) Effects of social interaction on well-being: developmental aspects. *Laboratory Animal Science* 41, 323–328.

Matthews, L.R. (1993) Deer handling and transport. In: Grandin, T. (ed.) *Livestock Handling and Transport*. CAB International, Wallingford, UK, pp. 253–272.

Matthews, L.R. and Ladewig, J. (1994) Environmental requirements of pigs measured by behavioural demand functions. *Animal Behaviour* 47, 713–719.

Maxwell, M.H., Hocking, P.M. and Robertson, G.W. (1992) Differential leucocyte responses to various degrees of food restriction in broilers, turkeys and ducks. *British Poultry Science* 33, 177–187.

McBride, G., Parer, I.P. and Foenander, F. (1969) The social behaviour and organization of feral domestic fowl. *Animal Behaviour Monographs* 2, 125–181.

McCay, C.M., Maynard, L.A., Sperling, G. and Barnes, L.L. (1939) Retarded growth, life span, ultimate body size, and age changes in the albino rat after feeding diets restricted in calories. *Journal of Nutrition* 18, 1–13.

McFarland, D. (1985) *Animal Behaviour: Psychology, Ethology and Evolution.* Longman Scientific and Technical, Harlow, UK.

McFarland, D. (1989) *Problems of Animal Behaviour.* Longman, Harlow.

McFarlane, J.M., Curtis, S.E., Shanks, R.D. and Carmer, S.G. (1989) Multiple concurrent stressors in chicks. 1. Effect on weight gain, feed intake, and behavior. *Poultry Science* 68, 501–509.

McFerran J.B. and Stuart, J.C. (1990) Adenoviruses. In: Jordan, F.T.W. (ed.) *Poultry Diseases.* Third Edition. Ballière Tindall, London.

McGlone, J.J. (1990) Olfactory signals that modulate pig aggressive behavior. In: Zayan, R. and Dantzer, R. (eds) *Social Stress in Domestic Animals.* Kluwer Academic Publications, Dordrecht, pp. 86–109.

McGlone, J.J. (1993) What is animal welfare? *Journal of Agricultural and Environmental Ethics* 6 (Supplement 2), 26–36.

McGlone, J.J. and Curtis, S.E. (1985) Behavior and performance of weanling pigs in pens equipped with hide areas. *Journal of Animal Science* 60, 20–24.

McGlone, J.J. and Hellman, J.M. (1988) Local and general anesthetic effects on behaviour and performance of two- and seven-week old castrated and uncastrated piglets. *Journal of Animal Science* 66, 3049–3058.

McGreevy, P.D., Cripps, P.J., French, N.P., Green, L.E. and Nicol, C.J. (1995) Management factors associated with stereotypic and redirected behavior in the thoroughbred horse. *Equine Veterinary Journal* 27, 86–91.

McGregor, P.K. and Ayling, S.J. (1990) Varied cages result in more aggression in male CFLP mice. *Applied Animal Behaviour Science* 26, 277–281.

McInerney, J.P. (1994) Animal welfare: an economic perspective. In: Bennett, R.M. (ed.) *Valuing Farm Animal Welfare.* Occasional Paper No. 3. Department of Agricultural Economics and Management, The University of Reading, UK, pp. 9–25. (Paper first presented at the Agricultural Economics Society Conference, Oxford, April 1993.)

McReynolds, P. (1962) Exploratory behavior: a theoretical interpretation. *Psychological Reports* 11, 311–318.

Mellor, D.J. and Murray, L. (1989) Effects of tail docking and castration on behaviour and plasma cortisol concentrations in young lambs. *Research in Veterinary Science* 46, 387–391.

Mench, J.A. (1992) The welfare of poultry in modern production systems. *Poultry Science Reviews* 4, 107–128.

Mench, J.A. and Stricklin, W.R. (1990) Consumer demand theory and social behavior: All chickens are not equal. *Behavioral and Brain Sciences* 13, 28.

Mendl, M. (1991) Some problems with the concept of a cut-off point for determining when an animal's welfare is at risk. *Applied Animal Behaviour Science* 31, 139–146.

Mendl, M. and Deag, J. (1995) How useful are the concepts of alternative strategy and coping strategy in applied studies of social behaviour? *Applied Animal Behaviour Science* 44, 119–137.

Mendl, M., Zanella, A.I. and Broom, D.M. (1992) Physiological and reproductive correlates of behavioural strategies in female domestic pigs. *Animal Behaviour* 44, 1107–1121.

Mepham, T.B. (1993) Approaches to the ethical evaluation of animal biotechnologies. *Animal Production* 57, 353–359.

Mérat, P. (1984) The sex-linked dwarf gene in the broiler chicken industry. *World's Poultry Science Journal* 40, 10–18.

Mercier, J.T. and Hill, W.G. (1984) Estimation of genetic parameters for skeletal defects in broiler chickens. *Heredity* 53, 193–203.

Meyer-Holzapfel, M. (1968) Abnormal behaviour in zoo animals. In: Fox, M.W. (ed.) *Abnormal Behavior in Animals*, Saunders, London, pp. 476–503.

Michell, A.R. (1987) What is stress? The physiology of malaise and malingering. In: Animal Disease – a Welfare Problem. *Proceedings of the 5th Symposium of the BVA Animal Welfare Foundation*, pp. 8–20.

Midgley, M. (1983) *Animals and Why They Matter*. University of Georgia Press, Athens, Georgia, USA.

Milinski, M. and Parker, G.A. (1991) Competition for resources. In: Krebs, J.R. and Davies, N.B. (eds) *Behavioural Ecology An Evolutionary Approach*, 3rd Edition. Blackwell Scientific Publications, Oxford, pp. 137–168.

Mill, J.M. and Ward, W.R. (1994) Lameness in dairy cows and farmers' knowledge, training and awareness. *Veterinary Record* 134, 162–164.

Mill, J.S. (1848) *Principles of Political Economy*. First Edn. Parker & Co., London.

Millan, M., Czlonkowski, A., Pilcher, C.W.T., Almeida, O.F.X. and Millan, M.H. (1987) A model of chronic pain in the rat: functional correlates of alterations in the activity of opioid systems. *Journal of Neuroscience* 7, 77–87.

Miller, B. and Stokes, C. (1994) The neonatal and postweaned pig. In: Wiseman, J., Cole, D.J.A. and Varley, M.A. (eds) *Principles of Pig Science*. Nottingham University Press, Nottingham, pp. 75–84.

Mills, A.D. (1983) Genetic analysis of strain differences in pre-laying behaviour in the fowl. PhD thesis, University of Edinburgh, UK.

Mills, A.D. and Faure, J.-M. (1989) Social attraction and the feeding behaviour of domestic hens. *Behavioural Processes* 18, 71–85.

Mills, A.D. and Faure, J.M. (1990) Panic and hysteria in domestic fowl: a review. In: Zayan, R. and Dantzer, R. (eds) *Social Stress in Domestic Animals*. Kluwer Academic Publishers, Dordrecht, pp. 248–272.

Mills, A.D. and Faure, J.M. (1991) Divergent selection for duration of tonic immobility and social reinstatement behavior in Japanese quail (*Coturnix coturnix japonica*) chicks. *Journal of Comparative Psychology* 105, 25–38.

Mills, A.D., Wood-Gush, D.G.M. and Hughes, B.O. (1985a) Genetic analysis of strain differences in pre-laying behaviour in battery cages. *British Poultry Science* 26, 187–197.

Mills, A.D., Duncan, I.J.H., Slee, G.S. and Clarke, J.S.B. (1985b) Heart rate and laying behavior in two strains of domestic chicken. *Physiology & Behavior* 35, 145–147.

Mills, A.D., Nys, Y. Gautron, J. and Zawadski, J. (1991) Whitening of brown shelled eggs: individual variation and relationships with age, fearfulness, oviposition interval and stress. *British Poultry Science* 32, 117–129.

Mills, A.D., Launay, F., Jones, R.B., Faure, J.M., Williams, J.B. and Turro, I. (1993a) Behavioural and physiological consequences of divergent selection for tonic immobility and social reinstatement behaviour in Japanese quail. In: Savory, C.J. and Hughes, B.O. (eds) *Proceedings of the Fourth European Symposium on Poultry Welfare*. Universities Federation for Animal Welfare, Potters Bar, UK, pp. 268–269.

Mills, A.D., Jones, R.B., Faure, J.M. and Williams, J.B. (1993b) Responses to isolation in Japanese quail selected for high or low sociality. *Physiology & Behavior* 53, 183–189.

Mills, A.D., Launay, F., Turro, I., Jones, R.B., Williams, J.B. and Faure, J.M. (1994) Sélection divergente sur la peur et la sociabilité chez la caille japonaise *Coturnix japonica*. Réponses et conséquences In: Picard, M., Porter, R. and Signoret, J.P. (eds) *Un point sur comportement et bien-être animal*. Institut National de la Recherche Agronomique, Paris, pp. 127–139.

Minton, J.E., Coppinger, T.R., Reddy, P.G., Davis, W.C. and Blecha, F. (1992) Repeated restraint and isolation stress alters adrenal and lymphocyte functions and some leukocyte differentiation antigens in lambs. *Journal of Animal Science* 70, 1126–1132.

Minton, J.E., Apple, J.K., Parsons, K.M. and Blecha (1995) Stress-associated concentrations of plasma cortisol cannot account for reduced lymphocyte function and changes in serum enzymes in lambs exposed to restraint and isoaltion stress. *Journal of Animal Science* 73, 812–817.

Mitchell, M.A. and Kettlewell, P.J. (1993) Catching and transport of broiler chickens. In: Savory, C.J. and Hughes, B.O. (eds) *Proceedings of the Fourth European Symposium on Poultry Welfare*. Universities Federation for Animal Welfare, Potters Bar, UK, pp. 240–241.

Mitchell, R.C. and Carson, R.T. (1989) *Using Surveys to Value Public Goods. The Contingent Valuation Method*. Resources for the Future, Washington DC.

Moberg, G.P. (ed.) (1985a) *Animal Stress*. American Physiological Society, Bethesda.

Moberg, G.P. (1985b) Biological response to stress: key to assessment of animal well-being? In: Moberg, G.P. (ed.) *Animal Stress*. American Physiological Society, Bethesda, pp. 27–49.

Moberg, G.P. (1985c) Influence of stress on reproduction: measure of well-being. In: Moberg G.P. (ed.) *Animal Stress*. American Physiological Society, Bethesda, pp. 245–267.

Mock, D.W., Lamey, T.C., Williams, C.F. and Pelletier, A. (1987) Flexibility in the development of heron sibling aggression: an interspecific test of the prey size hypothesis. *Animal Behaviour* 35, 1386–1393.

Mormède, P. (1988) Les réponses neuroendocriniennes de stress. *Recueil de Médecine Vétérinaire* 164, 723–741.

Morris, D. (1964) The response of animals to a restricted environment. Symposium of the Zoological Society of London 13, 99–118.

Morrison, W.D. and McMillan, I. (1985) Operant control of the thermal environment by chicks. *Poultry Science* 64, 1656.

Morrison, W.D., Bate, L.A., McMillan, I. and Amyot, E. (1987) Operant heat demand of piglets housed on four different floors. *Canadian Journal of Animal Science* 67, 337–341.

Morrison, W.D., Laforest, K.L. and McMillan, I. (1989) Effect of group size on operant heat demand of piglets. *Canadian Journal of Animal Science* 69, 23–26.

Morrow-Tesch, J.L., McGlone, J.J. and Salak-Johnson, J.L. (1994) Heat and social stress effects on pig immune measures. *Journal of Animal Science* 72, 2599–2609.

Morton, D.B. and Griffiths, P.H.M. (1985) Guidelines on the recognition of pain, distress and discomfort in experimental animals and an hypothesis for assessment. *Veterinary Record* 116, 431–436.

Muir, W.M. (1996) Group selection for adaptation to multi-hen cages: selection program and direct responses. *Poultry Science* 75, 447–458.

Muiruri, H.K., Harrison, P.C. and Gonyou, H.W. (1990) Preferences of hens for shape and size of roosts. *Applied Animal Behaviour Science* 27, 141–147.

Munck, A., Guyre, P.M. and Holbrook, N.J. (1984) Physiological functions of glucocorticoids in stress and their relation to pharmacological actions. *Endocrine Reviews* 5, 25–44.

Murphy, L.B. (1977) Responses of domestic fowl to novel food and objects. *Applied Animal Ethology* 3, 335–349.

Murphy, L.B. (1978) The practical problems of recognizing and measuring fear and exploration behaviour in the domestic fowl. *Animal Behaviour* 26, 422–431.

Murphy, L.B. and Duncan, I.J.H. (1978) Attempts to modify the responses of domestic fowl towards human beings. II. The effect of early experience. *Applied Animal Ethology* 4, 5–12.

Murray, K. and others (1995) A novel morbillivirus pneumonia of horses and its transmission to humans. *Emerging Infectious Diseases* 1, 31–34.

N.A.C. (1974) *Nutrients and Toxin Substances in Water for Livestock and Poultry.* National Academy of Sciences, Washington DC, USA.

Nakao, T., Sato, T., Moriyoshi, M. and Kawata, K. (1994) Plasma cortisol response in dairy cows to vaginoscopy, genital palpation per rectum and artificial insemination. *Journal of Veterinary Medicine* 41, 16–21.

Narveson, J. (1983) Animal rights revisited. In: Miller, H.B. and Williams, W.H. (eds) *Ethics and Animals*, Humana Press, Clifton New Jersey, pp. 45–59.

Nash, V.J. (1982) Tool use by captive chimpanzees at an artificial termite mound. *Zoo Biology* 1, 211–221.

Natelson, B.H., Ottenweller, J.E., Cook, J.A., Pitman, D. and McCarty, R. and Tapp, W.N. (1988) Effects of stressor intensity on habituation of the adrenocortical stress response. *Physiology & Behavior* 43, 41–46.

National Research Council (1992) *Recognition of Pain and Distress in Laboratory Animals.* National Academy Press, Washington DC, USA.

Neuringer, A.J. (1969) Animals respond for food in the presence of free food. *Science* 166, 399–401.

Newberry, R.C. (1995) Environmental enrichment: increasing the biological relevance of captive environments. *Applied Animal Behaviour Science* 44, 229–243.

Newberry, R.C. and Shackleton, D.M. (1997) Use of cover by domestic fowl: a Venetian blind effect? *Animal Behaviour* (in press).

Newberry, R.C., Wood-Gush, D.G.M. and Hall, J.W. (1988) Playful behaviour of piglets. *Behavioural Processes* 17, 205–216.

Newman, S. (1994) Quantitative – and molecular-genetic effects on animal well-being: adaptive mechanisms. *Journal of Animal Science* 72, 1641–1653.

Nicol, C.J. (1986) Non-exclusive spatial preference in the laying hen. *Applied Animal Behaviour Science* 15, 337–350.

Nicol, C.J. and Guilford, T. (1991) Exploratory activity as a measure of motivation in deprived hens. *Animal Behaviour* 41, 333–341.

Nicol, C.J. and Pope S.J. (1994) Social learning in small flocks of hens. *Animal Behaviour* 47, 1289–1296.

Nielsen, B.L., Lawrence, A.B. and Whittemore, C.T. (1995) Effect of group size on feeding behaviour, social behaviour and performance of growing pigs using single-space feeders. *Livestock Production Science* 44, 73–85.

Nienaber, J.A. and Hahn, G.L. (1984) Effects of water flow restriction and environmental factors on performance of nursery-age pigs. *Journal of Animal Science* 59, 1423–1429.

Niezgoda, J., Bobek, S., Wronska-Fortuna, D. and Wierzchos, E. (1993) Response of sympatho-adrenal axis and adrenal cortex to short-term restraint stress in sheep. *Journal of Veterinary Medicine* 40, 631–638.

Nilsson, C. (1992) Walking and lying surfaces in livestock houses. In: Phillips, C.J.C. and Piggins, D. (eds) *Farm Animals and the Environment*. CAB International, Wallingford, UK, pp. 93–110.

Noddings, N. (1984) *Caring – A Feminine Approach to Ethics and Moral Education*, Berkeley, University of California Press.

Nolan, A. and Reid, J. (1993) Comparison of the post-operative analgesic and sedative effects of carprofen and papaveretum in the dog. *Veterinary Record* 133, 240–242.

Ödberg, F. (1978) Abnormal behaviours (stereotypies), Introduction to the Round Table. In: *Proceedings of the First World Congress of Ethology Applied to Zootechnics*, Madrid, Editorial Garsi, Industrias Grafices Espana, Madrid, pp. 475–480.

Ödberg, F. O. (1987) The influence of cage size and environmental enrichment on the development of stereotypies in bank voles (*Clethrionomys glareolus*). *Behavioural Processes* 14, 155–173.

Ogunmodede, B.K. (1981) Vitamin A requirement of broiler chicks in Nigeria. *Poultry Science* 60, 2622–2627.

Oldham, J.D., Kyriazakis, I., Pine, A.R., Jessop, N.S. and Illius, A.W. (1993) Animal strategies for coping with inadequate nutrition. In: *Feeding Strategies for Improving Ruminant Productivity in Areas of Fluctuating Nutrient Supply*. IAEA, Vienna, pp. 7–17.

Ortman, L.L. and Craig, J.V. (1968) Social dominance in chickens modified by genetic selection: Physiological mechanisms. *Animal Behaviour* 16, 33–37.

Oxford English Dictionary (1973) *Shorter Oxford English Dictionary* (reprinted 1990). Oxford, Clarendon Press.

Packer, C. (1986) The ecology of sociality in felids. In: Rubenstein, D.J. and Wrangham, R.W. (eds) *Ecological Aspects of Social Evolution*. Princeton University Press, New Jersey, pp. 429–451.

Palya, W.L. and Zacny, J.P. (1980) Stereotyped adjunctive pecking by caged pigeons. *Animal Learning Behaviour* 8, 293–303.

Parrott, R.F. (1990) Physiological responses to isolation in sheep. In: Zayan, R. and Dantzer, R. (eds) *Social Stress in Domestic Animals*. Kluwer Academic Publications, Dordrecht, pp. 212–226.

Parrott, R.F. and Misson, B.H. (1989) Changes in pig salivary cortisol in response to transport simulation, food and water deprivation, and mixing. *British Veterinary Journal* 145, 501–505.

Parrott, R.F., Thornton, S.N. and Robinson, J.E. (1988) Endocrine responses to acute stress in castrated rams: no increase in oxytocin but evidence for an inverse relationship between cortisol and vasopressin. *Acta Endocrinol Copenhagen* 117, 381–386.

Parrott, R.F., Misson, B.H. and de la Riva, C.F. (1994) Differential stressor effects on the concentrations of cortisol, prolactin and catecholamines in the blood of sheep. *Research in Veterinary Science* 56, 234–239.

Pascoe, P.J. (1993) Analgesia after lateral thoracotomy in dogs: epidural morphine vs. intercostal bupivacaine. *Veterinary Surgery* 22, 141–147.

Perry, G.C. (ed.) (1990) Transport and Pre-slaughter Handling. *Applied Animal Behaviour Science* 28, special issue 1–2.

Peterse, D.J. (1986) Aetiology of claw disorders in dairy cattle. In: Wierenga, H.K. and Peterse, D.J. (eds) *Cattle Housing Systems, Lameness and Behaviour*. Martinus Nijhoff, The Hague.

Petherick, J.C. and Blackshaw, J.K. (1987) A review of the factors influencing the aggressive and agonistic behaviour of the domestic pig. *Australian Journal of Experimental Agriculture* 27, 605–611.

Petherick, J.C. and Rutter, S.M. (1990) Quantifying motivation using a computer-controlled push-door. *Applied Animal Behaviour Science* 27, 159–167.

Petherick, J.C., Duncan, I.J.H. and Waddington, D. (1990) Previous experience with different floors influences choice of peat in a Y-maze by domestic fowl. *Applied Animal Behaviour Science* 27, 177–182.

Petit, O. and Thierry, B. (1994) Aggressive and peaceful interventions in conflicts in Tonkean macaques. *Animal Behaviour* 48, 1427–1436.

Phillips, P.A., Thompson, B.K. and Fraser, D. (1988) Preference tests of ramp designs for young pigs. *Canadian Journal of Animal Science* 68, 41–48.

Phillips, P.A., Thompson, B.K. and Fraser, D. (1989) The importance of cleat spacing in ramp design for young pigs. *Canadian Journal of Animal Science* 69, 483–486.

Phillips, P.A., Fraser, D. and Thompson, B.K. (1991) Preference by sows for a partially enclosed farrowing crate. *Applied Animal Behaviour Science* 32, 35–43.

Phillips, P.A., Fraser, D. and Thompson, B.K. (1992) Sow preference for farrowing crate width. *Canadian Journal of Animal Science* 72, 745–750.

Phillips, P.A., Fraser, D. and Thompson, B.K. (1996) Sow preference for types of flooring in farrowing crates. *Canadian Journal of Animal Science* 76, 485–489.

Pitman, D.L., Ottenweller, J.E. and Natelson, B.H. (1990) Effect of corticoid responses in rats. *Behavioural Neuroscience* 104, 28–36.

Poole, T. (1996) Natural behaviour is simply a question of survival. *Animal Welfare* 5, 218.

Popilskis, S., Kohn, D.F., Laurent, L. and Danilo, P. (1993) Efficacy of epidural morphine versus intravenous morphine for post-thoracotomy pain in dogs. *Journal of Veterinary Anaesthesia* 20 (June), 21–28.

Potter, M.J. and Broom, D.M. (1986) The behaviour and welfare of cows in relation to cubicle house design. In: Wierenga, H.K. and Peterse, D.J. (eds) *Cattle Housing Systems, Lameness and Behaviour.* Martinus Nijhoff, The Hague, pp. 129–147.

Price, E.O. (1984) Behavioral aspects of animal domestication. *Quarterly Review of Biology* 59, 1–32.

Provenza, F.D., Lynch, J.J. and Cheney, C.D. (1995) Effects of flavour and food restriction on the response of sheep to novel foods. *Applied Animal Behaviour Science* 43, 83–93.

Pulliam, H.R. and Caraco, T. (1984) Living in groups: is there an optimal group size? In: Krebs, J.R. and Davies, N.B. (eds) *Behavioural Ecology An Evolutionary Approach,* 3rd Edition. Blackwell Scientific Publications, Oxford, pp. 122–147.

Rachels, J. (1983) *The Elements of Moral Philosophy.* New York, McGraw Hill.

Radostits, O.M., Blood, D.C. and Gay, C.C. (1994) *Veterinary Medicine.* Eighth Edition. Ballière Tindall, London.

Redbo, I. (1993) Stereotypies and cortisol secretion in heifers subjected to tethering. *Applied Animal Behaviour Science* 38, 213–225.

Regan, T. (1982) *All That Dwell Therein: Animal Rights and Environmental Ethics.* University of California Press, Berkeley and Los Angeles.

Regan, T. (1984) *The Case for Animal Rights.* Routledge, London.

Reid, J. and Nolan, A.M. (1991) A comparison of the postoperative analgesic and sedative effects of flunixin and papaveretum in the dog. *Journal of Small Animal Practice* 32, 603–608.

Reinhardt, V. (1990) Social enrichment for laboratory primates: a critical review. *Laboratory Primate Newsletter* 29, 7–11.

Reinhardt, V. (1991) Agonistic behavior responses of socially experienced, unfamiliar adult male rhesus monkeys (*Macaca mulatta*) to pairing. *Laboratory Primate Newsletter* 30, 5–7.

Reinhardt, V., Houser, D., Cowley, D., Eisele, S. and Vertein, R. (1989) Alternatives to single caging of rhesus monkeys (*Macaca mulatta*) used in research. *Zeitschrift für Versuchstierskunde* 32, 275–279.

Reite, M. (1985) Implantable biotelemetry and social separation in monkeys. In: Moberg, G.P. (ed.) *Animal Stress*. American Physiological Society, Bethesda, pp. 141–160.

Remignon, H., Desrosiers, V., Bruneau, A., Guémené, D. and Mills, A.D. (1996) Influence of an acute stress on muscle parameters in quail divergently selected for emotivity. In: *Proceedings of the XXth World's Poultry Science Conference*. World's Poultry Science Association, New Delhi, India.

Rempel, W.E., Lu, M., El Kanelgy, S., Kennedy, C.F.H., Irvin, L.R., Mickelson, J.R. and Louis, C.F. (1993) Relative accuracy of the halothene challenge test and a molecular genetic test in detecting the gene for Porcine Stress Syndrome. *Journal of Animal Science* 71, 1395–1399.

Renner, M.J. (1987) Experience-dependent changes in exploratory behavior in the adult rat (*Rattus norvegicus*): overall activity level and interactions with objects. *Journal of Comparative Psychology* 101, 94–100.

Renner, M.J. (1988) Learning during exploration: the role of behavioral topography during exploration in determining subsequent adaptive behavior. *The International Journal of Comparative Psychology* 2, 43–56.

Renner, M.J. and Rosenzweig, M.R. (1986) Object interactions in juvenile rats (*Rattus norvegicus*): effects of different experiential histories. *Journal of Comparative Psychology* 100, 229–236.

Renner, M.J. and Seltzer, C.P. (1991) Molar characteristics of exploratory and investigatory behavior in the rat (*Rattus norvegicus*). *Journal of Comparative Psychology* 105, 326–339.

Renner, M.J., Bennett, A.J. and White, J.C. (1992) Age and sex as factors influencing spontaneous exploration by preadult rats (*Rattus norvegicus*). *Journal of Comparative Psychology* 106, 217–227.

Riley, J.E. (1989) Recent trends in pig production: The importance of intake. In: Forbes, J.M., Varley, M.A. and Lawrence, T.L.J. (eds) *Voluntary Food Intake of Pigs*. BSAP, Edinburgh, pp. 1–5.

Robert, S., Matte, J.J. and Girard, C.L. (1991) Effect of feeding regimen on behaviour of growing-finishing pigs supplemented or not supplemented with folic acid. *Journal of Animal Science* 69, 4428–4436.

Robert, S., Matte, J.J., Farmer, C., Girard, C.L. and Martineau, G.P. (1993) High fibre diets for sows: effects on stereotypies and adjunctive drinking. *Applied Animal Behaviour Science* 37, 297–309.

Roberts, D. and Farrar, J. (1993) *The Economics of Egg Production 1992*. Special Studies in Agricultural Economics, Report No. 22. Department of Agricultural Economics, University of Manchester, UK, 90pp.

Rollin, B.E. (1990) *The Unheeded Cry*. Oxford University Press, Oxford, UK.

Rollin, B.E. (1992) *Animal Rights and Human Morality*. Revised edition. Prometheus Books, Buffalo, USA.

Rollin, B.E. (1993) Animal welfare, science and value. *Journal of Agricultural and Environmental Ethics* 6 (Supplement 2), 44–50.

Rollin, B.E. (1995) *The Frankenstein Syndrome: Ethical and Social Issues in the Genetic Engineering of Animals*. Cambridge University Press, Cambridge, UK.

Rolls, B.J. and Rolls, E.T. (1982) *Thirst*. Cambridge University Press, Cambridge, 194 pp.

Rolston, H. (1989) The value of species. In: Regan, T. and Singer, P. (eds) *Animal Rights and Human Obligations*, Prentice Hall, Englewood Cliffs, New Jersey, pp. 252–255.

Romeyer, A. and Bouissou, M.F. (1992) Assessment of fear reactions in domestic sheep, and influence of breed and rearing conditions. *Applied Animal Behaviour Science* 34, 93–119.

Rosales, A.G. (1994) Managing stress in broiler breeders: a review. *The Journal of Applied Poultry Research* 3, 199–207.

Rossellini, R.A. and Widman, D.R. (1989) Prior exposure to stress reduces the diversity of exploratory behavior of novel objects in the rat (*Rattus norvegicus*). *Journal of Comparative Psychology* 103, 339–346.

Rossitch, E.J. (1991) Experimental animal models of chronic pain. In: Nashold, J. and Nashold, J.O.L.B.S. (eds) *Deafferentation Pain Syndromes: Pathophysiology and Treatment*. Raven Press, New York, pp. 217–227.

Rots, N.Y., Cools, A.R., De Jong, J. and De Kloet, R. (1995) Corticosteroid feedback resistance in rats genetically selected for increased dopamine responsiveness. *Journal of Neuroendocrinology* 7, 153–161.

Rowan, A.N. (1988) Animal anxiety and animal suffering. *Applied Animal Behaviour Science* 20, 135–142.

Rumbaugh, D.M., Washburn, D. and Savage-Rumbaugh, E.S. (1989) On the Care of Captive Chimpanzees: Methods of Enrichment. In: Segal, E. (ed.) *Housing, Care and Psychological Wellbeing of Captive and Laboratory Primates*. Noyes Publications, Park Ridge, New Jersey, pp. 357–375.

Rushen, J. (1985a) Stereotypies, aggression and the feeding schedules of tethered sows. *Applied Animal Behaviour Science* 14, 137–147.

Rushen, J. (1985b) Stereotyped behaviour, adjunctive drinking and the feeding period of tethered sows. *Animal Behaviour* 32, 1059–1067.

Rushen, J. (1986a) Aversion of sheep to electro-immobilization and physical restraint. *Applied Animal Behaviour Science* 15, 315–324.

Rushen, J. (1986b) The validity of behavioural measures of aversion: a review. *Applied Animal Behaviour Science* 16, 309–323.

Rushen, J. (1987) A difference in weight reduces fighting when unacquainted newly weaned pigs first meet. *Canadian Journal of Animal Science* 67, 951–960.

Rushen, J. (1990) Social recognition, social dominance and the motivation of fighting by pigs. In: Zayan, R. and Dantzer, R. (eds) *Social Stress in Domestic Animals*. Kluwer Academic Publications, Dordrecht, pp. 135–143.

Rushen, J. (1993) Exploration in the pig may not be endogenously motivated. *Animal Behaviour* 45, 183–184.

Rushen, J. and de Passillé, A.M.B. (1992) The scientific assessment of the impact of housing on animal welfare: A critical review. *Canadian Journal of Animal Science* 72, 721–743.

Rushen, J. and de Passillé, A.M.B. (1995) The motivation of non-nutritive sucking in calves, *Bos taurus*. *Animal Behaviour* 49, 1503–1510.

Rushen, J., Lawrence, A.B. and Terlouw, E.M.C. (1993a) The motivational basis of stereotypies. In: Lawrence, A.B. and Rushen, J. (eds) *Stereotypic Animal Behaviour: Fundamentals and Applications to Animal Welfare*. CAB International Wallingford, UK, pp. 41–64.

Rushen, J., Schwarze, N., Ladewig, J. and Foxcroft, G. (1993b) Opioid modulation of the effects of repeated stress on ACTH, cortisol, prolactin, and growth hormone in pigs. *Physiology & Behavior* 53, 923–928.

Russell, P.A. (1983) Psychological studies of exploration in animals: a reappraisal. In: Archer, J. and Birke, L.I.A. (eds) *Exploration in Animals and Humans*. Van Nostrand Reinhold Inc., London, pp. 22–55.

Rutter, S.M. and Duncan, I.J.H. (1991) Shuttle and one-way avoidance as measures of aversion in the domestic fowl. *Applied Animal Behaviour Science* 30, 117–124.

Rutter, S.M. and Duncan, I.J.H. (1992) Measuring aversion in domestic fowl using passive avoidance. *Applied Animal Behaviour Science* 33, 53–61.

Ruzzante, D.E. (1994) Domestication effects on aggressive and schooling behavior in fish. *Aquaculture* 120, 1–24.

Sandøe, P. and Simonsen, H.B. (1992) Assessing animal welfare: Where does science end and philosophy begin? *Animal Welfare* 1, 257–267.

Sapolsky, R.M. (1990) Stress in the wild. *Scientific American* Jan., 106–113.

Satterlee, D.G. and Johnson, W.A. (1988) Selection of Japanese quail for contrasting blood corticosterone response to immobilization. *Poultry Science* 67, 25–32.

Savory, C.J., Seawright, E. and Watson, A. (1992) Stereotyped behaviour in broiler breeders in relation to husbandry and opioid receptor blockade. *Applied Animal Behaviour Science* 32, 349–360.

Savory, C.J., Maros, K. and Rutter, S.M. (1993) Assessment of hunger in growing broiler breeders in relation to a commercial restricted feeding programme. *Animal Welfare* 2, 131–152.

Savory, C.J., Hocking, P.M., Mann, J.S. and Maxwell, M.H. (1996) Is broiler breeder welfare improved by using qualitative rather than quantitative food restriction to limit growth rate? *Animal Welfare* 5, 105–127.

Scheurink, A., Steffens, A., Dreteler, G., Benthem, B. and Bruntink, R. (1989) Experience affects exercise-induced changes in catecholamines, glucose and FFA. *American Journal of Physiology* 256 (Regulatory Integrative Comparative Physiology 25) R169–R173.

Schjelderup-Ebbe, T. (1922) Beitrage zur Sozialpsychologie des Haushuhns. *Zeitschrift für Psychologie* 88, 225–252.

Schmidt, M. (1982) Abnormal oral behaviour in pigs. In: Bessei, W. (ed.) *Disturbed Behaviour in Farm Animals*. Eugen Ulmer, Hohenheimer Arbeiten, Stuttgart, pp. 115–121.

Schouten, W.G.P. (1986) Rearing conditions and behaviour in pigs. Doctoral thesis, Agricultural University, Wageningen, Netherlands.

Schouten, W. and Rushen, J. (1993) The role of endogenous opioids in stereotyped behaviour and in heart rate response in pigs. In: Parvizi, N. (ed.) *Opioids in Farm Animals*. Landwirtschaftverlag. GmbH, 4400 Munster-Hiltrup, 207–219.

Schouten, W., Rushen, J. and de Passillé, A.M. (1991) Stereotypic behavior and heart rate in pigs. *Physiology and Behaviour* 50, 617–624.

Sclafani, A. (1995) How food preferences are learned: laboratory animal models. *Proceedings of the Nutrition Society* 54, 419–427.

Scott, J.P. (1992) The phenomenon of attachment in human–nonhuman relationships. In: Davis, H. and Balfour, A.D. (eds), The Inevitable Bond: Examining Scientist–Animal Interactions, Cambridge University Press, Cambridge, pp. 72–92.

Seabrook, M.F. (1972a) A study to determine the influence of the herdsman's personality on milk yield. *Journal Agriculture Labour Science* 1, 45–59.

Seabrook, M.F. (1972b) A study of the influence of the cowman's personality and job satisfaction on milk yield of dairy cows. *Joint Conference of the British Society for Agriculture Labour Science and the Ergonomics Research Society*, National College of Agricultural Engineering, UK, September, 1972.

Seabrook, M.F. (1991) The influence of the personality of the stockperson on the behaviour of pigs. *Applied Animal Behaviour Science* 30, 187–188.

Selye, H. (1932) The general adaptation syndrome and the diseases of adaptation. *Journal of Clinical Endocrinology* 6, 117–152.

Selye, H. (1950) *Stress*. ACTA, Montreal, Canada.

Sen, A. (1987) *On Ethics and Economics*. Basil Blackwell, Oxford.

Shabalina, A.T. (1984) Dominance rank, fear scores and reproduction in cockerels. *British Poultry Science* 25, 297–301.

Shepherdson, D.J., Carlstead, K., Mellen, J.D. and Seidensticker, J. (1993) The influence of food presentation on the behaviour of small cats in confined environment. *Zoo Biology* 12, 203–216.

Short, C.E. and van Poznak, A. (1992) *Animal Pain*. Churchill Livingstone, New York.

Shutt, D.A., Fell, L.R., Connell, R. and Bell, A.K. (1988) Stress responses in lambs docked and castrated surgically or by the application of rubber rings. *Australian Veterinary Journal* 65, 5–7.

Siegel, P.B. (1975) Genetics of behaviour: Selection for mating ability in chickens. *Genetics* 52, 1269–1277.

Siegel, P.B. (1993) Behavior-genetic analyses and poultry husbandry. *Poultry Science* 72, 1–6.

Siegel, P.B. and Dunnington, E.A. (1990) Behavior genetics. In: Crawford, R.D. (ed.) *Poultry breeding and genetics. Developments in animal and veterinary science*. Volume 22. Elsevier, Amsterdam.

Singer, P. (1975) *Animal Liberation*. Jonathan Cape, London.

Singer, P. (1979) Killing humans and killing animals. *Inquiry* 22, pp. 145–156.

Singer, P. (1980) Animals and the value of life. In: Regan, T. (ed.) *Matters of Life and Death: New Introductory Essays in Moral Philosophy*. Random House, New York.

Singer, P. (1989) All animals are equal. In: Regan, T. and Singer, P. (eds), *Animal Rights and Human Obligations*. Prentice Hall, Englewood Cliffs, New Jersey, pp. 73–86.

Singer, P. (1990) *Animal Liberation*, 2nd edn. Avon Books, New York, USA.

Slatter, D.H. (1985) *Textbook of Small Animal Surgery*. First edition. Saunders, Philadelphia.

Slatter, D.H. (1993) *Textbook of Small Animal Surgery*. Second edition. Saunders, Philadelphia.

Smith, A. (1790) *The Theory of Moral Sentiments*, revised edition. T. Cadell, London. Republished in 1975 by Oxford University Press, Oxford.

Smith, P.K. and Dutton, S. (1979) Play and training in direct and innovative problem solving. *Child Development* 50, 830–836.

Sørensen, P. (1989) Broiler selection and welfare. In: Faure, J.M. and Mills, A.D. (eds) *Proceedings of the 3rd European Symposium on Poultry Welfare*. World's Poultry Science Association, Tours, pp. 45–58.

Sørensen, P. and Leenstra, F. (1986) Recent reports on breeding of meat production stocks. In: Larbier, M. (ed.) *Proceedings of the 7th European Poultry Symposium Volume 1*. French Branch of the World's Poultry Science Association, Paris, pp. 60–69.

Spedding, C.R.W. (1993) Animal welfare policy in Europe. *Journal of Agricultural and Environmental Ethics* 6, 110–117.

Spensley, J.C., Kyriazakis, I. and Cooper, S.D.B. (1993) Effect of nutrient density on the behaviour of individually penned growing sheep. *Proceedings of the Sheep Veterinary Society* 17, 242.

Spoolder, H.A.M., Burbridge, J.A., Edwards, S.A., Simmins, P.H. and Lawrence, A.B. (1995) Provision of straw as a foraging substitute reduces the development of excessive chain and bar manipulation in food restricted sows. *Applied Animal Behaviour Science* 43, 249–262.

Squires, V.R. and Wilson, A.D. (1971) Distance between food and water supply and its effect on drinking frequency, and food and water intake of Merino and Border Leicester sheep. *Australian Journal of Agricultural Research* 22, 283–290.

Stafleu, F.R., Grommers, F.J. and Vorstenbosch, J. (1996) Animal welfare: evolution and erosion of a moral concept. *Animal Welfare* 5, 225–234.

Statkiewicz, W.R. and Schein, M.W. (1980) Variability and periodicity of dustbathing behaviour in Japanese quail. *Animal Behaviour* 28, 462–467.

Stauffacher, M. (1992) Group housing and enrichment cages for breeding, fattening and laboratory rabbits. *Animal Welfare* 1, 105–125.

Steiger, A., Tschanz, B., Jacob, P. and Scholl, E. (1979) Verhaltensuntersuchungen bei Mastschweinen auf verschiedenen Bodenbelägen und bei verschiedener Besatzdichte. *Schweizer Archiv für Tierheilkunde* 121, 109–126.

Stephens, D.B. and Perry, G.C. (1990) The effects of restraint, handling, simulated and real transport in the pig (with reference to man and other species). *Applied Animal Behaviour Science* 28, 41–55.

Stephens, D.B., Bailey, K.J., Sharman, D.F. and Ingram, D.L. (1985) An analysis of some behavioural effects of the vibration and noise components of transport in pigs. *Quarterly Journal of Experimental Physiology* 70, 211–217.

Stephens, D.W. (1989) Variance and the value of information. *The American Naturalist* 134, 128–140.

Stevenson, M.F. (1983) The captive environment: its effect on exploratory and related behavioural responses in wild animals. In: Archer, J. and Birke, L.I.A. (eds) *Exploration in Animals and Humans*. Van Nostrand Reinhold Inc., London, pp. 176–198.

Stolba, A. and Wood-Gush, D.G.M. (1984) The identification of behavioural key features and their incorporation into a housing design for pigs. *Annales de Recherches Vétérinaires* 15, 287–298.

Stolba, A. and Wood-Gush, D.G.M. (1989) The behaviour of pigs in a semi-natural environment. *Animal Production* 48, 419–425.

Strickberger, M.W. (1976) *Genetics*. 2nd edn. Macmilllan Publishing Co. Inc. and Collier Macmillan Publishers, New York and London.

Suarez, S.D. and Gallup, G.G. (1982) Open-field behaviour in chickens: the experimenter is a predator. *Journal of Comparative and Physiological Psychology* 96, 432–439.

Sundin, O., Öhman, A., Palm, Th. and Ström, G. (1995) Cardiovascular reactivity, Type A behavior, and coronary heart disease: Comparisons between myocardial infarction patients and controls during laboratory-induced stress. *Psychophysiology* 32, 28–35.

Sylva, K., Bruner, J. and Genova, P. (1976) The role of play in the problem-solving of children 3–5 years old. In: Bruner, J., Jolly, A. and Sylva, K. (eds) *Play, its role in development and evolution*. Penguin, London.

Syme, L.A., Durham, I.H. and Elphick, G.R. (1981) Microprocessor control of sheep movement. In: *Proceedings 2nd Conference on Wool Harvesting Research and Development*. Australian Wool Corporation, pp. 237–245.

Tachibana, T. (1982) A comment on confusion in open-field studies: Abuse of null hypothesis significance test. *Physiology & Behavior* 25, 159–161.

Tannenbaum, J. (1991) Ethics and animal welfare: The inextricable connection. *Journal of the American Veterinary Medical Association* 198, 1360–1376.

Tauson, R. and Abrahamsson, P. (1994) Foot and skeletal disorders on laying hens. Effects of perch design, hybrid, housing system and stocking density. *Acta Agriculturæ Scandinavica*, Section A, 44, 110–119.

Taylor, G.B. (1972) One man's philosophy of welfare. *Veterinary Record* 91, 426–428.

Taylor, P. (1985) Analgesia in the dog and cat. *In Practice* 17, 5–13.

Terlouw, E.M.C., Lawrence, A.B. and Illius, A.W. (1991) Influences of feeding level and physical restriction on development of stereotypies in sows. *Animal Behaviour* 42, 981–991.

Terlouw, E.M.C., Lawrence, A.B., Koolhaas, J. and Illius, A.W. (1992) Relationship between amphetamine and environmentally induced stereotypies in pigs. *Pharmacology Biochemistry and Behavior* 43, 347–355.

Terlouw, E.M.C., Wiersma, A., Lawrence, A.B. and MacLeod, H.A. (1993) Ingestion of food facilitates the performance of stereotypies in sows. *Animal Behaviour* 46, 939–950.

Terlouw, C., Kent, S., Dantzer, R. and Monin, G. (1994) L'hyperthermie induite par le stress: données préliminaires. In: Picard, M., Porter, D. and Signoret, J.P. (eds) *Comportement et adaptation des animaux domestiques aux contraintes de l'élevage: bases techniques du bien-être animal*. INRA, Paris, pp. 191–201.

Terlouw, E.M.C., Kent, S., Cremona S. and Dantzer, R. (1996) Effect of intracerebroventricular administration of vasopressin on stress-induced hyperthermia in rats. *Physiology & Behavior* 60, 417–424.

Thompson, S.E. and Johnson, J.M. (1991) Analgesia in dogs after intercostal thoracotomy – a comparison of morphine, selective intercostal nerve block, and interpleural regional analgesia with bupivacaine. *Veterinary Surgery* 20, 73–77.

Thorp, B.H. and Maxwell, M.H. (1993) Health problems in broiler production. In: Savory, C.J. and Hughes, B.O. (eds) *Proceedings of the Fourth European Symposium on Poultry Welfare. Universities Federation for Animal Welfare*, Potters Bar, UK, pp. 208–218.

Thorpe, W.H. (1965) Appendix III. The assessment of pain and distress in animals. In: Brambell, F.W.R. (chairman) *Report of the Technical Committee to Enquire into the Welfare of Animals kept under Intensive Livestock Husbandry Systems*. Her Majesty's Stationery Office, London, UK, pp. 71–79.

Thurmon, J.C., Tranquilli, W.J. and Benson, G.J. (1996) *Lumb and Jones' Veterinary Anesthesia*. Third edition. Williams and Wilkins, Baltimore.

Tinbergen, N. (1951) *The Study of Instinct*. Clarendon Press, Oxford, UK.

Tinbergen, N. (1963) On aims and methods of ethology. *Zeitschrift für Tierpsychologie* 20, 410–433.

Toates, F.M. (1983) Exploration as a motivational and learning system: a cognitive incentive view. In: Archer, J. and Birke, L.I.A. (eds) *Exploration in Animals and Humans*. Van Nostrand Reinhold Inc., London, pp. 55–72.

Toates, F.M. (1986) *Motivational Systems*. Cambridge University Press, Cambridge.

Toates, F.M. and Jensen, P. (1990) Ethological and psychological models of motivation – towards a synthesis. In: Meyer, J.A. and Wilson, S. (eds) *From Animals to Animats*. MIT Press, Cambridge, Mass., pp. 194–205.

Tolkamp, B.J., Burger, M., Kyriazakis, I., Oldham, J.D., Dewhurst, R.J. and Newbold, J. (1996) Diet selection in dairy cows: effect of training on choice of dietary protein level. *Animal Science* 62, 637.

Townsend, P. (1987) A survey of the use of opiate analgesics in dogs. Dissertation, Royal Veterinary College, London.

UKCCCR (1988) *UKCCCR Guidelines for the Welfare of Animals in Experimental Neoplasia*. UKCCCR, London.

Utting, J.E. (1984) Commentaries. In: Lunn, J.N. (ed.) *Quality of Care in Anaesthetic Practice*. Macmillan, London.

Valentino, R.J., Cha, C.I. and Foote, S.L. (1986) Anatomic and physiologic evidence for innervation of noradrenergic locus coeruleus by neuronal corticotropin-releasing factor. *Society of Neuroscience Abstracts* 12, 1003.

van den Broek, F.A.R., Klompmaker, H., Bakker, R. and Beynen, A.C. (1995) Gerbils prefer partially darkened cages. *Animal Welfare* 4, 119–123.

van Oers, J.W., Hinson, J.P., Binnekade, R. and Tilders, F.J. (1992) Physiological role of corticotropin-releasing factor in the control of the adrenocorticotropic-mediated corticosterone release from the rat adrenal gland. *Endocrinology* 130, 282–288.

van Putten, G. (1982) Welfare in veal calf units. *Veterinary Record* 111, 437.

van Putten, G. and van de Burgwal, J.A. (1990) Vulva biting in group-housed sows: preliminary report. *Applied Animal Behaviour Science* 26, 18–186.

van Rooijen, J. (1982) The value of choice tests in assessing welfare of domestic animals. *Applied Animal Ethology* 8, 295–299.

Veasey, J.S., Waran, N.K. and Young, R.J. (1996) On comparing the behaviour of zoo housed animals with wild conspecifics as a welfare indicator, using the giraffe (*Giraffa camelopardalis*) as a model. *Animal Welfare* 5, 139–153.

Vehrencamp, S.L. (1983) A model for the evolution of despotic versus egalitarian societies. *Animal Behaviour* 31, 667–682.

Verstegen, M.W.A. and Close, W.H. (1994) The environment and the growing pig. In: Cole, D.J.A., Wiseman, J. and Varley, M.A. (eds) *Principles of Pig Science*. Nottingham University Press, Nottingham, pp. 333–353.

Vestergaard, K. (1982) Dust-bathing in the domestic fowl: diurnal rhythm and dust deprivation. *Applied Animal Ethology* 8, 487–495.

Vestergaard, K.S., Kruijt, J.P. and Hogan, J.A. (1993) Feather pecking and chronic fear in groups of red junglefowl: their relationships to dustbathing, rearing environment and social status. *Animal Behaviour* 45, 1127–1140.

Visalberghi, E. and Anderson, J.R. (1993) Reasons and risks associated with manipulating captive primates' social environments. *Animal Welfare* 2, 3–15.

von Borell, E. and Hurnik, J.F. (1991) Stereotypic behaviour, adreno-cortico function and open field behaviour of individually-confined gestating sows. *Physiology & Behavior* 49, 709–714.

von Borell, E. and Ladewig, J. (1989) Altered adrenocortical response to acute stressors or ACTH (1-24) in intensively housed pigs. *Domestic Animal Endocrinology* 6, 299–309.

von Borell, E. and Ladewig, J. (1992) Relationship between behaviour and adreno-cortical response pattern in domestic pigs. *Applied Animal Behaviour Science* 34, 195–206.

von Holst, D. (1986) Vegetative and somatic components of tree shrews' behaviour. *Journal of the Autonomic Nervous System*, supplement, 657–670.

Wahlstrom, R.C., Taylor, A.R. and Seerley, R.W. (1970) Effects of lysine in the drinking water of growing swine. *Journal of Animal Science* 30, 368–373.

Waring, G.H. (1983) *Horse Behaviour. The Behavioural Traits and Adaptations of Domestic and Wild Horses, Including Ponies*. Noyes Publications, Park Ridge, New Jersey, USA, pp. 235–250.

Warriss, P.D., Bevis, E.A., Brown, S.N. and Ashby, J.G. (1989) An examination of potential indices of fasting time in commercially slaughtered sheep. *British Veterinary Journal* 145, 242–248.

Wathes, C. and Charles, D. (eds) (1994) *Livestock Housing*. CAB International, Wallingford, UK.

Weary, D.M. and Fraser, D. (1995a) Calling by domestic piglets: reliable signals of need? *Animal Behaviour* 50, 1047–1055.

Weary, D.M. and Fraser, D. (1995b) Signalling need: costly signals and animal welfare assessment. *Applied Animal Behaviour Science* 44, 159–169.

Webster, A.J.F. (1994) Comfort and injury. In: Wathes, C.M. and Charles, D.R. (eds) *Livestock Housing*. CAB International, Wallingford, UK.

Webster, A.J.F. (1995) *Animal Welfare – A Cool Eye towards Eden*. Blackwell Science, Oxford.

Webster, J., Saville, C. and Welchman, D. (1986) *Improved Husbandry Systems for Veal Calves*. Farm Animal Care Trust, London, UK.

Weiss, J.M. (1970) Somatic effects of predictable and unpredictable shock. *Psychosomatic Medicine* 32, 397–408.

Weiss, J.M. (1971) Effects of coping behaviour with and without a feedback signal on stress pathology in rats. *Journal of Comparative and physiological Psychology* 77, 22–30.

Welker, W.I. (1956) Some determinants of play and exploration in Chimpanzees. *Journal of Comparative and Physiological Psychology* 49, 84–89.

Welker, W.I. (1961) An analysis of exploratory and play behaviour in animals. In: Fiske, D. and Maddi, S. (eds) *Functions of Varied Experience*. Dorsey Press, Illinois.

Wemelsfelder, F. (1993) The concept of animal boredom and its relationship to stereotyped behaviour. In: Lawrence, A.B. and Rushen, J. (eds) *Stereotypic Animal Behaviour: Fundamentals and Applications to Welfare*. CAB International, Wallingford, UK, pp. 65–95.

White, R.W. (1959) Motivation reconsidered: the concept of competence. *Psychological Review* 66, 297–333.

Whittington, C.J. and Chamove, A.S. (1995) Effects of visual cover on farmed red deer behaviour. *Applied Animal Behaviour Science* 45, 309–314.

Wiedenmayer, C. (1997) Causation of the ontogenetic development of stereotypic digging in gerbils. *Animal Behaviour* 53, 461–470.

Wiepkema, P.R. and Koolhaas, J.M. (1993) Stress and animal welfare. *Animal Welfare* 2, 195–218.

Wiepkema, P.R. and Schouten, W.G.P. (1990) Mechanisms of coping in social situations. In: Zayan, R. and Dantzer, R. (eds) *Social Stress in Domestic Animals*. Kluwer Academic Publications, Dordrecht, pp. 8–24.

Wiepkema, P.R., van Hellemond, K.K., Roessingh, P. and Romberg, H. (1987) Behaviour and abomasal damage in individual veal calves. *Applied Animal Behaviour Science* 18, 257–268.

Williams, J.M., Zurawski, J., Mikecz, K. and Glant, T.T. (1993) Functional assessment of joint use in experimental inflammatory murine arthritis. *Journal of Bone and Joint Surgery* 11, 172–180.

Wohlt, J.E., Allyn, M.E., Zajac, P.K. and Katz, L.S. (1994) Cortisol increases in plasma of Holstein heifer calves from handling and method of electrical dehorning. *Journal of Dairy Science*, 77, 3725–3729.

Wood, G.N., Molony, V. and Fleetwood-Walker, S.M. (1991) Effects of local anaesthesia and intravenous naloxone on the changes in behaviour and plasma concentrations of cortisol produced by castration and tail docking with tight rubber rings in young lambs. *Research in Veterinary Science* 51, 193–199.

Wood-Gush, D.G.M. (1959) A history of the domestic chicken from antiquity to the 19th century. *Poultry Science* 38, 321–326.

Wood-Gush, D.G.M. (1963) The control of nesting behaviour of the domestic hen. I. The role of the oviduct. *Animal Behaviour* 11, 293–299.

Wood-Gush, D.G.M. (1972) Strain differences in response to sub-optimal stimuli in the fowl. *Animal Behaviour* 20, 72–76.

Wood-Gush, D.G.M. (1975) The effect of cage floor modification on pre-laying behaviour in poultry. *Applied Animal Ethology* 1, 113–119.

Wood-Gush, D.G.M. and Gilbert, A.B. (1964) The control of nesting behaviour of the domestic hen. II. The role of the ovary. *Animal Behaviour* 12, 451–453.

Wood-Gush, D.G.M. and Gilbert, A.B. (1973) Some hormones involved in the nesting behaviour of hens. *Animal Behaviour* 21, 98–103.

Wood-Gush, D.G.M. and Vestergaard, K. (1989) Exploratory behavior and the welfare of intensively kept animals. *Journal of Agricultural Ethics* 2, 161–169.

Wood-Gush, D.G.M. and Vestergaard, K. (1991) The seeking of novelty and its relation to play. *Animal Behaviour* 42, 599–606.

Wood-Gush, D.G.M. and Vestergaard, K. (1993) Inquisitive exploration in pigs. *Animal Behaviour* 45, 185–187.

Wood-Gush, D.G.M., Duncan, I.J.H. and Fraser, D. (1975) Social stress and welfare problems in agricultural animals. In: Hafez, E.S.E. (ed.) *The Behaviour of Domestic Animals*, 3rd edition. Baillière Tindall, London, pp. 183–200.

Wood-Gush, D.G.M., Vestergaard, K. and Petersen, V. (1990) The significance of motivation and environment in the development of exploration in pigs. *Biology of Behaviour* 15, 39–52.

Woodworth, R.S. (1958) *Dynamics of Behavior*. Holt, Reinhart and Winston, New York.

Wurbel, H., Stauffacher, M. and von Holst, D. (1996) Stereotypies in laboratory mice – quantitative and qualitative description of the ontogeny of wire-gnawing and jumping in ICR and ICRnu mice. *Ethology* 102, 371–385.

Yang, T.S., Howard, B. and MacFarlane, W.V. (1981) Effects of food on drinking behaviour of growing pigs. *Applied Animal Ethology* 7, 259–270.

Yeomans, M.R. and Savory, C.J. (1989) Altered spontaneous and osmotically induced drinking for fowls with permanent access to quinine. *Physiology & Behavior* 46, 917–922.

Young, R.J. and Lawrence, A.B. (1994) Feeding behaviour of pigs in groups monitored by a computerised feeding system. *Animal Production* 58, 145–152.

Young, R.J., Carruthers, J. and Lawrence, A.B. (1994) The effect of a foraging device (the 'Edinburgh Foodball') on the behaviour of pigs. *Applied Animal Behaviour Science* 39, 237–247.

Yoxall, A.T. (1978) Pain in small animals – its recognition and control. *Journal of Small Animal Practice* 19, 423–438.

Zeuner, F.E. (1963) *A history of domesticated animals*. Harper and Row, New York.

Zhang, S.H., Hennessy, D.P., Cranwell, P.D., Noonan, D.E. and Francis, H.J. (1992) Physiological responses to exercise and hypoglycemia stress in pigs of differing adrenal responsiveness. *Comparative Biochemistry and Physiology* 103, 695–703.

Ziegler, J.S., Sing, Y., Corcoran, K.P., Nie, L., Mayrand, P.E., Hoff, L.B., McBride, L.J., Kronick, M.N. and Diehl, S.R. (1992) Application of automated DNA sizing technology for genotyping microsatellite loci. *Genomics* 14, 1026–1031.

Zuidhof, M.J., Robinson, F.E., Feddes, J.J.R. and Hardin, R.T. (1995) The effects of nutrient dilution on the well-being and performance of female broiler breeders. *Poultry Science* 74, 441–456.

Zulkifli, I. and Siegel, P.B. (1995) Is there a positive side to stress? *World's Poultry Science Journal* 51, 63–76.

Zulkifli, I., Dunnington, E.A. and Siegel, P.B. (1995) Age and psychogenic factors in response to food deprivation and refeeding in White Leghorn chickens. *Archiv für Geflügelkunde* 59, 175–181.

INDEX